Focusing on Relationships
An Effort That Pays

Parent–Child Relationship
Competencies-Based Assessment,
Treatment Planning, Documentation, and Billing

Maria Seymour St. John

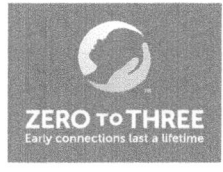

ZERO TO THREE
Early connections last a lifetime

Washington, DC

Published by

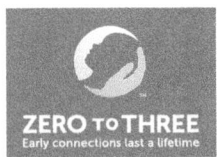

ZERO TO THREE
1255 23rd St., NW., Ste. 350
Washington, DC 20037
(202) 638-1144
Toll-free orders (800) 899-4301
Fax: (202) 638-0851
Web: http://www.zerotothree.org

Copyedited by Tyler Krupa.

Book design and composition: K Art & Design, Inc.

10 9 8 7 6 5 4 3 2 1

ISBN 0978-1-938558-65-8

TABLE OF CONTENTS

FOREWORD

This very complex and illuminating volume is constructed to include history, process, practical application, and vivid examples of the infant, parent, and clinician's work. It also represents the broad diversity of families and their unique and individual structures. It is theoretical and practical, and the perspective is consistently viewed through an essential and unique multicultural lens, which enriches and informs everything.

The clinical work is presented through a series of compelling, representative, and varied vignettes. They illustrate the many challenges and the careful efforts of mental health clinicians. In addition, and utterly unique, each vignette is linked to its appropriate and critical source of funding. This feature confronts the dilemma of what that mysterious source might be. This novel solution to a chronically aggravating problem will surely prove deeply welcome to everyone.

How you are in engaging with families should always clearly convey that they are in possession of all the relevant information and that you will patiently explore with them what they are experiencing; whether parent, infant, toddler, or caregiver.

Clearly, we all owe a debt of gratitude to the pioneering work of Selma Fraiberg in this field, and this new volume is a splendid and comprehensive contribution to it. It is beautifully written and brilliantly conceived. It has needed to be written and it is here.

Jeree H. Pawl, PhD
Former Director of the Infant-Parent Program

PREFACE

This book is about the magnetic strength of parent–child relationships and how mental health professionals can tap that power to support family well-being. I write as a psychotherapist with many years of experience working with individuals and families around relationship questions and challenges; I also write as a parent and as the grown child of parents. I work in two practice settings: one public and the other private. In my public practice, I am part of a community mental health clinic serving expectant parents and families of children from birth through 5 years old who are struggling with relationship and mental health challenges. In my private practice, I work with adults, children, and families—addressing relationship questions, life transitions, paths to parenthood and family formation, and caregiving challenges—supporting people to find their own right balance among individual pursuits and family and community connections.

The Parent–Child Relationship Competencies (PCRCs) framework is a tool that I developed to help my students, trainees, and colleagues over the years to conceptualize and translate (to families, to one another, and to funders) the complex and often elusive nature of relationship-focused clinical intervention. It is important to state from the outset that the PCRCs are a tool, not a measure. They have not been standardized or validated, and they are not to be used as a yardstick against which to measure the adequacy of any parent, child, or relationship. Instead, they are to be used as a framework for thinking, planning, organizing, and tracking the work of the *practitioner*.

The content of the PCRCs is not my invention. Each PCRC encapsulates the collective wisdom of many parents and professionals regarding specific elements of parenting, child development, and family life. What I offer with this framework is a synthesis of the work of many other people whose contributions have enriched my understanding and my practice. This book also contains many concrete examples of the application of this framework in planning for and documenting clinical work that can be hard to capture in words.

There is nothing absolute about there being 20 PCRCs. The list evolved in my mind and practice over the years. At first there were 10 competencies, which seemed like a nice tidy number, but then more emerged from the vibrancy and variability of the families I worked with, and so I added them. Sometimes I came to realize that two PCRCs were so overlapping that it was not helpful to keep them separate, and so I merged them into a single one. As a result, some competencies are more streamlined and sparse, whereas others are quite elaborate and multifaceted. Colleagues with whom I have shared the PCRCs have reported that some of them are very salient in their work, whereas others do not come into focus for them at all. I imagine that in the future I may add or subtract or otherwise revise the framework, and I certainly welcome readers to use the PCRCs as a springboard for their own work rather than as a constraining or limiting frame.

This book is focused on clinical work with parents of children from birth through 5 years old. The PCRCs emerge spontaneously under "ordinary good enough" conditions during the first few years of life, and they may be supported to "come on line" through clinical intervention when circumstances have mitigated against their spontaneous emergence. However, relationships between parents and children are animated, supported, and fueled by the PCRCs throughout all phases of family life, with meaningful variations and elaborations sometimes taking shape as parents age and adult children assume caregiving roles in relation to them.

At the time of this writing, I am in the astounding position of parenting two people, one who is 21 years old and the other who is in her first year of life. Both of these amazing individuals are teaching me more about the PCRCs every day, as are my partner, parents, stepparents, and parents-in-law. Therefore, although I hope that this book will be immediately useful for clinicians working with families of children from birth through 5 years old, I imagine that it might also resonate for clinicians attuned to the relational world who work with people of all ages and stages of life.

Contact information for the author may be found at MariaSeymourStJohn.com.

ACKNOWLEDGMENTS

It takes a village to write a book. My queer, transracial, multigenerational, blended, extended family is nested in a vibrant community of friends, relations, neighbors, comrades, and co-workers. I cherish my multiple roles within these communities, and this book would not exist without the inspiration, challenge, and sustaining contributions of this network. Some of you are specifically named here. Many are not.

I want to thank first and foremost the people who have entrusted me as a psychotherapist with their intimate struggles. You have met with me in the context of my private practice and the public clinic and at times welcomed me for home visits. I have learned from and been moved by each one of you, and while none of your stories are directly represented in these pages, each has contributed something absolutely unique to the understandings I have sought to articulate here.

Many thanks to ZERO TO THREE for hosting my first national training on the Parent–Child Relationship Competencies in 2011 and to Editor Stefanie Powers for subsequently publishing them in the *ZERO TO THREE Journal*. And heartfelt thanks to Julia Richards and Jennifer Moon Li for their expert shepherding of this project.

To my colleagues at the University of California, San Francisco Infant-Parent Program, I am deeply grateful, both for thinking through parent–child relationship issues with me over many years, and for bearing with me when I reduced my time at the program to open up a writing life. Janelle Albanes, Leslie Baxter, Lea Brown, Maria Cristina Borges Cruz, Benjamin Fife, Amee Jaiswal, Kadija Johnston, Elizabeth Lujan, Livia Ondi, Kristin Reinsberg, Andrea Scott, Miriam Silverman, Anna Spielvogel, Meghan Spyker, Adriana Taranta, Blanca Valle, and Abby Waldstein: Thank you. Thanks also to the many trainees who taught me so much over the years, and to the colleagues who journeyed with us in the program in the past, especially Sandra Willard, who insisted many years ago that I "just write it down!"

I am also grateful to the Community Psychoanalysis Committee: Barbara Blasdel, Judy Blumenfeld, Loni Chow, David Cushman, Nancy Drooker, Francisco Gonzalez, Shubha Herlekar, Betsy Kassoff, Julie Leavitt, Mary Margaret McClure, Molly Merson, Marlene Milikan, Rachael Peltz, Lee Slome, Annika Sridharan, Kara Swedlow, and Alla Volovich. Community psychoanalysis lives, and it is wonderful to be part of this committed group of practitioners striving to represent, sustain, learn from, and teach it. Our passionate project has informed how I wrote this book.

Being part of the collaborative group that forged and disseminates the *Diversity-Informed Tenets for Work With Infants, Children and Families* (© Irving Harris Foundation) has been an honor and an inspiration. The Tenets are not only represented in this book, they have been the wind in my sails as I have traversed tumultuous waters. I thank my Tenets Working Group comrades Ana Arbel, Nicola Brown, Karen Frankel, Nucha Isarowong, Ayannakai Nalo, Carmen Rosa Noroña, Rebecca Shahmoon-Shanok, Tonia M. Spence, Alison Steier, and Gregory Tate. Special thanks are owed to Amanda Hwu and Phyllis Glink of the Irving Harris Foundation and to our tireless leader in the Tenets Initiative, Kandace Thomas.

The two past directors of the Infant-Parent Program (who sustained and nurtured it after the untimely death of the original director, Selma Fraiberg) have been treasured mentors throughout my entire adult life: Judith Pekarsky and Jeree Pawl. My roving—yet keenly pertinent—conversations with Dr. Pawl throughout the writing of this book are the gift of a lifetime.

I acknowledge and thank my ancestors (biological, intellectual, political, and spiritual) and hope this book pleases you in its usefulness. I thank my dear family of origin—father, mother, and three brothers—and my contemporary family, and I am grateful that (through marriages, divorces, non-dominant unions, reproductive ingenuity, gender transitions, births, and adoptions) these are continuous and expanded! Special thanks to Cornelia St. John for your love, nurturance, and friendship throughout this writing process and always. Lydia Adkins, Frances Roma Adkins, and Noah Pawl Silverman St. John: you bring me so much joy and then you bring me...more joy.

INTRODUCTION

The setting was the family kitchen or the living room. The patient who couldn't talk was always present at the interviews—if she wasn't napping. The patient who could talk went about her domestic tasks or diapered and fed the baby. The therapist's eyes and ears were attuned to both the nonverbal communications of the baby and the mother's verbal communications. Everything that transpired between mother and baby was in the purview of the therapist and in the center of the therapy.

—Selma Fraiberg (1980, p. 171)

It Pays to Focus on Relationships

"Relationships matter." This ZERO TO THREE motto encapsulates decades of professional wisdom and groundbreaking research around early development. Every domain of development is affected by the quality and nature of the caregiving relationships in which the child is nested— relationships with parents and other caregiving adults. Caregiving relationships are directly influential in shaping infants' and young children's experiences and emerging selves. They can be inherently nurturing, can act as a conduit linking the child to growth-promoting experiences and resources offered by the world surrounding them, and can constitute a powerful protective factor shielding the child from harm and promoting resilience in the face of stress. The power of caregiving relationships cuts both ways, however. Serious problems in caregiving relationships can be triply costly to infants and young children: depriving them of needed nurturing experiences, limiting their access to growth-promoting connections and experiences, and undermining their resilience.

The assertion that "focusing on relationships is an effort that pays" has several meanings. It pays to focus on caregiving relationships when serving infants and young children because these are foundational in determining the child's capacity to thrive. The potential merits of any intervention on behalf of an infant or young child may be enhanced or undermined by these influential relationships. When there is a problem that is negatively affecting an infant or young child, exclusive focus on either the infant or child as an individual or the caregiver as an individual without regard for the relationship is insufficient, wasteful, and potentially harmful. Relationship-focused intervention, by contrast, pays off through the reverberating effects as gains are solidified through ongoing family life.

It also pays to focus on caregiving relationships because the costs to society of failing to support early caregiving relationships are far greater than the costs associated with supporting them.

Finally, "it pays to focus on relationships" means that people can—and should—get paid for doing relationship-focused work on behalf of infants and young children. However, the fact that it is ethical to intervene at the level of the relationship does not mean that it is easy to do. In addition, it is not easy to document relationship-focused work to facilitate reimbursement. On the contrary, this documentation can be quite challenging. Many practitioners who have mastered the challenge of providing relationship-focused intervention nonetheless struggle with how to represent this work in ways that facilitate remuneration. This book offers a framework for conceptualizing and documenting relationship-focused work to facilitate getting paid for it.

The Parent–Child Relationship Competencies (PCRCs)

This book introduces the PCRCs, a set of 20 culturally varied yet universal capacities developed during the first few years of life that enhance family well-being across the life span (see Appendix A). They are bidirectional: parent-to-child and child-to-parent. The PCRCs emerge spontaneously under ordinary circumstances, but they may be strained, impaired, or absent in conditions of stress. These conditions may include trauma, adversity, or developmental or mental health difficulties on the part of the parent, the child, or both. PCRC-focused assessment, formulation, and treatment planning aid infant and early childhood mental health workers in identifying the relevant sources of strain and critical targets of intervention to support child development, adults' functioning in their parental roles, and family well-being.

Because expression of the PCRCs is culturally varied, it is critical that infant mental health (IMH) workers apprehend families through a lens sensitive to sociocultural variance (Costa & Noroña, 2019; Lewis, 2005). The *Diversity-Informed Tenets for Work With Infants, Children, and Families* (© 2012 Irving Harris Foundation; hereafter, "the Tenets"; see www.diversityinformedtenets.org) provide a framework that guides practitioners in working with families in ways that are maximally responsive to issues of diversity, equity, and inclusion—recognizing that the social location of the practitioner must be taken into consideration together with the social location of the family (St. John & Nalo, 2016; St. John, Thomas, & Noroña, 2012; K. Thomas, Noroña, & St. John, 2019). The full text of each Tenet is included in Chapter 1. The Tenets taglines are:

Tenet # 1: Self-Awareness Leads to Better Services for Families

Tenet # 2: Champion Children's Rights Globally

Tenet # 3: Work to Acknowledge Privilege and Combat Discrimination

Tenet # 4: Recognize and Respect Non-Dominant Bodies of Knowledge

Tenet # 5: Honor Diverse Family Structures

Tenet # 6: Understand That Language Can Hurt or Heal

Tenet # 7: Support Families in Their Preferred Language

Tenet # 8: Allocate Resources to Systems Change

Tenet # 9: Make Space and Open Pathways

Tenet # 10: Advance Policy That Supports All Families

The Tenets are discussed in Chapter 1. Throughout the book, Tenets taglines appear in the margins wherever the PCRC material under discussion pertains to a particular Tenet. Readers are encouraged to consider how the Tenets might aid them in bringing a diversity, inclusion, or equity lens to their PCRC-focused work.

The word "parent" stirs powerful associations and feelings for most people. These feelings can range from sorrow and anger (related to ways we may have felt failed, abandoned, or harmed by our parents) to gratitude, fortitude, and joy (related to love, protection, or care that we received from parenting figures). The word "parent" is complex and political. The legal status of parenthood is regulated by societies in ways that are sometimes at odds with people's experiences of parenthood. Adults are influenced in their parenting experiences by political forces. Sometimes experiences of having been parented are connected to caregivers who were not recognized as parents. Thus, in this book, *parent* is defined inclusively in keeping with the definition offered by the National Research Council and Institute of Medicine (2000):

> *We use the term "parenting" to capture the focused and differentiated relationship that the young child has with the adult (or adults) who is (are) most emotionally invested in and consistently available to him or her. Usually this is a birth or adoptive parent (thus the use of the term "parenting"), but sometimes it is a grandparent, a foster parent, or another primary caregiver.* **Who** *fills this role is far less important than*

the quality of the relationship she or he establishes with the child. The hallmark of this important relationship is the readily observable fact that this special adult is not interchangeable with others. (p. 226)

The PCRCs define "parent" in this inclusive, psychologically determined sense.

Infant Mental Health (IMH)

This book emerges from the field of IMH and is intended to be used as a tool for clinical assessment, treatment planning, and documentation by those whose practice involves working with parents and young children together to treat developmental, emotional, behavioral, and relational difficulties in infants and young children and the adults involved. The field of IMH is part of the broader "prenatal to age 5" field, which also includes early intervention, early care and education, physical health, and social services or child welfare. A core contribution from early intervention is the recognition that parents are children's first and most influential teachers; thus, the role of the provider is to collaborate with parents in ways that support them to interact with their children in growth-promoting ways and to ally with parents in pursuing their goals for their child and family. IMH practitioners respect the self-righting and self-healing capacities of infant–parent relationships, and they direct efforts at removing impediments to families' self-healing and self-determination.

ZERO TO THREE's (2017) *Cross-Sector Core Competencies for the Prenatal to Age 5 Field* (P-5 Competencies) define the "knowledge, skills and attitudes held in common among professionals working with expectant parents, young children birth to 5 years old, and their families" (p. 1). Although the PCRCs are competencies that parents and children hold, it is important that those who serve parents and children bring our own professional competency to this work. Therefore, ZERO TO THREE's *Cross-Sector Core*

Competencies are linked throughout this book to discussions of IMH work aimed at supporting the PCRCs. The P-5 Competencies consist of eight domains, each entailing related knowledge, skills, and attitudes (see Figure 1):

P-5 ① Early Childhood Development

P-5 ② Family-Centered Practice

P-5 ③ Relationship-Based Practice

P-5 ④ Health & Developmental Protective & Risk Factors

P-5 ⑤ Cultural & Linguistic Responsiveness

P-5 ⑥ Leadership to Meet Family Needs & Improve Services & Systems

P-5 ⑦ Professional & Ethical Practices

P-5 ⑧ Service Planning, Coordination, & Collaboration

These eight P-5 Competency domains are referenced throughout this book wherever they are most pertinent to the discussion.

Figure 1. P-5 Competency Domains

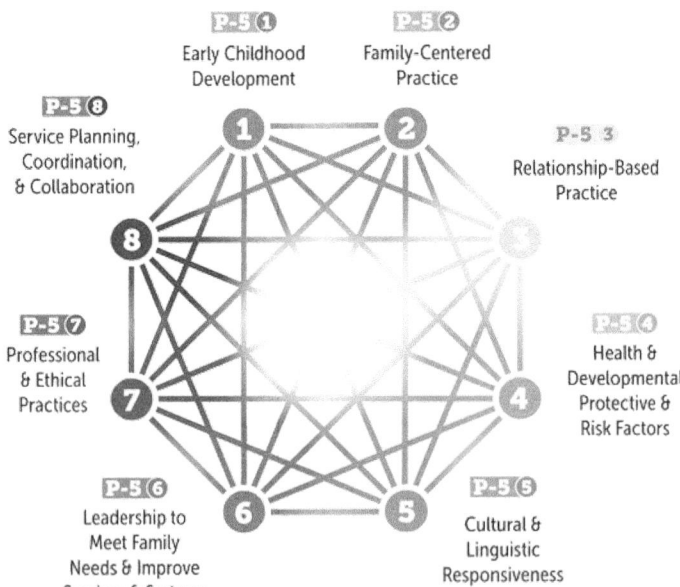

The P-5 Competencies also provide a foundation for ZERO TO THREE's Critical Competencies for Early Childhood Educators™ (Reschke, LeMoine, Greene, & Macasaet, 2017), which define the specific evidence-based teaching methods that support and nurture young children's development and learning in three overarching areas: social–emotional, cognitive, and language and learning (see Figure 2). Because parents interact with children in ways that further these critical developmental phenomena, the Critical Competencies are referenced throughout the book wherever a vignette illustrates how a parent might be helped to hone these specific skills for supporting their child's development.

The Critical Competencies for Early Childhood Educators include:

SE-1 Building Warm, Positive, and Nurturing Relationships

SE-2 Providing Consistent and Responsive Caregiving

SE-3 Supporting Emotional Expression and Regulation

SE-4 Promoting Socialization

SE-5 Guiding Behavior

SE-6 Promoting Children's Sense of Identity and Belonging

C-1 Facilitating Exploration and Concept Development

C-2 Building Meaningful Curriculum

C-3 Promoting Imitation, Symbolic Representation, and Play

C-4 Supporting Reasoning and Problem Solving

LL-1 Promoting Communication Exchange

LL-2 Expanding Expressive and Receptive Language and Vocabulary

LL-3 Promoting Early Literacy

The field of IMH is interdisciplinary, drawing on the expertise of all mental health disciplines and all of the prenatal to age 5 sectors. The field is also informed and enriched by

Figure 2.
Critical Competencies Areas

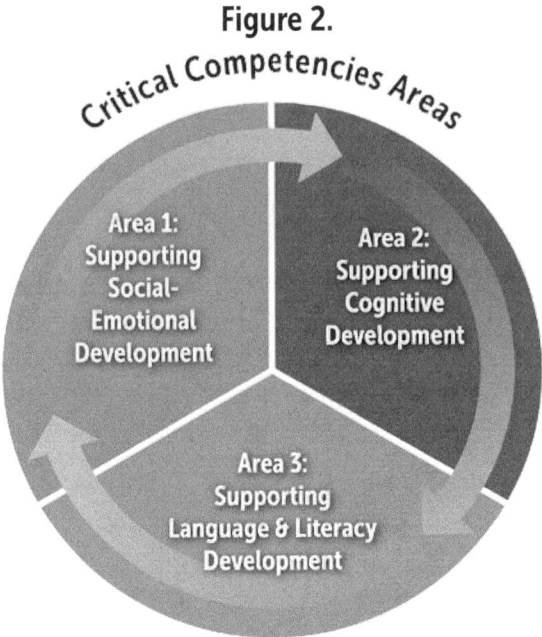

Critical Competencies Sub-Areas

🔵 Area 1: Supporting Social-Emotional Development

- **SE-1** Building Warm, Positive, and Nurturing Relationships
- **SE-2** Providing Consistent and Responsive Caregiving
- **SE-3** Supporting Emotional Expression and Regulation
- **SE-4** Promoting Socialization
- **SE-5** Guiding Behavior
- **SE-6** Promoting Children's Sense of Identity and Belonging

🔵 Area 2: Supporting Cognitive Development

- **C-1** Facilitating Exploration and Concept Development
- **C-2** Building Meaningful Curriculum
- **C-3** Promoting Imitation, Symbolic Representation, and Play
- **C-4** Supporting Reasoning and Problem Solving

🔵 Area 3: Supporting Language & Literacy Development

- **L&L-1** Promoting Communication Exchange
- **L&L-2** Expanding Expressive and Receptive Language and Vocabulary
- **L&L-3** Promoting Early Literacy

any work in the social sciences or the humanities that takes infants, young children, parents, and caregivers as its subject. Moreover, the field is most profitably (though rarely) defined in yet broader ways, including social movements aimed at combatting injustice and ameliorating conditions for all families. These movements include the people's health movement, the reproductive health and justice movement, the disabilities rights movement, the food justice movement, and racial justice movements.

This book understands the field to be broad and far-reaching, yet it is a tool to be used in the context of mental and behavioral health service provision. This book does not describe or advocate a particular modality of intervention, although it is weighted toward infant–parent and child–parent psychotherapy in the tradition of Selma Fraiberg, as discussed later. Rather, it supports those who are already working in the field of infant and early childhood mental health who include the parent–child relationship as the compass for their work, to document this relationship-focused work in ways that will be recognizable and meaningful to families, colleagues, and third-party reviewers.

The term *IMH worker* is used to designate the person providing mental or behavioral health intervention to the child and parent. The IMH worker might be a family therapist, a social worker, a psychiatrist, a psychologist, or another kind of therapist who is qualified to provide mental or behavioral health services where they practice. States, systems of care, and agencies vary regarding licensure and practice requirements for delivering mental and behavioral health services. IMH workers are responsible for understanding their scope of practice and competence and using the PCRC framework accordingly.

Translating IMH Work to Others

Part of being an IMH worker involves explaining IMH work to others. It is painful to think about an infant or young child suffering emotional pain—having a broken heart, for instance. In general, people prefer to imagine infancy and childhood as a sheltered zone characterized by tenderness, innocence, and playfulness. However, infants and young children do experience broken hearts as well as terror, fury, despair, and other emotions that bring grown-ups to our knees...and hopefully into mental health treatment that helps us to cope, heal, and restore our lives to the most promising trajectory possible. IMH workers offer treatment that helps infants, young children, and caregivers to cope, to heal, and to restore their lives in the most promising trajectory possible—together. By intervening at the inclusive level of the parent–child relationship, IMH workers draw on and support the most powerfully influential element of the child's life, addressing impediments to its functioning in

P-5 2 protective and growth-promoting ways. When carried out in this spirit—intervention in the service of supporting and strengthening the parent–child relationship—the impact of IMH treatment reverberates throughout a child's life. It is a

P-5 6 wonderfully hopeful message to bring to the wide world.

This good news is challenging to articulate, however, be-cause systems and societies tend to be organized around individuals rather than relationships. For example, many competent mental health providers serving adults who are parents of infants or young children would listen to ac-counts of conflict in the relationship between their client and their client's child without recommending a referral for IMH treatment. They focus on the meaning of the conflict to the parent who is their patient. This method is problematic because although excellent progress in the parent's men-tal health difficulties may be made over time, in the words of Selma Fraiberg (1980), the baby cannot wait. Because of the furious rate of development in the first few years of life, a baby's time counts differently. They will benefit from services now, and IMH workers have to ensure that parents, colleagues, systems, and societies understand and support

P-5 6 this concept. The PCRC framework is a key to translating between the foreign languages of the individually focused systems versus relationship-focused intervention so that families can understand what might most help them. The PCRC framework can also help professionals of all kinds understand IMH intervention, when it might be indicated, and how to collaborate to support it; systems can recalibrate to facilitate this work, and funders can pay for it.

This book puts the PCRCs in the hands of those who already have the tools to treat infants, young children, and parents but who can benefit from support in translating their work. Short chapters illustrated by vignettes guide IMH workers through an approach to clinical assessment, formulation, treatment planning, and documentation. Chapters describe the functioning of each PCRC when all is well and offer examples of each PCRC under strain. Vignettes are systematically articulated with the *DC:0–5™: Diagnostic Classification of Mental Health and Developmental Disorders of Infancy and Early Childhood* (DC:0–5; ZERO TO THREE, 2016), the *Diagnostic and Statistical Manual of Mental Disorders* (5th ed.; DSM–5; American Psychiatric Association, 2013), and the *10th Revision of the International Classification of Diseases* (ICD–10; World Health Organization, 1992), demonstrating how particular diagnoses may lead to functional impairments in family roles and how strengthening corresponding PCRCs can lead to symptom reduction and enhanced well-being. Sample objectives and interventions point the way to documenting clinical work such that billing for these services is straightforward.

Learning to See and Describe Relationships

Relationships exist and have indisputable material and emotional consequences, but they are themselves largely invisible. Yet, they are both experienced and inferred. Potent IMH paradigms, such as Edward Tronick's (2007) Still Face, attest to the significant, powerful existence of relationships. In this brief experiment, an infant is in an infant seat, and his parent is situated face-to-face and instructed to play and interact as they normally would. Then the parent is instructed to stop interacting and be still—to remain sitting before the baby but to maintain a blank expression—for 1 minute. This protocol allows us to see how energetically and persistently infants will work in an attempt to reengage the responses of the parent, and how distressing and disorganizing it is for the infant when these attempts fail.

The Still Face allows us to see many important things about infant–parent relationships. The protocol is difficult for the parents and for most people to watch because it is common to empathically experience the distress that the child seems clearly to manifest. Typically, the relationship between the parent and the infant can be hard to perceive in all of its complexity in the ordinary flow of daily life. However, when the "flow" is impeded and disrupted by design, it becomes clear just how powerful it is. The PCRC framework helps IMH workers to see and describe parent–child interaction and relationships by highlighting and describing dynamics that are so ordinary as to go unnoticed in the usual flux and flow.

Often when an IMH worker enters a family system, she is met with a confusing panoply of impressions and competing demands for her attention. They may include environmental risks, material needs, multiple players, and high emotions. Because she is a human being, she also brings to the mix her own unique social location, biases, personality, vulnerabilities, and foibles. It can be challenging in this context to formulate a cohesive understanding of the family's strengths and difficulties, isolate discreet areas in need of clinical intervention, prioritize among these areas, and forge reasonable objectives. The PCRCs aid in

Tenet # 1:
Self-Awareness Leads to Better Services for Families

this process by describing features of parent–child relationships that are universally present when all is going well enough, such that the IMH worker can pinpoint both areas of strength and health in the relationship that she is assessing and areas that are fraught or may not be developed.

It is important to emphasize that the PCRCs are deliberately descriptive and impressionistic rather than objective or measurable. Two different competent IMH workers might well come away from a clinical assessment of the same parent–child relationship with two different understandings of how particular PCRCs are functioning. This outcome is unproblematic because the PCRC framework is deliberately a tool to facilitate *IMH workers' clinical thinking and communication*, not a test that marks or measures families in any way. Therefore, the two competent IMH workers imagined here might actually conduct two different treatments, both of which would presumably be of benefit to the family. The PCRCs help IMH workers and parents collaborate around treatment goals and objectives, provide internal coherence to the treatment, and help render the 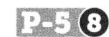 treatment equally coherent to collateral providers and third-party payers.

The PCRCs and Assessment Toward Treatment Planning

The PCRC framework is not an assessment in and of itself. It is assumed that the IMH worker is already trained and competent in an approach to mental or behavioral health assessment that is appropriate for their scope of practice. (For an excellent assessment resource, see Frankel, Harrison, & Wanjiku's, 2019, *Clinical Guide to Psychiatric Assessment of Infants and Young Children*. See also the summary of assessment tools specific to infancy and early childhood in Speranza & Mayes, 2017.) The PCRCs supplement the IMH worker's assessment repertoire and help with the problem of how individually focused many assessment instruments are. They do not supplant these important instruments but instead offer a roadmap to relationship-focused intervention and documentation that makes use of all available assessment information.

PCRCs usually emerge spontaneously under "ordinary good enough" circumstances. This phrase was introduced by D. W. Winnicott (1956, 1966) to describe the impressive fact that, despite the enormous complexity and intensity of caregiving demands with which parents of infants and young children are faced, they usually find the wherewithal to meet these demands in their own right way. The phrase is not intended to arbitrate what is "good enough," but rather to recognize and honor what transpires in the preponderance of instances.

PCRCs are bidirectional. Both the parent and the child make a contribution, and each PCRC cannot be said to be functioning well if only one partner in the relationship is doing their part. Picture again the Still Face paradigm described earlier. In the first part of the experiment, we might say that PCRC 4—*Parent is able to be* **emotionally attuned** *to/empathize with child AND child is able to experience and express a developmentally expectable range of human emotion*—is well established. Parent and child are mutually attuning and communicating emotionally in a nuanced, back-and-forth flow. However, during the chilling Still Face minute, the child seems to experience a bewildering, confusing, dismaying loss of a sense of effectiveness and agency. (In a classroom reconstruction of this protocol, participants playing the part of the parent reported how excruciating it was for them to refrain from acting on their empathy, to withhold comfort, and to stay "in role" while the child became distressed.) During this part of the experiment, we would have to say that the parent is not doing their part of PCRC 4, although the child is certainly making their contribution. If an IMH worker meets with a similar pattern actually occurring between a parent and child, such as may happen when a parent becomes depressed (e.g., during the postpartum period) and is unable to muster the capacity for emotional attunement, the worker would identify PCRC 4 as a competency in need of strengthening.

Each PCRC may be assessed to be functioning well, or it may be strained, impaired, or absent (see Appendix B). These are impressionistic, descriptive distinctions, not quantifiable categories. They constitute a conceptual continuum in the mind of the IMH worker. They help with dyadic clinical assessment, disciplined reflection, and collaborative treatment planning. A relevant reflective question is, "How worried am I about this PCRC?" The range of answers might be as follows:

- 0—"The relationship is functioning well in this area. I am not worried at all—this PCRC is clearly in evidence to the benefit of both members of the dyad."

- 1—"The relationship seems strained in this area. I am a little worried. One or both members of the dyad struggles with this PCRC, and they are not benefiting from it quite as much as they might. I am probably not going to propose targeting it for treatment, but I will keep an eye on it."

- 2—"The relationship is impaired here. I am worried about this PCRC. It is not functioning well for this dyad, to the detriment of one or both members. I believe it should be a target of treatment (unless strengthening other PCRCs is more pressing at the moment)."

- 3—"There seems to be a serious problem in this area. I am very worried about this PCRC. It does not seem to be in evidence at all. Striving to ignite and foster this PCRC should be a high priority of treatment."

Because these distinctions are impressionistic on the part of the IMH worker and are made in the mind of the IMH worker, it is very important that the worker have access to reflective supervision or consultation during the clinical assessment process (see Chapter 21).

P-5 ⑦

As the time comes to move from an assessment phase toward the treatment planning phase (this time frame varies by practice setting), the IMH worker will engage in collaborative conversations with the parent(s), sharing whatever impressions seem clinically useful and developing together a conceptualization of how treatment might benefit the family by lending support to particular PCRCs. The IMH worker will use clinical judgment regarding how detailed or explicit to be with the parent(s) about the language of the

PCRCs. Returning to the earlier example involving a parent suffering from depression with postpartum onset negatively affecting PCRC 4, the IMH worker might share and discuss PCRC 4 with the parent explicitly and propose that strengthening this PCRC be a goal of treatment. Conversely, the IMH worker might assess that the parent's vulnerability to guilt is too extreme currently such that this discussion would be injurious. In that case, the IMH worker would choose not to use the explicit language of the PCRC but might instead say, "You have shared with me that your depression leaves you feeling isolated and cut off from other people and keeps you from feeling the things you wish you could feel about and with your baby. I think a goal of our working together could be finding ways to lift your mood and increase the things that you can experience about and with your baby. I think this would be helpful to you and your baby and that the three of us could plan to work together on this."

The PCRCs and Identified Clients and Collateral Partners

"Who is the patient?" asked Alicia Lieberman and Jeree Pawl (1993) in a chapter describing infant–parent psychotherapy. They continued, "Beginning practitioners of infant–parent psychotherapy often find themselves grappling with the question: who are we treating, the parent or the baby? The briefest answer is: Both" (Lieberman & Pawl, 1993, p. 427). They further explained that "neither the parent nor the infant is the sole and ultimate focus of intervention. The focus is rather on the relationship, which is created through the interactional expression of each of their unique characteristics" (p. 428).

Often, however, IMH services are provided in the context of systems in which one member of the parent–child dyad must be selected as the "identified client" for purposes of treatment, documentation, and billing. The PCRC framework allows IMH workers to determine which partner makes more sense to designate as the identified client for these purposes.

The other person may be identified as the "collateral partner"—a family member who will be centrally involved in the treatment to support the utilization of services, receive direct support from the services in relation to the identified client's difficulties, and participate in the process of improving functioning or resolving problematic conditions.

In the process of assessing how the PCRCs are functioning, for example, the IMH worker may notice that several PCRCs are strained primarily because of difficulties that a child has in playing their role in the partnership. In other instances, it will become clear that certain PCRCs have failed to develop for the dyad primarily because of the parent's inability. No matter who the identified client is, both partners are negatively affected. The PCRC framework advocates steady attention to how both partners in the dyadic relationship are experiencing and contributing to the difficulty, and intervention is aimed at healing via strengthening the PCRCs. Regardless of who may be designated as the identified client, both parent and child have active roles in treatment, and treatment is geared to benefit both of them. It is, after all, as Fraiberg (1980) has told us, the relationship that is the target of all of our efforts. Resulting strengths in the relationship will then support the parent and child well beyond the time frame of the treatment.

For example, imagine a family who is referred for IMH treatment because of a finding of child abuse. A clinical assessment process including the consideration of PCRCs reveals that several PCRCs are strained or impaired. It is also revealed that the child displays some symptoms of trauma but does not meet full criteria for a diagnosis of Posttraumatic Stress Disorder or any other condition meeting medical necessity (see p. 21). The parent, however, suffers from symptoms meeting criteria for a diagnosis of Intermittent Explosive Disorder. In this instance, it would make sense for the parent to be the identified client for purposes of documentation and billing, and the case formulation would link the parent's diagnosis and symptoms with impairments in their role functioning as a parent. This procedure would include the acting out that constituted the child abuse. It would also articulate why involving the child in the IMH treatment as a collateral partner will be critical: so that treatment directly benefits the child, directly affects the parent's role-functioning difficulties, and mitigates against future abuse by promoting safety in parent–child interactions. The overarching aim will be to strengthen the PCRCs so that the resulting parent–child relationship is protective, nurturing, and growth promoting.

If, by contrast, the same assessment process pinpointed the same PCRCs as strained or impaired but found that the child's symptoms did meet full criteria for a diagnosis of Posttraumatic Stress Disorder, it might make sense to designate the child as the identified client regardless of whether the parent also met criteria for a diagnosis. The clinical formulation would then presumably link the child's symptoms with the incidents or patterns of abuse and would clearly state why the parent's involvement in treatment as collateral partner would be vitally important: to support the client's healing from the trauma, offer opportunities for reparation, and develop together patterns of interaction that are protective and nurturing for the client. The overarching aim will be exactly the same: to strengthen the PCRCs so that the parent–child relationship is protective, nurturing, and growth promoting.

The PCRC framework can help the IMH worker and the parent arrive at a clear understanding together about what the difficulties are and what might help as well as who will play what role in the treatment. Whether the IMH worker explicitly introduces the PCRC framework to the parent is a matter of clinical judgment. It may make more clinical sense simply to share the impression that the dyad seems to need support in strengthening their capacity to do one thing or another together that they are currently finding difficult or impossible. The IMH worker can readily translate the relevant PCRCs so that they are clear and meaningful to the parent and discuss how meeting together may help. The understanding developed with the parent regarding the

PCRCs that are the target of treatment and the roles to be played by each person (identified client or collateral partner) will be clearly stated in the clinical formulation. This method sets the stage for ongoing collaboration and clarity with documentation, billing, and review of progress toward goals and objectives (see p. 24).

The PCRCs and Diagnosis

In many systems of care and practice settings, arriving at a diagnosis is a necessary step in moving from the assessment process into providing treatment. As the earlier discussion of the "identified client" and "collateral partner" illustrated, the same PCRC may be strained, impaired, or absent because of a diagnosable condition on the part of the parent or the child. Chapter by chapter, therefore, each PCRC is described and then illustrated via two vignettes in which the PCRC in question is strained, impaired, or absent. In one vignette, a diagnosable condition on the part of the *parent* contributes to or is exacerbated by the difficulty in that PCRC; in the other vignette, a diagnosable condition on the part of the *child* contributes to or is exacerbated by the difficulty. In all cases, if the PCRC can be strengthened, this outcome helps ameliorate or resolve the problem. DSM–5 diagnoses are offered for parents, and DC:0–5 diagnoses cross-walked to the DSM–5 are offered for children. Associated ICD–10 codes are also provided. (See Appendix H. For a supplemental diagnostic framework that includes a comprehensive summary of assessment tools specific to infancy and early childhood, see Speranza & Mayes, 2017.)

Assigning diagnoses can be uncomfortable for some IMH workers concerned about the dangers of pathologizing people, and especially infants and young children, whose presentation is usually so profoundly shaped by the nature of their caregiving relationships.

The DC:0–5 articulates the purpose of diagnosis in this system:

> Diagnosis *is the identification and classification of specific infant/young child disorder....The primary purpose of classification of disorders is so that professionals—including clinicians, researchers, and policy makers—can communicate clearly about descriptive syndromes. Having a shared and standard nosology allows clinicians to link their observations to a growing body of knowledge concerning etiology, pathogenesis, the course of a disorder, and expectations concerning treatment. Using the common language of a diagnostic classification system facilitates the connection of individuals to existing services and thus can aid in the mobilization of appropriate systems of mental health care.* (ZERO TO THREE, 2016, p. 7)

In this book, it is assumed that the IMH worker is trained and qualified to make determinations regarding diagnosis or is working closely with a supervisor who is responsible. What is offered here is a way of understanding how both parent and child conditions may be affecting or affected by difficulties in the PCRCs. The PCRCs draw clinical attention away from siloed adult-versus-child systems of care and approaches to treatment, and they help us work at the heart of the difficulty—in the critical, dynamic space ongoing between the parent and child.

Note that each PCRC is followed by two vignettes, each involving one diagnostic picture. These vignettes are merely offered as illustrations. No association is implied between difficulty in a particular PCRC and susceptibility to a particular diagnosis. In theory, every PCRC could be affected by every imaginable diagnosable condition, and vice versa. That would make this a very long book. The reader can rely on their own expertise to determine how a client's own symptoms are affecting or affected by particular PCRCs. (For further details regarding diagnosis, symptoms, and impairments, see Appendices D and E.)

Establishing Medical Necessity: PCRC-Focused Relational Clinical Formulation

In many systems of care, intervention can be funded only if it is established that the service is medically necessary. Funding streams, third-party payers, and systems of care vary with respect to medical necessity benchmarks, types of service rendered, and other parameters of reimbursable services. In many systems, however, a qualifying mental health diagnosis is one necessary element permitting mental health intervention to be reimbursed, together with a clear description of how the diagnosable condition is creating problems for the individual and how these problems may be responsive to treatment.

Some of the diagnoses in the illustrative vignettes in these chapters may not meet criteria for service qualification or reimbursement within particular practice settings, systems, or locales. Some may fall outside of the mission of particular agencies or the scope of practice or competence of individual IMH workers. Moreover, agencies may be contracted to provide some services and use some billing codes (e.g., collateral treatment) but not others (e.g., family therapy). In addition, some systems may require that the duration and intensity of treatment be specified (e.g., "Weekly infant–parent psychotherapy is recommended for a period of 6 months, at which time client's and family's needs should be reassessed"). Some of the relational clinical formulations in this book omit some of these elements. It is assumed that the IMH worker is clear about their own scope of practice and competence, is familiar with the relevant parameters in their practice setting, and has access to reflective supervision or consultation to sort out any questions along these lines.

It is critical that IMH workers help systems and societies know when conceptual, political, or bureaucratic constraints hinder best practice. For example, it is inappropriate for a mental health system to purport to serve children from birth to 5 years old if parents cannot be designated as identified clients within that system. Often, it is the parent who

P-5 ⑦ suffers from a diagnosable condition that puts the child's development and well-being at risk, and the child needs to be directly included in the treatment to benefit immediately. In recognition of this, the U.S. Department of Health and Human Services (2016) offered the following guidance regarding Medicaid eligibility and dyadic service provision:

> *Mothers who are not Medicaid eligible may receive some benefit from diagnostic and treatment services directed at treating the health and well-being of the child (such as family therapy services) to reduce or treat the effects of the mother's condition on the child. Consistent with current policy regarding services provided for the "direct benefit of the child," such diagnostic and treatment services must actively involve the child, be directly related to the needs of the child and such treatment must be delivered to the child and mother together, but can be claimed as a direct service for the child.* (p. 4)

The National Center for Children in Poverty (2018) conducted a national survey and issued a report documenting a range of ways that states use Medicaid funds to cover infant and early childhood mental health services. IMH workers **P-5 ⑥** can help programs, systems of care, and states understand where they are on this map and articulate where they want to be.

IMH workers must advocate to make sure that services that truly are necessary to restore or promote the healthy development and well-being of infants and young children are recognized within the funding structures that exist to ensure care. There is often a role for reflective supervisors and consultants in supporting IMH workers in identifying such points of policy and opportunities for engagement. **Tenet # 10: Advance Policy That Supports All Families** Additionally, they need to support the allocation of resources for advocacy so that systems of care and society at large may benefit. It is vital that the voices of families and frontline IMH workers be heard.

To illustrate the process of establishing medical necessity, each vignette is followed by a relational clinical formulation linking the diagnosis (including some of the symptoms demonstrating that criteria for this diagnosis are met) to functional impairments related to the child's development and functioning or to the adult's functioning as a parent. Impact on the family more broadly is described in some instances, and either member of the dyad's functioning in other settings— child care, school, work, community, and so forth—may be outlined. Sociocultural factors affecting the difficulty in positive or negative ways may be included. Family strengths and vulnerabilities, as well as ameliorating and exacerbating factors, are often listed here, and the dyad's orientation to the difficulty and to services may be described. A succinct case is made for relationship-focused clinical intervention aimed at strengthening a particular PCRC to decrease the client's symptoms or enhance functioning. Each formulation suggests how intervention will aim to do one or more of the following:

1. *Correct or ameliorate* the diagnosable condition,

2. *Resolve* the signs or symptoms that indicated the need for treatment,

3. *Resolve* the circumstances giving rise to or exacerbating the condition,

4. Significantly *diminish* the functional impairment,

5. *Prevent* significant deterioration in functioning, or

6. *Allow for* the child to progress developmentally as individually appropriate.

Each formulation also includes a clear justification for and description of the role of the relationship partner (parent or child) as collateral partner in the treatment. (For further details regarding elements of clinical formulation, see Appendix C.)

PCRC-Derived Goals, Objectives, and Interventions

(For further details regarding goals, objectives, and interventions, see Appendices F and G.)

In each chapter, the relational clinical formulation is followed by a sample goal keyed to the PCRCs and several sample treatment objectives (referred to in some systems as "expected behavioral changes") that are measurable and observable. *Goals* are overarching aims of treatment; *objectives* are the concrete changes that demonstrate that progress toward the goal is in evidence. The process of articulating goals and objectives and forging a treatment plan must be a meaningful, collaborative exchange with parents in which understanding is shared regarding the nature of the problem, the hoped-for change, the signs of progress, and the roles that family members and the IMH worker will play.

In some systems and practice settings, it is necessary to identify a baseline against which change will be measured and a planned interval of time within which this change will be measured (e.g., "within 3 months, incidents of emotional dysregulation at morning drop-off will be reduced from 5 times per week to 0–1 times per week"). It is also often important to note how this will be determined (e.g., "per parent's report," "as observed by IMH worker," "per report of child care provider during collateral meeting with IMH worker"). Some sample objectives offered in this book are more impressionistic and some baselines more descriptive than what may be accepted as adequate in particular service settings, so it is important for IMH workers to be in conversation with those responsible for utilization review or quality assurance within their system of care to be sure that standards are met.

Readers will notice that the vignettes often point to several PCRCs that may need strengthening, and realistically, treatment would call for more than one goal. In practice, IMH workers will often arrive at several goals collaboratively with parents. For simplicity's sake, each of the 40 vignettes in these pages is linked to a single goal with several attendant sample objectives.

Objectives are things that clients and their collateral partners will demonstrate, achieve, or manifest. Sometimes objectives are articulated in keeping with a stages-of-change framework as described in Taubman's (2007) guide to treatment planning and Copeland's (2000) wellness recovery action plan. This approach articulates the following sequence for objectives:

1. Client [or collateral partner] will acknowledge the problem.

2. Client [or collateral partner] will be able to describe the problem accurately.

3. Client [or collateral partner] will identify strengths, resources, and strategies available to resolve the problem.

4. Client [or collateral partner] will act on identified strengths, resources, and strategies to resolve the problem.

5. Client [or collateral partner] will manifest ultimate outcomes.

Treatment planning also involves identifying interventions— things IMH workers will do and ways they will bring their expertise to bear in supporting clients toward realizing their goals and meeting their objectives. The PCRC framework emerged in the context of many decades of clinical work "in the Fraiberg tradition"—that is, work that grew out of the pioneering IMH programs, intervention modalities, and theories developed by Selma Fraiberg and her colleagues (e.g., Fraiberg, 1980). This tradition includes infant–parent psychotherapy (Fraiberg, 1980; Lieberman, Silverman, & Pawl, 2000; St. John & Pawl, 2000) and child–parent psychotherapy (Lieberman, Ghosh Ippen, & Van Horn, 2015; Lieberman & Van Horn, 2008).

Selma Fraiberg was a social worker and a psychoanalyst. Key features of clinical work in the Fraiberg tradition include the triadic influence of social work practice, psychodynamic formulation and technique, and a developmental orientation; a deep appreciation for the influence of attachment relationships; a readiness to deliver services in families' homes or communities; an ethic of disciplined learning through clinical experience; and a commitment to clinical research, writing, and training. This tradition challenges the conventional opposition posited between psychoanalytic or psychodynamic versus cognitive–behavioral approaches because it is focused on the behavioral manifestations in the parent–child relationship and material impact on the family environment of intra- and intersubjective dynamics.

At the core of this tradition is the conviction that it is parents who are the authorities on their children, and IMH workers must earn parents' permission to contribute their expertise; they also must develop understandings of the child's and family's difficulties collaboratively with parents. This method involves having a wide-angle focus because tangles in a parent–child relationship involve threads leading in many directions—to current and historical political issues, social and economic forces, parental history, ancestral traditions, and so forth.

Work in the Fraiberg tradition also means a commitment to teaching and training that is rooted in service delivery so that the lessons learned come first and foremost from the families served. This book is steeped in this tradition, as the clinical vignettes will illustrate. Appendix G offers sample relationship-focused clinical interventions drawn primarily from this tradition. However, this volume is not intended as an introduction to these modalities of intervention. Rather, it is hoped that the IMH worker, regardless of training, affiliation, or orientation, will find these pages useful in bringing the parent–child relationship into focus and making their approach clear to families and funders. The PCRCs framework is a tool that supports clinicians in efficiently translating each family's unique needs and strengths into terms that will be recognizable by funding structures and by providers across spheres of practice, freeing up clinicians' time for responsive, creative, and healing relationship-focused clinical work with infants, young children, and families.

A Note Regarding Vignettes

Each PCRC is illustrated via two vignettes, one in which a diagnosable condition on the part of a parent contributes to or is manifest in a PCRC needing strengthening, and the other depicting a situation in which a child meets criteria for a diagnosable condition that contributes to or is manifest in the PCRC-related difficulty. Many of the vignettes include sociocultural details about the family and the IMH worker. These are included in order to illustrate the integration of a diversity-informed approach in assessment, formulation, treatment planning, and documentation. Appendix I (Questions to Guide Reflection) offers discussion prompts to support reflection about this material.

It is critical that the reader understand that the vignettes are purely illustrative and that no correlation is suggested between:

- particular PCRCs and vulnerability to particular diagnoses

- particular family constellations and troubles with particular PCRCs

- particular areas of parent–child relationship difficulty and particular sociocultural groups

All vignettes are constructed for illustrative purposes. Although these examples are informed by elements of real families' experiences, the vignettes are fictive.

After each vignette throughout this book, the diagnoses and codes listed refer to the following three sources:

- *DC:0–5™: Diagnostic Classification of Mental Health and Developmental Disorders of Infancy and Early Childhood* (DC:0–5; ZERO TO THREE, 2016)

- *Diagnostic and Statistical Manual of Mental Disorders* (5th ed.; DSM–5; American Psychiatric Association, 2013)

- *International Classification of Diseases, 10th Revision, Clinical Modification* (ICD–10–CM; World Health Organization, 1992)

CHAPTER 1

Multicultural Practitioner and Family Realities: The *Diversity-Informed Tenets for Work With Infants, Children, and Families*

The Parent–Child Relationship Competencies (PCRCs) belong to parents and children. They are spontaneously occurring, bidirectional, dynamic systems unfolding in the interactions and intersubjective space between parents and children. They are galvanizing, organizing, and growth promoting for families. They are universally present when all is going well enough, yet their individual expression is in each instance entirely unique. Understanding the PCRCs means appreciating both their universal features and the awesome diversity of their lived expression.

Along with other prenatal to age 5 professionals, infant mental health (IMH) workers are well positioned by virtue of training, expertise, scope of practice, and professional ethics to recognize and support families in strengthening PCRCs as needed. To do this, IMH workers must be equipped to recognize and respond to both the universal features of the PCRCs and how they manifest in ways that are individually and socioculturally variable and meaningful. In short, it is not possible for an IMH worker to appropriately support families around the PCRCs unless this effort is diversity informed.

The *Diversity-Informed Tenets for Work With Infants, Children, and Families*[1.1] (© 2012 Irving Harris Foundation; hereafter, "the Tenets"; see www.diversityinformedtenets.org) help practitioners focus on diversity, equity, and inclusion in all spheres of practice. The developers of the Tenets intended them to be "a set of guiding principles that could

---

[1.1] The Tenets were collaboratively generated by a Working Group of the Harris Professional Development Network. They are reproduced with permission from the Tenets Initiative and the Irving Harris Foundation (© 2012 by the Irving Harris Foundation).

be used as a navigational tool to ensure that while immersed in their day-to-day work [early childhood] professionals [are] steering toward a more equitable, inclusive, and socially just world for all infants, children, and families" (K. Thomas et al., 2019, p. 46). This chapter introduces the Tenets, which were collaboratively developed and are collaboratively revised and disseminated by the Tenets Working Group,[1,2] and offers examples of their potential application by IMH workers engaged in PCRC-focused assessment, treatment, and documentation. Much of the material in this chapter was generated collaboratively by members of the Tenets Working Group through an iterative process of refinement. The Tenets are referenced throughout the later chapters as they come into play in relation to specific PCRCs.

The Tenets are influenced by several bodies of thought and practice, including intersectionality theory (Collins, 1991; Collins & Bilge, 2016; Crenshaw, 1989), which contends that multiple systems of oppression collectively affect all individuals. In her pioneering essay on intersectionality, Kimberly Crenshaw (1989) argued that the specific and collective struggles of Black women are consistently obscured when racism and sexism are examined separately. She wrote, "because the intersectional experience is greater than the sum of racism and sexism, any analysis that does not take intersectionality into account cannot sufficiently address the particular manner in which Black women are subordinated" (p. 140). Intersectionality theorist Patricia Hill Collins (1991) argued further that systems of oppression— such as racism, classism, sexism, able-ism, homophobia, and xenophobia—are interlocking such that "each system needs the others in order to function" (p. 222) and that "all groups possess varying amounts of penalty and privilege in one historically created system" (p. 225). This framework sees individuals as positioned in complex ways such that many axes of identity—race, class, gender, ability status, sexuality,

---

[2] Current members of the Tenets Working Group include the following: Ana Arbel, Nicola Brown, Karen Frankel, Nucha Isarowong, Ayannakai Nalo, Carmen Rosa Noroña, Rebecca Shahmoon-Shanok, Tonia M. Spence, Alison Steier, Maria Seymour St. John, Gregory Tate, and Kandace Thomas—with Amanda Hwu of the Irving Harris Foundation.

nationality, and others—intersect, and one may experience penalty along one axis and privilege along another. IMH workers must be sensitive to dynamics of penalty and privilege as these play out in families' lives, in programs and systems of care, and in individual relationships between IMH workers and families.

The Tenets are also grounded in postcolonial theory (e.g., Fanon, 1952/2008), critical pedagogy (e.g., Freire, 1974/2007), and liberation psychology (e.g., Martín-Baró, 1996). These influences call for attention to the ways that human beings are indoctrinated into historical and sociopolitical contexts in which the interests of particular groups are furthered at the expense of others. It is squarely within the purview of IMH workers to analyze how these indoctrination processes shape—at the most profound levels imaginable—our sense of who we are, who others may be, and how the world works. IMH workers engage with families at a potent time in family life: on the occasion of a new baby entering the family and the world. Society at large has vested interests in this family affair, whether in the direction of celebrating and privileging this new member of society or, conversely, in the direction of devaluation and disregard. In all likelihood, a complex, multipronged process of elevation and denigration along various axes will be busily underway, with possibilities of "being" for the baby and the family rapidly foreclosing as perceptions, projections, and identifications take shape. IMH workers can intervene to call attention to and alter these processes, strengthening parents' sense of agency, protecting possibilities of being for the baby, and supporting family self-determination. To do this task, IMH workers must attend to the historical and sociopolitical realities that shape their own experiences and the experiences of the families they serve.

Doing so has not historically been common practice. For example, in a volume that marked the emergence of the IMH field, Selma Fraiberg (1980) told the story of an adolescent mother, Beth, and her 4-month-old infant, Trudy, who was "starving." She wrote, "Trudy has dropped far below the third percentile on her growth chart and all evidence shows that Beth is unable to feed her baby...Beth has refused all help at our hospital....The situation is critical" (p. 29). The clinical intervention that Fraiberg described unearthed the story of Beth's own early childhood trauma and worked to interrupt its intergenerational transmission and repetition. She wrote, "Beth had been a war orphan, found abandoned at an unknown age on the streets of a war-torn country. She was starving when she was admitted to an orphanage. She was still in a state of severe nutritional inadequacy when she was adopted by an American family at age 2½" (pp. 30–31). Fraiberg described poignantly the healing therapeutic work that ensued, putting the painful memories and feelings from Beth's past into words so that they were no longer played out in action with Trudy in turn playing the part of the starving and neglected baby.

The therapeutic pathways Fraiberg and colleagues opened up were revolutionary, ushering in decades of clinical innovation, research, and advances in early childhood policy. However, these passages also exemplify a problematic lack of historical and sociopolitical specificity that is characteristic of a great deal of professional writing and reflective of a similar common pattern of avoidance at the level of clinical practice (K. Thomas, 2019). From a diversity-informed practice perspective, the following questions must be asked: From which "war-torn country" did Beth hail? What were the politics of the war? What dispossessed group was she likely a member of? What might have composed her ancestry? What was her native tongue? What was the ethnicity of the American family who adopted her? How did they understand their parenting role? Did they find ways of forging links to her homeland and history? Did they strive to learn her language? How did they enfold her membership in their family? Where are they now? Exploring these questions is critical to developing a sufficient diversity-informed understanding of Beth's and Trudy's struggles.

A diversity-informed inquiry would also entail analysis of the clinician as a person who has an influential professional role with Beth and Trudy and who is herself situated along multiple axes of identity. What has the clinician ("Mrs. Adelson") been taught about Beth's country of origin? What are her thoughts and feelings about the fact that Beth is "17½, an unwed mother" (Fraiberg, 1980, p. 29)? What are her views regarding orphans, adolescence, marriage, adoption, and war—and what contributed to shaping her thoughts and feelings about such matters? The fact that none of this information is disclosed is in keeping with conventions of professional writing. Such conventions produce a representation of the practitioner as disembodied—an objective authority figure who is herself above the fray of intersectionality.

In addition to situating families' and practitioners' experiences in nuanced understandings of sociopolitical influences, a diversity-informed practice approach entails examining programs and systems of care through the same lens. Fraiberg (1980) noted that Beth had refused all help at the hospital, and she suggested that this refusal reflected her psychological vulnerability. From a diversity-informed practice perspective, one would ask who benefits from the use of the word "refusal" and what this refusal says not only about Beth but also about the hospital. What definition of "help" prevails at this hospital? What messages are sent by the architecture, signage, décor, personnel, and engagement and care delivery processes? What efforts are made to make Beth feel expected, seen, welcome, understood, respected, and empowered here? Whose time is valued? Whose languages are spoken? What healing practices are shared?

Is the hospital "for" healing those who are patients there, or is it also or mostly "for" furthering the careers of those who work there, containing public health risks, generating profit for the pharmaceutical industry, fueling the medico-research industrial complex, and so forth? In all likelihood, the truthful answer is "all of these," but only the first is openly acknowledged; the hospital professes mainly to traffic only in healing and the promotion of well-being. From a diversity-informed approach, it would be countertherapeutic to pretend that Beth's refusal was indicative only of Beth's pathology. Instead, it would be important to embrace Beth's refusal as, in part, an apt critique-in-action of the ways that the hospital also represents and reproduces forces of oppression that are actively dangerous to her and her baby (Boggs, 2011; Ghosh-Ippen, & Lewis, 2011). From this understanding, an IMH worker could support Beth in appraising whether the hospital also has something to offer of which she would wish to avail herself.

The Tenets support IMH workers in keeping questions such as these in mind. They also suggest pathways for intentional critical self-reflection and action. What follows is the text of each of the 10 Tenets (www.diversityinformedtenets.org) followed by a brief discussion and a list of sample actions that an IMH worker might take toward upholding the Tenet.

Tenet # 1:
Self-Awareness
Leads to Better
Services for
Families

1. Self-Awareness Leads to Better Services for Families: "Working with infants, children, and families requires all individuals, organizations, and systems of care to reflect on our own culture, values, and beliefs, and on the impact that racism, classism, sexism, able-ism, homophobia, xenophobia, and other systems of oppression have had on our lives in order to provide diversity-informed, culturally attuned services."

Tenet #1 undergirds all other Tenets. It calls on IMH workers to engage in intentional reflection regarding the impact of intersecting systems of oppression on one's personal and professional experiences. It asserts that the embodied and socially located personhood of the IMH worker matters to the work they do and the families they serve. Actions that an IMH worker might take toward upholding Tenet #1 include the following:

- Make use of reflective supervision to expand awareness of the IMH worker's social location and personal experiences as these come into play in serving families (Hardy & Bobes, 2017; Hernández

& McDowell, 2010; Noroña, Heffron, Grunstein, & Nalo, 2012);

- Create a personal cultural genogram (Hardy & Leszloffy, 1995);

- Undergo disciplined "self-observation" and inventory through reflective writing on "how one reacts when stressed in moments of racial conflict" (Stevenson, 2014, p. 41) and conflict around other "isms";

- Register and reflect on countertransference responses to explore whether they provide information about the IMH worker, client's family, or both;

- Note how working with children in different developmental phases and families of various sociocultural contexts may stir different issues from the IMH worker's personal history;

- Question assumptions, and elicit the family's experience;

- Evaluate continuities and discontinuities between the IMH worker and the family's social location;

- Research aspects of family culture with which the IMH worker is unfamiliar;

- Without placing undue burden on professionals from underrepresented groups, make links with and seek consultation from colleagues more knowledgeable regarding family culture;

- Consider IMH worker power and privilege as this affects family and work (DiAngelo, 2011; McIntosh, 1989);

- Be alert to and accountable around IMH worker microaggressions toward family (Sue et al., 2007);

- Disclose personal responses in ways that may be useful to the IMH worker–family relationship; and

- Expand capacity to "stay engaged," "tolerate discomfort," and "expect and accept non-closure" (Singleton, 2015, pp. 71–75) without withdrawal or retaliation.

Tenet # 2:
Champion
Children's
Rights Globally

2. Champion Children's Rights Globally: "Infants and children are citizens of the world. The global community is responsible for supporting parents/caregivers, families, and local communities in welcoming, protecting, and nurturing them."

Tenet #2 asserts that children have human rights that may supersede particular families' or societies' ideas. Children's rights have been pondered, debated, and asserted internationally. For example, the UN Convention on the Rights of the Child was drafted in 1989 and went into force in 1990. Although this is the most widely ratified treaty in history, the United States has yet to ratify it. Tenet #2 calls on IMH workers to take a global, human rights–based view of children rather than basing IMH work in a more narrow, perhaps nationalist, stance. Simultaneously, Tenet #2 recognizes the importance of ancestry, homeland, culture, and community, and it demands that parents/caregivers, families, and local communities be supported in caring for their children. Actions that IMH workers might take toward upholding Tenet #2 include the following:

- Become familiar with the UN Convention on the Rights of the Child;

- Become familiar with the World Association for Infant Mental Health's (2016) position paper on the rights of infants;

- Remain informed regarding developments in human rights, intergenerational justice, reproductive health and justice, birth justice, disabilities rights, people's health, food justice, and racial justice movements nationally and internationally;

- Challenge infractions against children's and families' rights;

- Inquire about and affirm families' roots, ties, commitments, and resources beyond national borders;

- Support parents in advocating for children's and families' rights;

- Take steps to remove impediments to parental, family, and community capacities to welcome, protect, and nurture their children;

- Recognize that children's love crosses all borders, and take steps to protect connections and facilitate contact among separated family members (Ghosh Ippen, Noroña, & Thomas, 2012);

- Think of the earth as all children's birthright, and ensure children's access to recreation, education, physical activity, play, and natural environments and resources, now and into the future;

- Speak up when a society makes decisions or takes actions that will have negative consequences for children;

- Advocate to safeguard children's health and well-being in the present and the future;

- Raise public awareness regarding the needs and rights of children;

- Raise public awareness regarding the adverse effects of criminalizing families for their migration decisions; and

- Work to expand opportunity for all children.

3. **Work to Acknowledge Privilege and Combat Discrimination:** "Discriminatory policies and practices that harm adults harm the infants and children in their care. Privilege constitutes injustice. Diversity-informed practitioners acknowledge privilege where we hold it, and use it strategically and responsibly. We combat racism, classism, sexism, able-ism, homophobia, xenophobia, and other systems of oppression within ourselves, our practices, and our fields."

> **Tenet # 3:**
> Work to Acknowledge Privilege and Combat Discrimination

Tenet #3 calls on IMH workers to keep in mind Leena Banerjee Brown's (2007) insight that "privilege and discrimination are made possible because of one another. Both are products of a paradigm and a mindset defined by hierarchy and exclusion, in which value is afforded to the few at the expense of many" (p. 19). IMH workers must monitor how dynamics of privilege and discrimination play out in their places of work, their relationships with coworkers and families served, and society. Society needs the expertise of IMH workers to understand the impact of policies and practices that may intentionally or inadvertently cause harm to infants, children, and families. An IMH worker might do the following:

- Expand awareness of racism, classism, sexism, ableism, homophobia, xenophobia, and other systems of oppression through personal inquiry, research, and conversations in reflective supervision;

- Track via disciplined observation, and document via reflective writing, how privilege operates in the workplace;

- Deploy one's privilege to expand access to resources for a family;

- Rather than exercising privilege in a given moment, call attention to the injustice inherent in being afforded the privilege (e.g., speak up or weigh in when others with less privilege are not considered or consulted);

- Challenge discriminatory workplace practices through speaking up, filing grievances, and so forth;

- Support colleagues who take risks to combat discrimination;

- Create spaces and structures where privileged subgroups can learn together and support one another around accountability (e.g., White caucuses) so that the onus is not on less privileged groups to teach, challenge, and facilitate growth;

- Take risks where others with less privilege may not be able to;

- Engage in organizing and advocacy around policies that harm families;

- Raise public awareness through writing and public speaking;

- Confront colleagues who interact with families or coworkers in harmful ways; and

- Escalate the matter when efforts to end discriminatory practices are unsuccessful.

4. Recognize and Respect Non-Dominant Bodies of Knowledge: "Diversity-informed practice recognizes non-dominant ways of knowing, bodies of knowledge, sources of strength, and routes to healing within all families and communities."

Tenet # 4: Recognize and Respect Non-Dominant Bodies of Knowledge

Tenet #4 challenges the notion that help, healing, knowledge, and resources flow from providers to families, asserting instead that these things are endogenous to families and that it is incumbent on IMH workers to acknowledge, recognize, and respect family expertise. Often, this is a challenging attitudinal shift for IMH workers, who may have spent many years acquiring specialized skills and knowledge precisely because they want to be helpful! However, when helping professionals rush in with zeal, they can fail to see the family's strength and sometimes damage important capacities held by families (Fadiman, 1997). Tenet #4 encourages IMH workers to engage in a collaborative process with families so that the perspectives and expertise of both the family and the IMH worker may be marshaled to further the family's goals. Actions that IMH workers might take toward upholding Tenet #4 include the following:

- Factor family strengths into assessment, formulation, and treatment planning;

- Identify and work to dismantle institutional policies and practices that exclude or denigrate non-dominant ways of knowing and healing;

- Examine and expose how professionalization processes embed disparaging and delegitimizing representations of non-dominant practices;

- Inquire about family's construal of areas of strengths and challenges;

- Explore what solutions family members might offer, perhaps including how ancestors might have tackled such challenges;

- Demonstrate to children respect for parental authority and efficacy;

- Look and listen for narratives, themes, and images of strength and healing in family discourse, actions, and environment;

- Consult cultural authorities about illness and healing in family culture; and

- Support linkage to community resources if this is welcome by the family.

Tenet # 5:
Honor Diverse Family Structures

5. Honor Diverse Family Structures: "Families decide who is included and how they are structured; no particular family constellation or organization is inherently optimal compared to any other. Diversity-informed practice recognizes and strives to counter the historical bias toward idealizing (and, conversely, blaming) biological mothers while overlooking the critical child-rearing contributions of other parents and caregivers including second mothers, fathers, kin and felt family, adoptive parents, foster parents, and early care and educational providers."

Tenet #5 challenges IMH workers to think critically about inherited notions of family and to make sure to find out directly from families themselves how they hold family contours and ties. It also seeks to redress historical biases in the field by pointing out ways in which the field has tended to be "matri-centric" to the detriment of all. This bias in the field runs very deep, as is reflected in such terms as "maternal-child health," "mommy and me" or "mother–baby" programs, "maternal deprivation," "maternal sensitivity," and so forth. This bias sets biological mothers up for intense idealizations and de-idealizations, and it leaves other parents and caregivers marginalized. In keeping with Tenet #5, IMH workers might do the following:

- Ask at outset and again later who the members of the infant's or child's family are;
- Collaborate with family about best treatment constellation and consider shifts over time;
- Ask whether the infant or child has more than one household;
- Evaluate collaboratively with family how current division of caregiving labor is working for everyone and whether shifts would be useful;
- Actively inquire about whether there are people who may be "felt family" (e.g., play cousins, chosen family);
- Experience infant or child in the context of a range of important relationships;
- Challenge parent's gatekeeping behaviors that may be undermining or hindering the child's access to relationships with other important caregivers;
- Consider using phone calls, video conferencing, letter writing, and so forth to include caregivers who may remain in home countries or be incarcerated, deported, or otherwise unable to attend sessions (Noroña, 2011);
- Analyze with parents how the myths of the "good mother" and the "bad mother" may negatively affect their family;

- Make space without the child for adults to work through animosity toward one another;

- Assist adults who hold animosity toward one another to bear and honor the importance of each to the child;

- Support multiple caregivers in clarifying one another's roles and contributions to child rearing;

- Be sure your behavior demonstrates to the child the IMH worker's respect for the authority of parents and caregivers;

- Actively affirm non-dominant family structures to counter discrimination and oppression;

- Share research findings with families that counter discriminatory myths regarding adverse child outcomes linked to non-dominant family structures; and

- Raise public and professional awareness about family diversity.

Tenet # 6:
Understand That
Language Can
Hurt or Heal

6. Understand That Language Can Hurt or Heal:

"Diversity-informed practice recognizes the power of language to divide or connect, denigrate or celebrate, hurt or heal. We strive to use language (including body language, imagery, and other modes of nonverbal communication) in ways that most inclusively support all children and their families, caregivers, and communities."

Tenet #6 cautions IMH workers to critically examine professional language and to recognize that a great deal is conveyed through images, architecture, and so forth. Silence and invisibility send messages too. Adreinne Rich wrote, "When someone with the authority of a teacher, say, describes the world and you're not in it, there's a moment of psychic disequilibrium, as if you looked into a mirror and saw nothing" (cited in Burt, Gelnaw, & Lesser, 2010, p. 97). The field of IMH is dedicated to representing not just some but *all* infants and families—to making sure that all families find themselves respectfully represented. Tenet #6 draws on the spirit of the Americans with Disabilities Act of 1990, which called for universal inclusion of people with disabilities. It is not acceptable (or legal) to discriminate against people with disabilities either overtly or by omission. Their/our active participation in public life must be anticipated and protected through the presence and availability of needed accommodations. Despite this monumental advance in disabilities rights, a tremendous amount of discrimination persists, including intense discrimination against parents with disabilities (see the National Council on Disability's [2012] report *Rocking the Cradle: Ensuring the Rights of Parents With Disabilities and Their Children*). This Tenet calls on IMH workers to look at who is finding their way to services, and who may be excluded, and to create the infrastructure that clearly communicates to all families that they belong. Toward upholding this Tenet, an IMH worker might do the following:

- Imagine that parents and families read every word written in assessments, progress notes, and reports and then ask whether they would find this material respectful;

- Imagine that parents and families hear every word spoken about them in conferences, collateral meetings, and case reviews and then ask whether they would they find this material respectful;

- Inquire of family members how they would like to be addressed;

- Review intake forms and so forth to analyze whether families are likely to feel respected and welcomed by them;

- Review layout, décor, signage, visual imagery, and so forth in service sites with an eye to how welcome, comfortable, and respected children and families are likely to feel in the space;

- Consider unspoken rules about personal comport-ment and interpersonal interaction in the workplace (e.g., are particular cultural mores and modes of expression deemed more acceptable than others?);

- Become familiar with the resources of Welcoming Schools (www.welcomingschools.org);

- Consider what one's own attire and comportment might convey to families;

- Challenge professional language and other conventions that may be disrespectful toward families;

- Challenge professional language and other conventions that naturalize and aggrandize institutional oppression;

- Exercise caution in using the language of "risk" (e.g., "high-risk populations" or "at-risk child"), because this language is often associated with stigma, blame, and profiling;

- Avoid labeling people (e.g., "autistic child" or "schizophrenic mother"), and instead identify conditions as needed (e.g., "child with autism" or "woman who meets criteria for a diagnosis of Schizophrenia");

- Research dynamics of stigma related to client groups served;

- Cultivate clinical sensitivity to behavioral signs of shame; and

- Look for behavioral signs (e.g., client withdrawal or angry acting out) indicating that one's words or actions may have landed in a hurtful way, and then inquire about this reaction.

Tenet # 7:
Support Families in Their Preferred Language

7. Support Families in Their Preferred Language: "Families are best supported in facilitating infants' and children's development and mental health when services are available in their native languages."

Tenet #7 makes a distinction between "native" language and "preferred" language because it is important that families who are bilingual have the ability to choose which language they wish to use and when. A great wealth of professional literature documents the salience of language in mental health treatment. Often, the need for bilingual IMH workers outstrips the capacity of programs and systems of care. This Tenet demands that this deficit be critically examined. Given that professional ethics mandate that mental health treatment be available in clients' native languages, what are the structural barriers to workforce development perpetuating the injurious status quo? Often, the forces of oppression that conspire to actively maintain this status quo are obscured, and the state of affairs is simply passively lamented. IMH workers can do the following:

- Advocate for expansion of bilingual or multilingual services;

- Contribute to workforce development efforts to support a pipeline of bilingual IMH workers;

- Ensure that multiple languages can be comfortably spoken in the workplace;

- Support families in accessing services and resources in their native languages;

- Share information with parents regarding the benefits for children of growing up bilingual and how bilingualism can be supported;

- Raise public awareness to counter damaging myths regarding adverse outcomes for children raised bilingually;

- Describe themselves as monolingual when this is the case (one frequently hears non-English-speaking clients referred to as "monolingual," but one rarely hears English-speaking professionals referred to in this way, although they tend to be);

- Make shifts in distribution of labor to relieve bilingual IMH workers of undue burden;

- Avoid asking fellow IMH workers to serve as translators—instead, professional interpreters should be accessed;

- Ensure that interpreters receive appropriate training and support for their role and experiences;

- Avoid asking children or other family members to serve as translators—instead, professional interpreters should be accessed; and

- Work to ensure that reflective supervision is available for bilingual IMH workers in their native languages and the languages in which they are delivering services.

8. Allocate Resources to Systems Change:

"Diversity and inclusion must be proactively considered when doing any work with or on behalf of infants, children, and families. Resource allocation includes time, money, additional/alternative practices, and other supports and accommodations, otherwise systems of oppression may be inadvertently reproduced. Individuals, organizations, and systems of care need ongoing opportunities for reflection in order to identify implicit bias, remove barriers, and work to dismantle the root causes of disparity and inequity."

Systems of oppression are reproduced continually via institutional and discursive practices bearing material consequences. Some policies and practices are blatantly oppressive or patently unjust. However, many policies and practices exist for perfectly good reasons, further reasonable ends, and seem innocuous; nevertheless, they may contribute in complex ways to perpetuating an unjust status quo. Tenet #8 recognizes that such processes must be actively interrupted, and it assigns responsibility to all IMH workers to participate in intentional disruption of the status quo and rerouting of resources toward social justice. From this perspective, all IMH workers—regardless of the degree of organizational power or authority they may hold—serve as resource gatekeepers. This notion means that all

IMH workers have the power to engage or not engage with families in ways that are respectful and meaningful to the family, to include or exclude families, to represent them in a positive or negative light to others, to increase or limit their access to resources and services, and also to shine a critical light on workplace practices—asking how things might be changed toward advancing social justice. However, individual IMH workers cannot do this alone.

Tenet #8 calls on programs and systems of care to embed reflective supervision or other structures to support reflection and to institutionalize reflective practice to ensure that resources are expended in ethical directions. This practice is akin to the "time out" in the Universal Protocol for Patient Safety in Surgery, wherein the surgeon must take a time out before initiating a planned procedure in the operating room to ensure that the cut they are about to make is the right one. Before money is spent, before someone new is hired, before a case is dismissed, before a new project is undertaken, IMH workers should pause and ask, "Is this in the service of positive change on behalf of infants, children, and families?" In furtherance of Tenet #8, an IMH worker might do the following:

- Remember—and help others remember—that "resources" include time, money, space, material goods, and human attention and then ask whether all of these resources are being expended in ways that further social justice;

- Analyze and perhaps work to change decision-making processes so that families' interests are prioritized;

- Review the agenda prior to a staff meeting with an eye to what or who is being prioritized or sidelined;

- Convey to program leadership what issues are most affecting the families served;

- Identify programmatic and systemic barriers to supporting families in optimal ways;

- Seek to understand and perhaps challenge how budgetary decisions are made;

- Compile a list of concrete changes collaboratively with coworkers that would signify progress toward particular social justice-informed goals, track and celebrate progress, and note to others when progress is slow or nonexistent; and

- Raise public awareness regarding systemic barriers.

Tenet # 9:
Make Space
and Open
Pathways

9. Make Space and Open Pathways: "Infant, child, and family-serving workforces are most dynamic and effective when historically and currently marginalized individuals and groups have equitable access to a wide range of roles, disciplines, and modes of practice and influence."

Tenet #9 extends the "interrupt and disrupt" principle discussed in connection to Tenet #8 to the child and family-serving workforce. Employment patterns fall out in this field, as in most others, along entirely predictable race- and gender-stratified lines. Systemic barriers tend to bar people of color from the access, safety, security, and mobility afforded to White people. Women tend to be subjected to discrimination, exposed to violence, and burdened with disproportionate caregiving responsibilities, leaving men at an employment and advancement advantage. The barriers and penalties mount for those who are on the "down side" of power along multiple axes of oppression. Often within systems, institutions, agencies, and teams, those on the down side of power along more axes of oppression have less decision-making power, autonomy in their jobs, and status in the workplace than their more privileged counterparts. Tenet #9 enjoins IMH workers to do the following:

- Make use of reflective supervision to analyze one's role in the workplace and relationships with coworkers through the lens of the "make space and open pathways" concept;

- Practice "make space/take space"—pushing oneself to take space and speak up if this is challenging and, conversely, to make room for others to do so if this option is more challenging;

- Take stock of how systems of oppression affect employment patterns and interpersonal dynamics in the workplace (e.g., how some people's contributions may be recognized and responded to, whereas others are ignored, blocked, or stolen);

- Use reflective writing to articulate observed patterns;

- Take steps to interrupt such patterns;

- Draw attention to culture-bound gaps and biases in professional literature, research protocols, and intervention approaches;

- Advocate for explicit conversations about race with coworkers;

- Make changes to division of labor so that underrepresented voices can be heard;

- Devise and demand equitable decision-making structures;

- Make contributions to workforce development efforts to nurture a pipeline of diverse professionals;

- Raise public and professional awareness regarding the benefits to children and families of being able to access practitioners reflective of their culture; and

- Assess whether a professional opportunity is best seized, shared, or surrendered to another.

10. Advance Policy That Supports All Families:

"Diversity-informed practitioners consider the impact of policy and legislation on all people and advance a just and equitable policy agenda for and with families."

Tenet # 10:
Advance Policy
That Supports
All Families

Tenet #10 draws attention to the importance of working "upstream" to influence legislation and public policy that affect children and families. It also encourages IMH workers to view inherited policies suspiciously; sometimes what is taken for policy is merely conventional practice, perhaps bolstered by its congruence with prevailing systems of oppression. IMH workers can do the following:

- Discuss in reflective supervision matters of law and public policy that affect families served;

- Research matters of law and public policy that affect children and families (see ZERO TO THREE's state-by-state policy resources: www.zerotothree.org/resources/states);

- Create spaces in the workplace to collectively engage and share resources around matters of law and policy affecting families served;

- Engage in advocacy efforts;

- Be alert to opportunities to usefully engage with clients around significant matters of law and policy;

- Use IMH expertise to raise public and professional awareness regarding important matters of law and policy;

- Challenge system of care and workplace policies that are harmful to some children and families (Roberts, 2002); and

- Vote.

Exploring and upholding the Tenets is a lifelong process. This chapter has offered a few preliminary thoughts and possible action steps. In the chapters that follow, the Tenets are cited as they relate to particular PCRCs.

CHAPTER 2

PCRC 1—The Deceptively Simple Concept of Need

There was before you, and then there was after, and in this after, you were the God I'd never had. I submitted before your needs, and I knew then that I must survive for something more than survival's sake. I must survive for you.

—Ta-Nehisi Coates (2015, p. 67)

PCRC 1: Parent is able to register and respond effectively to child's **needs** AND child is able to signal needs clearly in keeping with age level.

Parent–Child Relationship Competency (PCRC) 1 describes the most fundamental feature of the parent–child relationship: the powerful capacity of even newborn infants to convey to their caregivers what is vital for them to survive and thrive and the monumental efforts parents make to provide these things. D. W. Winnicott (1965c) introduced the term the "facilitating environment," which refers to the entire surroundings that parents and caregivers provide to a child to support their existence and development. All that parents do globally and in sustained ways to provide shelter, sustenance, and experiences that protect and enrich the child—as well as specifically and immediately in responding to such things as fluctuations in a baby's temperature, state of alertness, appetite for stimulation, or inclination for interaction—constitute provisions of the facilitating environment. These facilitating environments look very different from one culture to the next and one household to the next, and parents have varying degrees of access to resources or control over their circumstances. Still, even in conditions of extreme deprivation or intrusion, such as when families are homeless, in refugee camps, or in detention centers, parents tend to marshal any resources at their disposal to respond to their children's perceived needs.

"Need" as a construct is complex and contested. Drawing lines between needs and desires, or connecting the dots between needs and rights, always involves political actions. Societies make consequential decisions about resource allocation that affect diverse constituents differently, perpetuating social injustice.

Tenet # 2:
Champion
Children's
Rights Globally

In light of such disparities, the World Association of Infant Mental Health (2016) issued a global call to action to protect infants' rights that was grounded in a set of assertions regarding infants' needs. The preamble states, "there are unique considerations regarding the needs of infants during the first three years of life which are highlighted by contemporary knowledge, underscoring the impact of early experience on the development of human infant brain and mind" (World Association for Infant Mental Health, 2016, p. 1). The needs identified in this document are framed as universal human rights. For example, the declaration states the following:

> *Caregiving relationships that are sensitive and responsive to infant needs are critical to human development and thereby constitute a basic right of infancy. The Infant therefore has the right to have his/ her most important primary caregiver relationships recognized and understood, with the continuity of attachment valued and protected—especially in circumstances of parental separation and loss. This implies giving attention to unique ways that infants express themselves and educating mothers, fathers, caregivers and professionals in their recognition of relationship-based attachment behaviors.* (World Association for Infant Mental Health, 2016, p. 2)

Need is thus a human rights issue. Need is an ideological issue as well. Political theorist Jean Baudrillard (1981) wrote about the ways that ideas and convictions regarding needs are produced from the outside rather than emanating uncontrovertibly from the inside. Baudrillard asserted that "there are only needs because the system needs them" (p. 82). He was referring to the system of consumer culture (or perhaps it is more appropriate to say "producer culture") in which productivity depends on people perceiving that we have needs that must be met through consumption. Disposable diapers are a good example of this phenomenon. Many parents raising babies in a social context in which this practice is the norm perceive disposable diapers to be a basic need. However, in fact, disposable diapers are historically and geographically specific, and the fact that we feel we "need" them results from a good deal of successful marketing on the part of the booming industry that produces them. In Baudrillard's words, the diaper industry needs us to need these diapers.

Human infants cannot survive without a great deal of care, including care around excretion and hygiene. Cultures, communities, and families care for infants in wide-ranging successful ways—including whether to use diapers. The important thing with respect to this PCRC is that the need signaled by the child and registered and responded to by the parent is particular to this child and parent in this moment in the context of their family, community, and culture. All human infants experience and express hunger, but what is needed—cereal, formula, breast milk, broth—is personal, interpersonal, and cultural. This notion means that when a practitioner is assessing the degree to which this PCRC is established for a particular parent and child, the practitioner must suspend her own culturally informed notions of what it is that children need. She must not, for example, import the idea that diapers are needed and miss the excellent functioning of this PCRC when an infant conveys to his caregiver that he is about to urinate and the caregiver provides a bucket.

Tenet # 1:
Self-Awareness Leads to Better Services for Families

Tenet # 4:
Recognize and Respect Non-Dominant Bodies of Knowledge

Because children are dependent on adult care for many years to survive, early parenting is steeped in powerful experiences related to need. Paradoxically, because early development is so rapid, infants' and toddlers' needs are constantly changing. This rapid development means that parents need a tremendous amount of support from their communities and sometimes from infant mental health (IMH) providers. Those supporting parents around early caregiving must be able to register, tolerate, and respond to these powerful and evolving needs.

P-5 ③ As with any PCRC, this one emerges spontaneously under ordinary conditions, and it may be strained, impaired, or absent as a result of difficulties affecting the dyad. IMH intervention may be indicated to establish or strengthen this PCRC. The first vignette below illustrates how a diagnosable disorder on the part of an infant impedes the functioning of PCRC 1; in the second vignette, the difficulty originates in a diagnosable condition on the part of the parent.

Vignette 1.1

A monolingual English-speaking White pediatrician at the county hospital refers Paula, a 4-month-old infant of Mexican descent, to the IMH clinic. The doctor reports that the baby rarely demonstrates interest when presented with a bottle, feeds inconsistently, spits up a lot, fusses a lot, and is not gaining weight in keeping with expectations. The pediatrician is concerned and has assigned a designation of nonorganic failure to thrive. A bilingual/bicultural Columbian IMH worker responds to the referral and confers with the Spanish-speaking White (non-Hispanic) nurse practitioner at the pediatric clinic. The nurse practitioner states that this child's mother, Anna, who is a Mexican immigrant, cannot tell when her baby may be hungry and probably feels frustrated and incompetent. She reports that the mother and infant cannot relax into feeding episodes, and the mother is trying constantly to get the baby to feed. The mother did not attend the most recent scheduled pediatric visit, stating that she was too busy to bring the infant in because her own mother was visiting from out of town. The IMH worker met with the dyad in their home four times over the course of 2 weeks to develop an understanding and a plan collaboratively with this mother. The baby's grandmother was present for two of these meetings. Because the mother expressed feeling supported by the grandmother, she was included in the planning process, too.

DC:0–5 diagnosis: Undereating Disorder

DSM–5 diagnosis: Unspecified Feeding or Eating Disorder

> ***Note to readers:*** After each vignette throughout this book, the diagnoses and codes listed refer to the following three sources:
>
> • *DC:0–5™: Diagnostic Classification of Mental Health and Developmental Disorders of Infancy and Early Childhood* (DC:0–5; ZERO TO THREE, 2016)
>
> • *Diagnostic and Statistical Manual of Mental Disorders* (5th ed.; DSM–5; American Psychiatric Association, 2013)
>
> • *International Classification of Diseases, 10th Revision, Clinical Modification* (ICD–10–CM; World Health Organization, 1992)

ICD–10–CM code: F50.9

Relational Clinical Formulation

The identified client, a 4-month-old infant of Mexican descent, meets criteria for a DC:0–5 diagnosis of Undereating Disorder, as evidenced by her concerning low weight and slow rate of weight gain without identifiable organic cause, her apparent lack of interest in and refusal of the bottle, the resulting lack of efficacy experienced by her mother, and the general distress this lack of efficacy causes her mother. Together, these issues negatively affect the client's developmental functioning and the mother's functioning as a parent. The difficulties are exacerbated by immigration-related stress experienced by client's mother and communication challenges as mother has relied on monolingual providers. These difficulties are best addressed in the context of the infant–parent relationship, as feeding interactions are central. This dyad will benefit from IMH services aimed at strengthening PCRC 1, with client's mother participating as a collateral partner. The client's mother experiences her own mother, who is visiting from Mexico for an extended time, as supportive, so she too may take part in treatment on client's behalf.

Goal: Client will achieve a developmentally expectable weight via strengthening PCRC 1.

Sample collaboratively generated objectives include the following:

1. At present, the client's mother reports that the client refuses the bottle nine out of 10 times it is offered. The client will accept the bottle when offered three times out of four within the next 2 weeks per the parent's report.

2. At present, the client's mother reports trying "constantly" to get the client to take the bottle. The parent will report refraining from trying to interest the client in feeding for longer than 5 minutes at a time during each waking hour for the next 2 weeks.

3. The parent will, per her own report, enlist the client's grandmother's support in identifying signs of hunger in the client at least 5 times per day while the grandmother is in town for the next few weeks. (Baseline zero: The client's mother reports being too worried at present to be able to wait for signs of hunger.)

4. The parent will, during weekly meetings with the IMH worker over the next 2 months, notice out loud at least one thing other than hunger that the client seems to be experiencing in the moment. (Baseline zero: The client's mother reports being so focused on getting the client to feed that it is hard for her to direct attention to anything else.)

5. Client's mother's agitation, which contributes to stressful feeding interactions, is exacerbated by immigration- and acculturation-related challenges. Client's mother will identify family needs so that a plan can be developed during weekly home-base IMH meetings to meet these one-by-one.

Vignette 1.2

A home visiting public health nurse is concerned when she visits a 35-year-old woman 2 weeks postpartum and finds her preoccupied with frenzied cleaning of her apartment and talking with urgency about the importance of foiling the ants that tend to march across her kitchen floor when it rains. Although her infant is crying in his crib, the information this mother wants from the nurse pertains to ant-control measures rather than infant care. She denies having any questions about the baby. When asked how she is feeling, she states, "Never better. I don't know what everyone complains about. Since he was born, I've gotten more accomplished than in the past 9 months." The public health nurse makes a referral to an IMH worker for a mental health assessment. The IMH worker meets with the dyad in their home several times. With the public health nurse's consent, she explains to the parent that they both have concerns that her long-standing struggle with emotional difficulty may be exacerbated by the physiological, psychological, material, and relational stresses connected with the transition to parenthood. She also states that she believes that a psychiatrist may be an important member of the team helping with this transition. She is clear with the mother that she has concern for both her and the baby's safety. The mother agrees that more support may be beneficial, and they collaborate on a plan of care.

DSM–5 diagnosis: Bipolar II Disorder
ICD–10–CM code: F31.81

Relational Clinical Formulation

The identified client is a 35-year-old woman and first-time mother with a history of depression who presents at this time with hypomania expressed through elevated energy and confidence, reporting not being troubled by lack of sleep related to newborn care and being focused on housekeeping to the exclusion of responding to her infant's distress. These symptoms meet criteria for a diagnosis of Bipolar II Disorder with peripartum onset. This condition puts the client's infant at risk because it interferes with the client's capacity to register or respond to the baby's needs. The client is at risk of losing custody of the infant if she is not able to manage her symptoms and shift her focus to caring for the baby. At present, the condition is preventing the client from functioning effectively as a parent. A collateral referral for medication evaluation is indicated. In addition, the client will benefit from IMH intervention that includes her baby so that the detrimental impact of symptoms may be mitigated and the infant's well-being may be monitored in conjunction with the client's treatment. Dyadic intervention aimed at increasing parental functioning via strengthening PCRC 1 is recommended.

Goal: Client's condition will be stabilized such that PCRC 1 is in evidence.

Sample collaboratively generated objectives include the following:

1. The client reports having avoided following up on a medication evaluation referral despite recognizing that this evaluation might be helpful because of being "too busy." The client will follow through with the medication evaluation referral within 1 week.

2. The client will, during each weekly IMH meeting, identify verbally at least three things her baby appears to be needing and experiencing. (Baseline zero: The client reports being too preoccupied with keeping the apartment clean to be able to consider the baby.)

3. At present, the client reports that she lets her baby cry in his crib for long stretches every day because "babies cry," and she feels she must prioritize other things. The client will report during weekly IMH meetings experimenting with having soothing interactions with her baby when he cries at least three times per day.

CHAPTER 3

PCRC 2—People's Health Matters

Death from starvation suddenly became a distinct possibility...."My children are going to die," Laila said. "Right before my eyes." "They are not," Miriam said. "I won't let them. It's going to be all right, Laila jo. I know what to do."

—Khaled Hosseini (2007, p. 306)

PCRC 2: Parent is able to maintain his or her own **health and well-being**, promote child's health, and access pediatric (or other culturally meaningful) care as needed AND child is able to grow in keeping with developmental expectations and maintain physical health.

Parent–Child Relationship Competency (PCRC) 2 describes the mutual influence of parents' and children's states of health, the relational dynamics that foster physical health, and the wherewithal that is required to access and make use of help from healing arts practitioners as needed. PCRC 2 rises to the fore as an appropriate focus of intervention when health-related issues are straining the parent–child relationship or when dynamics in the relationship compromise physical health.

Health is a matter of social justice. As the People's Charter for Health (2000) states,

> Health is a social, economic and political issue and above all a fundamental human right. Inequality, poverty, exploitation, violence and injustice are at the root of ill-health and the deaths of poor and marginalized people. Health for all means that powerful interests have to be challenged, that globalization

has to be opposed, and that political and economic priorities have to be drastically changed. (p. 2)

The deleterious effects of social forces of oppression are evident in the grossly disproportionate mortality rates for specific groups of infants and mothers. Solomon (2018) noted, for example, that African American women and their babies are dying at alarming rates. According to Solomon, Black mothers are 3–4 times more likely to die in childbirth than their White, non-Hispanic counterparts, and the death rate for infants born to Black mothers is more than twice that of infants born to White, non-Hispanic infants. Solomon identified a range of contributing factors but emphasized the deeply entrenched structures of racism that constitute a "constant toxin" endangering the lives of Black women and infants. Infant mental health (IMH) workers must be alert to the impact of forces of oppression on the health of the families they serve, including the manifestation of these forces within their own practice settings. Vignette 2.1 provides an example of addressing the impact of racism in family health treatment planning.

Tenet # 3:
Work to Acknowledge Privilege and Combat Discrimination

Tenet # 8:
Allocate Resources to Systems Change

Isolating health-related issues can be challenging in IMH work because experience and learning for infants and young children are largely body-based, and bodily experiences loom large. Infants require a great deal of physical care. The way a baby is handled—fed, comforted, cleaned, and so forth—is relational and largely feeling based. Parents frequently experience caregiving challenges in the body-based realms of infant feeding, excretion, sleep, and grooming. Because it takes time to sort out the contributing factors to signs of infant distress, it can be difficult to isolate the source of the difficulty. With respect to a feeding difficulty, for example, it can be hard to know whether the food is disagreeing with the baby or whether there is something in the feeding exchange that is not going well.

For parents, many lifetime factors have contributed to their current state of health, and illness may, of course, befall any of us at any time. From a PCRC perspective, all individuals bring to life and to relationships with others an innate capacity for health and healing, and intimate caring relationships have a beneficial effect on physical health. When PCRC 2 is functioning well, parents manage to attend to their own health and well-being while also promoting the health of the child, and the child's healthy development nourishes the parent. A grandmother raising her grandson commented as she hurried after him toward the climbing structure at the park, "He keeps me active. He keeps me young!"

PCRC 2 is also functioning well when parents and infants navigate illness and disability in healthy ways. In their research with infants blind from birth, Fraiberg and colleagues (1977) found that infant blindness per se, although challenging for families, had no universal adverse effects on parent–child attachment relationships or on infant development. Indeed, they concluded that when infant blindness did constitute an obstacle to healthy development, a mental health difficulty was the mediating factor. This recognition encouraged Fraiberg and colleagues to develop infant–parent psychotherapy as a particular dyadic modality of intervening when a mental health difficulty interferes with the self-righting function that most frequently supports families in navigating challenges of various sorts.

Healthy dyads develop ingenious adaptations in response to disability. A woman whose disability prevented the use of her left arm was unable to lift her baby from the crib in the conventional manner, so the baby slept in the crib on a pad with handles. Whereas other infants might reach up to participate in being lifted from the crib, this baby curled readily into a fetal position when his mother approached in her wheelchair. This act facilitated her gathering the corners of his pad and lifting him out of the crib and into her lap, where he then uncurled and engaged actively with her.

Tenet # 4:
Recognize and Respect Non-Dominant Bodies of Knowledge

Parents likewise often adapt successfully to children's disabilities and may or may not require the support of an

Tenet # 3:
Work to
Acknowledge
Privilege
and Combat
Discrimination

IMH worker in this process. When IMH support is needed in relation to either a parent or child disability, there is often an important advocacy element of this intervention because able-ism encountered by families across systems frequently compounds any difficulty presented by the disability itself.

One health-related challenge that frequently negatively affects parent–child relationships and that requires IMH intervention is substance use (*ZERO TO THREE Journal*, 2018). From the PCRC perspective, all parents use substances of some kind to sustain themselves and to self-regulate: at least food and often medication, sugar, caffeine, nicotine, or alcohol, if not criminalized substances. The food justice movement calls for universal access to healthy food, air, and water free of environmental contaminants. Short of this goal (and we are, at present, quite drastically short of it), all parents use substances that take a toll on their bodies and on the environment by exposing them to pathogens of various kinds, making a harm-reduction approach a necessary element of health promotion. This approach may mean peeling fruits and vegetables with permeable outer membranes if organic produce is not available, learning to drink water where the soda industry has successfully infiltrated and exploited thirst, reducing caffeine or sugar consumption as needed to promote well-being, and so forth. Substance use may be an appropriate focus of IMH intervention when parents' challenges in this area negatively affect their relationship with their child. Substance abuse treatment approaches are often very individually focused, excluding the infants and young children who may be profoundly affected by their parents' struggles. When a parent struggles with addiction, IMH intervention focused on promoting the well-being of the child in the context of the parent's recovery is usually needed. Vignette 2.2 provides an example of IMH intervention addressing parental substance abuse.

Whether a child or a parent is facing a health challenge, the question of who helps with the healing is important. An immigrant woman overheard by a nurse in the waiting room of a pediatric clinic was advising a new immigrant mother regarding what not to tell the doctor. She clearly had the experience of being judged and criticized for practices that differed from those promoted by her child's pediatrician. It is incumbent on health care providers to be open to, and educated regarding, health practices that may be unfamiliar to them and even counter to their training. Providers must practice extreme caution in judging a culturally specific child-rearing practice to be harmful. There is often an important role for the IMH worker in supporting families in identifying what healing practices are right for the family, accessing needed health services, navigating complex medical systems, and providing medical advocacy on behalf of children and families.

Tenet # 4:
Recognize and Respect Non-Dominant Bodies of Knowledge

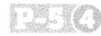

Vignette 2.1

Felicia, a 20-year-old African American woman with a 3-year-old son, is in her second trimester of a new pregnancy. She is referred for perinatal mental health treatment by a hospital social worker in the obstetrics clinic where she was seen recently for the first time. The social worker made the referral because Felicia had a concerning score on a depression screener and was reluctant to schedule another prenatal visit. In the early visits with the perinatal mental health worker (IMH worker), Felicia disclosed that when she was pregnant with her son at 17 years old, she had felt judged and shamed by many people, including medical providers. She described experiences of being ignored or not taken seriously on the one hand and intruded upon on the other hand. Although there had been no medical concerns throughout the pregnancy, the delivery had been induced for reasons she did not understand, and the labor had been a frightening and alienating experience for her. She stated, "I don't want to go see those people until I have to." Felicia struggles with fatigue and isolation, explaining that she does not have time to socialize because of her

parenting responsibilities. She did not graduate from high school, which she also attributes to her parenthood, stating, "I liked school, but people are harsh." She regrets not having completed high school and does not believe that obtaining rewarding employment is a possibility for her. She is worried that the presence of the new baby may be overwhelming for her and challenging for her son, explaining, "I know he will probably be jealous. It's been just us two all this time." The African American home visiting IMH worker meets with Felicia and her son several times, engaging her in reflective conversations regarding her experiences as a mother and her feelings and concerns about the impending birth of her second child. Together, they identify past and present difficulties and potential supports.

DSM–5 diagnosis: Persistent Depressive Disorder with peripartum onset

ICD–10–CM code: F34.1

Relational Clinical Formulation

The identified client is a 20-year-old pregnant African American woman who meets criteria for a diagnosis of Persistent Depressive Disorder with peripartum onset, as evidenced by experiences of low mood, low self-esteem, low energy, and difficulty feeling hopeful about her future, which originated around the birth of her child 3 years ago. The client reports experiencing stigma as an adolescent mother, which was likely exacerbated by racism. She also suffered medical trauma in the form of disempowerment around labor and delivery, resulting in avoidance of prenatal care at the present time. She is a conscientious parent, and the idea of her son experiencing distress causes her guilt. Because parental depression negatively affects children, and because the 3-year-old will likely need support around the coming family transition, treatment directly involving the 3-year-old is recommended, alongside individual meetings preparing for the birth of the new baby, with a transition to including the baby in treatment following delivery. Medical advocacy will be an important collateral element. The client and family will likely benefit from treatment aimed at strengthening PCRC 2.

Goal: Reduce depressive symptoms and increase health by strengthening PCRC 2.

Sample collaboratively generated objectives include the following:

1. At present, the client's depression-based tendency toward internalization and avoidance prevent her from identifying racial trauma she suffered in the past, leading to avoidance of medical care now. The client will describe during IMH sessions negative interactions with helping professionals during her first pregnancy that may have been shaped by interpersonal or institutional racism by [date].

2. Depression-based difficulty advocating for herself has prevented the client from being proactive about her medical care. The client will generate a set of interview questions for prenatal providers by [date].

3. Previous traumatic medical experiences have led to the client's avoiding planning for her care, increasing the chances of repeated negative experiences with the coming labor and delivery. The client will make a birth plan by [date], which includes identified support people who will advocate for her during labor.

4. Depression-based withdrawal has prevented the client from talking with her son about the coming baby, which sets them up for a likely difficult adjustment. The client will construct a developmentally meaningful narrative about the coming delivery and share it with her son in a treatment session by [date].

Vignette 2.2

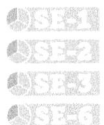

Joy is an 18-month-old White girl who is referred for IMH treatment by her child welfare worker as part of a reunification plan. Joy's parents, Sam and Sonja, have struggled with opioid addiction for many years. When they discovered that Sonja was pregnant, they both entered drug treatment, which included a methadone maintenance program. Joy was born methadone dependent and spent her first month of life in the hospital where she was weaned off methadone. She was discharged home to her parents, who maintained their sobriety for a little over a year before they relapsed. At this time, the whole family was involved in a car accident. Joy was injured and hospitalized, but she was discharged to emergency foster care after 24 hours because her injuries were minor. Her parents were both arrested on the scene of the accident and charged with child endangerment. These charges were dropped when they entered residential substance abuse treatment programs and a voluntary drug treatment–focused court program.

Joy was placed in foster care, where she exhibited symptoms of trauma, including resisting sleep, waking from sleep screaming, and being upset at getting into a car seat. Visits with her parents were delayed for a time while they were in a mandatory "blackout" (i.e., no contact with anyone outside of the drug treatment program) phase. The foster mother reported that every time the doorbell rang, Joy would ask, "Mama? Papa?" She also did not like anything to be out of place in the foster home, for example, attempting to push the vacuum back into the closet when it was left in the living room.

An African American IMH worker who is also a certified substance abuse counselor conducts an assessment. In initial IMH meetings with her parents, Joy has presented with a remarkably bright mood, but she engages in caregiving behaviors with her parents and the IMH worker (e.g., feeding everyone pretend food) and moves from one play activity to another in a frenzied manner. She becomes suddenly despondent and dysregulated at the end of sessions. The IMH worker discusses her thoughts and impressions with Sam and Sonja, and together they develop a plan of care.

DC:0−5 diagnosis: Generalized Anxiety Disorder

DSM−5 diagnosis: Generalized Anxiety Disorder

ICD−10−CM code: F41.1

Relational Clinical Formulation

The identified client is an 18-month-old White girl who meets criteria for a diagnosis of Generalized Anxiety Disorder, as evidenced by difficulties with sleep, chronic worry about loss of love reflected in solicitous behavior toward caregivers, and fears about loss of control reflected in a need to have things in the environment be "just so." Symptoms of anxiety prevent the client from benefiting from play, relating, or learning opportunities because she tends to move from one activity to another in a frenzied manner. The client suffered a multifaceted trauma and exhibited some stress responses secondary to this behavior, but her symptoms do not meet criteria for Posttraumatic Stress Disorder at this time. The client's parents both struggle with addiction and are in early recovery. Because substance abuse undermines parental health and compromises parents' capacities to protect and respond optimally to children's needs, it will be important to involve parents as collateral partners in client's care. Triadic treatment focused on improving the quality of interactions between the client and her parents in the context of the parents' recovery is warranted as a path toward reducing the client's anxiety. The family will likely benefit from IMH services aimed at strengthening PCRC 2 (among others).

Goal: Decrease client's anxiety by strengthening PCRC 2 and securing parents' recovery and health.

Sample collaboratively generated objectives include the following:

1. The client's parents' recovery, critical to the client's potential to reduce anxiety, is jeopardized by their avoiding talking about potential triggers to use. The client's parents will each identify during each weekly IMH meeting one parenting-related experience that occurred during the preceding week that threatened their recovery.

2. The client's parents' recovery program does not integrate parenting experiences in the conceptualization of recovery, leaving them alone with figuring out how to address the client's needs while maintaining their recovery. The client's parents will each identify during each weekly IMH meeting one parenting-related experience that occurred during the preceding week that supported their recovery.

3. At present, the client often engages in role reversal and caregiving of her parents, suppressing her own need for nurturance, which exacerbates her anxiety. The client's parents will respond to the client's caregiving overtures during each IMH session with assurances that they are healthy now and can take care of (e.g., feed, comfort) themselves and the client.

4. At present, the client's constant worry prevents her from relaxing into growth-promoting play experiences. The client will demonstrate confidence in her parents' wellness by relaxing into an interlude of calm, focused play lasting at least 10 minutes as observed by an IMH worker during weekly clinic-based sessions by [date].

CHAPTER 4

PCRC 3—Attachment, Caregiving, and the Interpersonal Nature of Safety

My hands reach down, trembling in anger, reach toward the needy child, but instead of roughly managing her they close gently as a whisper on her body. As though I am somehow physically enlarged, I draw her to me, breathing deeply. The tension drops away. At this moment, I am invested not with my own thin, worn, endurance, but with my mother's patience. This is a gift she has given to me from far away. Her hands have poured it into me. The hours she soothed me and the deep quiet in which I watched her rock, nurse, and comfort my younger brothers and sisters have passed invisibly into me.

—Louise Erdrich (1995, pp. 70–71)

PCRC 3: Parent has the capacity to provide **safety, protection, and comfort** for child AND child seeks out and accepts comfort and protection from parent and has a developmentally expectable ability to register security, anxiety, and fear.

Many volumes have been devoted to documenting and theorizing this Parent–Child Relationship Competency (PCRC). Indeed, it could be said that the identification of PCRC 3 gave rise to the entire, multifaceted field of attachment theory and research.

Parents do countless things to support the development of important capacities in their children. However, the distinguishing characteristic of the PCRCs is their bidirectionality. Under ordinary circumstances, they emerge in tandem; it is as though each partner draws the reciprocal capacity from the other, including seeking and invitational behaviors that inspire and invite response. The attachment and caregiving behavioral motivational systems epitomize this process. Unless something has gone awry, a young child is intrinsically motivated to seek protection from the caregiver, and the caregiver is intrinsically motivated to protect the child from harm. Also, children are endowed with attributes and strategies designed to elicit protective and nurturing actions from their parents, and parents are primed at the level of the body to act accordingly. Louise Erdrich (1995) described the first weeks of her daughter's life:

> *Our baby's cries are not monotonous. They seem quite purposeful, though hard to describe. They are a language that changes every week, one so primal that the meaning I gather is purely physical. I do what she "tells" me to do—feed, burp, change, amuse, distract, hold, help, look at, help to sleep, reassure—without consciously choosing to do it. I take her instructions without translating her meaning into words, but simply bypass straight to action.* (p. 56)

In the passage that opens this chapter, Erdrich pays homage to the transmissions from her own mother that paved the way for her own receptivity and responsiveness to her daughter's bids for protection and comfort, even at a moment when she is bitterly tired and irrationally—though understandably—enraged.

Monumental as such feats of caregiving truly are, they are also, as D. W. Winnicott (1966) emphasized, absolutely "ordinary." A lot must have gone wrong or be going wrong for a parent to consciously or unconsciously refuse protection when their child is truly endangered, or for a child to encounter perceived danger without seeking protection from their parent. Of course, a lot can and does go wrong all too frequently. The life-course impact attests to the profound gravity of attachment and caregiving injuries.

Although attachment patterns are influential and abiding, even intergenerational patterns of problematic attachment can be interrupted. A parent's attachment wounds can be healed and need not be inflicted on their child. Especially if supported by a sensitive, supportive practitioner, a child's love can be the balm that makes this possible. As Selma Fraiberg (1980) described, "The baby...provides a powerful motive for positive change in his parents. He represents their hopes and deepest longings; he stands for renewal of the self; his birth can be experienced as a psychological rebirth for his parents" (pp. 53–54).

Powell, Cooper, Hoffman, and Marvin (2014) noted that attachment has plasticity: "Even parents from the most insecure, threatening backgrounds can 'earn' security—through secure relationships later in life, through the self-reflection processes that create new internal working models and override childhood insecurity" (p. 18). Powell and colleagues went on to note that this type of change is possible because of parents' "innate desire to do the best for their children" and to "become the parents they wish they had had" (p. 18). PCRC 3 is central to this redemptive possibility offered by parenthood. There is often a role for infant mental health (IMH) workers in helping parents to bring to awareness some of the emotional pain they experienced around attachment failures or injuries in their own care so that these may be resolved, freeing the parent to respond protectively to their child rather than repeating the worst of their experience. Toward this end, it is critical that IMH workers attend assiduously to the interpersonal experience of safety in the parent–IMH worker relationship. **P-5 3**

This practice is both a necessary condition of intervention and also a source of information about the specific challenges to achieving a sense of interpersonal safety and security with which this particular parent struggles.

Tenet # 1:
Self-Awareness
Leads to Better
Services for
Families

It is critical to note in this context, however, that families are systematically unevenly exposed to and protected from overt dangers. Factors such as race, class, ethnicity, gender, sexual orientation, nationality, and ability status may be mapped in predictable ways onto the likelihood of a person being exposed to or shielded from dangers such as police violence and criminal justice system involvement, community violence, interpersonal violence, forced separation, and targeting. IMH workers factor these sociopolitical realities into assessment and treatment planning in relation to

Tenet # 3:
Work to
Acknowledge
Privilege
and Combat
Discrimination

PCRC 3, refraining from blaming parents for society's crimes and failures that affect them. IMH work in the realm of PCRC 3 commonly involves supporting families in accessing protective resources as needed and advocating on behalf of families when systems fail or harm them. IMH workers also continue to support parents' growth and the reality of their experience.

Vignette 3.1

Billy is a 2½-year-old White toddler who is referred by his child welfare worker for relationship-focused therapy with his foster mother, who hopes to adopt him. "We made every mistake," the worker laments during the intake conversation. "Three CPS [child protective services] reports were filed by relatives during his first year of life because his mother kept leaving him with people and disappearing. Each time it was investigated, it seemed he was not in imminent danger, and he was with family who seemed committed to him, so no case was opened. Next time, he would be with a different person, but same story. He came into emergency care at 14 months because a policeman found him on the street outside a liquor store—the cousin who was caring for him was intoxicated and had not noticed that he had wandered out of the store. His mother was out of state, and his father was not identifiable, so at this point he went to foster care. The first placement failed because the foster mother got sick. The second one failed because they found him too challenging. He is quiet most of the time, but tantrums with no identifiable reason and can be reckless and bolt in public places. This foster mother—who hopefully will adopt him—is gifted in dealing with that kind of thing, but she is worried because she feels he is hard to please and doesn't show any signs of needing or caring about her. She needs help understanding how dangerous and frightening it feels to him to expose himself to possible disappointment and abandonment."

DC:0–5 diagnosis: Reactive Attachment Disorder

DSM–5 diagnosis: Reactive Attachment Disorder

ICD–10–CM code: F94.1

Relational Clinical Formulation

The identified client is a 30-month-old White toddler who has suffered multiple relationship losses and changes in caregiving environment throughout his life. He meets the criteria for a diagnosis of Reactive Attachment Disorder on the basis of his history of relationship deprivation together with his limited capacity to enjoy interactions with others or to seek comfort from caregivers. He is prone to reckless behavior, moving away from caregivers in dangerous settings (e.g., into the street), and he exhibits emotional distress and dysregulation without identifiable provocation. The client's adoptive mother feels he does not enjoy, need, or care about her. It is important that these challenging but understandable difficulties be addressed in the context of the caregiving re- lationship. Intensive dyadic treatment aimed at strengthening PCRC 3 is recommended, with auxiliary individual meetings with the adoptive mother to support the adoptive mother, elicit and accept her concerns, and evaluate progress.

Goal: Establish a secure attachment with the adoptive mother as reflected in strengthening PCRC 3.

Sample collaboratively generated objectives include the following:

1. At present, the client rarely seeks or accepts comfort from the mother. The client will accept comfort from the

mother (e.g., settle into physical holding) at least once each day per the mother's report by [date].

2. The client's mother finds the client's help-rejecting behavior hurtful and often withdraws, leaving his emotional needs unmet. Over the next 3 months, the client's mother will, with the guidance of the IMH worker, identify miscues (moments when the client's behavior likely communicates the opposite of his emotional needs) during each weekly infant–parent psychotherapy session.

3. The client's mother has waited a long time to adopt a child and worries that expressing negative thoughts or feelings might undermine her chances of being approved for adoption, which leaves her and the client alone with these challenging experiences. The client's mother will express fears, ambivalences, and misgivings regarding adopting the client during regularly scheduled individual meetings with the IMH worker over the next 6 months.

4. Incidents of the client's dangerous bolting (which presently occur, on average, once a week) will cease by [date].

Vignette 3.2

 Brenda, a 33-year-old Chinese American woman who has carried a diagnosis of Schizophrenia for many years, is referred to the IMH clinic together with her 11-month-old daughter, Jenna, as part of the step-down plan as she transitions out of the subacute residential facility where she has resided since the end of her pregnancy. Brenda is on disability, having been hospitalized repeatedly during her late adolescence and in her 20s but then having been fairly stable and consistent with care in the years leading up to her pregnancy. The case worker who makes the referral says, "Brenda has done really well here. I wish she could stay on, but we are a 6-month placement, and we just can't extend beyond a year." The case worker reports that Brenda

is medication compliant and will continue to be followed by the psychiatrist she has been seeing. She is also active with a patients' rights organization.

The IMH worker meets with Brenda and Jenna in their new apartment several times for an assessment. Brenda is able to attend to Jenna's physical needs, but she tends to respond to emotional needs with physical ministrations (e.g., offering a bottle or attempting a diaper change when Jenna may be signaling an interest or impulse for interaction). Brenda does not talk with Jenna, and she finds the worker's inquiry about this matter a bit silly, explaining, "She can't talk yet!" Brenda has a hard time finding the energy to follow through with the home-making tasks she wishes to accomplish, so the dyad's belongings remain in the suitcases and boxes they arrived in, and some furniture (including Jenna's crib) remains unconstructed. Instead, the two sleep in a mattress on the floor. The clutter, together with Brenda's low level of energy and slow responsiveness, presents something of a safety hazard because Jenna is an active crawler who is also beginning to cruise. In addition, in the course of the month-long assessment period, the building manager reports with irritation that Brenda has set off the smoke alarm repeatedly by leaving pots on the stove and forgetting about them.

DSM–5 diagnosis: Schizophrenia, multiple episodes, currently in full remission

ICD–10–CM code: F20.9

Relational Clinical Formulation

The identified client has a history of delusions, suicidality, and grossly disorganized behavior leading to multiple hospitalizations and meeting criteria for a diagnosis of Schizophrenia. The client's symptoms are well managed. She works collaboratively with a psychiatrist with whom she has a long-standing relationship, and she is active with a patients' rights organization that provides a rewarding social network. At present, the client is living independently for the first time since the birth of her infant daughter, and her current symptoms of psychomotor retardation, difficulty reading social–emotional cues, and disorganization put her daughter's development and safety at risk.

Goal: Increase physical and emotional safety by strengthening PCRC 3.

Sample collaboratively generated objectives include the following:

1. The client's challenges with organization have led to her burning things on the stove, triggering the building's smoke alarm approximately one time per week. Incidents of triggering the smoke alarm will cease.

2. The client's low energy level makes it hard to keep up with her busily locomoting baby, resulting in the baby often getting into things that might endanger her. With the building manager's cooperation, the client will implement childproofing measures in her apartment by [date].

3. The client's strategies for responding to her baby's cries are limited primarily to feeding and diapering. During each weekly home-based IMH session over the course of the next 6 months, the client will practice a new strategy for responding that is geared to providing comfort and support social–emotional development, such as singing, talking, or playing.

CHAPTER 5

PCRC 4—"I Feel You": Attunement and Human Emotion

In the nighttime
the wind brings night whispers,
so I follow them...
past my toybox...
and out my door...
then down the hall.
Night whispers all around.
At last Daddy's holding me
warm and safe
and we listen together
to the night whispers

Angela Johnson (1994, pp. 1–10)

PCRC 4: Parent is able to be **emotionally attuned** to/ empathize with child AND child is able to experience and express a developmentally expectable range of human emotion.

Most Parent–Child Relationship Competencies (PCRCs) contain a miniature "theory of mind" or hypothesis about how particular child-rearing practices or parental capacities give rise to corresponding capacities in developing children. This attribute is true of PCRC 4. It posits that when developing children have the experience of adults accurately perceiving and resonating with or sharing in their emotional experiences, this emotional connectedness supports those children in being able to experience and express a full range of emotion going forward. It suggests, by contrast, that when parents are unable to allow themselves to feel what infants and young children are feeling, this occurrence may introduce difficulties for the child that results in certain realms of emotional experience being cordoned off and inaccessible to them. This would not mean that these realms would disappear entirely but that they would be experienced as foreign and probably dangerous territory. It is not necessary, possible, or desirable for a parent to experience exactly what an infant experiences. However, it is important that an infant is cared for in an interpersonal context in which adults recognize that infants have internal experiences and that the adults are working to make sense of the child's experience.

P-5 3

Infants' and young children's capacities to experience states of emotion are present from birth, although these are initially inextricable from physiological states. With time, emotions become increasingly nuanced. It typically comes quite naturally to most people to register and wonder about infants' emotional expressions. When an infant cries in a restaurant, for example, most heads will turn in his direction. All of those diners have instinctively engaged in the first steps in the process of attunement. If the infant persists in crying, his father may take him out of the restaurant and dedicate himself wholeheartedly to the project of attuning—feeling his way into his son's state in an effort to gather information about how to calm him. When PCRC 4 is functioning well, parents go about their business and meanwhile attune to their baby, matching a signal of sleepiness with a lowering of the voice or noticing a state of receptivity for play and becoming silly while folding laundry.

Sometimes, attuning to infants' states is destabilizing for parents as a result of emotional difficulties with which the parents struggle. That is, parents may be called to feel startling things from two directions simultaneously—the vulnerable infant in their arms and the awakened defenseless infant inside themselves, long since equipped with the dignifying trappings of maturation such as language, a sense of time, an understanding of the difference between inside and outside, and so forth. Early parenthood is "undoing" of the adult self for this reason, which can be frightening.

Many early childhood researchers and clinicians believe that there is no short cut—that is, no less emotionally demanding avenue—for supporting children to become emotionally integrated and securely attached. Dan Siegel (2001), for example, wrote that "sharing...nonverbal expressions of primary emotion...allows for the most direct connection of one mind to another" (p. 84). He further stated that "it is in this manner that emotionally attuned communication, the resonant sharing of nonverbal signals, allows for the child to 'feel felt' and to create a secure attachment with that connecting adult" (p. 84). Because this part of the job is hard at times for most parents, and profoundly disturbing for some, there is often an important role for infant mental health (IMH) workers in supporting parents in understanding and valuing this part of parenting.

P-5 (2)

It is important to be clear that supporting parents in this process necessitates a parallel openness to feeling on the part of the IMH worker. This requires a high degree of self-awareness, as IMH workers must be able to monitor and reflect on their own emotional processes. Wright (1992) described some of the countertransference challenges that IMH workers can face, including attuning to painful feelings in infants. Wright wrote, "the therapist must not only acknowledge, but sustain these troublesome feelings" (p. 128) to be able to reflect on them in developing an understanding of what may be happening for the parent and child. For this reason, among many others, it is critical that IMH workers have available to them ongoing access to reflective supervision and consultation.

Tenet # 1:
Self-Awareness Leads to Better Services for Families

Tenet # 8:
Allocate Resources to Systems Change

P-5 (7)

Although it is necessary for parents to be able to register and resonate with the raw emotional experiences that their infants are "asking" them to help them manage, it is also important that parents be able to keep one foot on dry land. If an infant is feeling that her hunger pangs mean that she is being sliced through at the middle and the parent gets this feeling and panics, the infant's terror may be doubled. As S. I. Greenspan and Greenspan (2003) wrote,

> *The capacity for balanced empathy on the part of the nurturing figure—that is, the ability to be indulgent, giving, loving, and protective and at the same time to experience emotionally something of what the infant experiences—is essential. A mother with balanced empathy is both in tune with her infant and able to distinguish her own needs from her infant's needs.* (p. 243)

Such a parent registers (perhaps without conscious recognition) the intensity of the physical and emotional experiences associated with acute hunger but simultaneously takes practical steps to feed the baby, conveying both that the feelings are understandable and that the need is meetable.

As with all PCRCs, when this one is functioning well, it is largely invisible. To an onlooker, the exchanges described in the previous paragraph—a baby crying and an adult preparing a bottle and offering it—would probably seem quite banal. The high drama posited here can be a very quiet one, hard to catch with the naked eye. Indeed, important innovations in the microanalysis of filmed interactions between infants and caregivers have offered access to some of the nuanced exchanges heretofore theorized rather than directly observed (Beebe, Cohen, & Lachmann, 2016). Often, it would be news to parents that any high-drama interaction had transpired. It is important to emphasize the fact that what is being described here happens all the time in parent–child relationships and has little to do with a parent's conscious attitudes or beliefs. As the vignettes in this chapter illustrate, parents who think a great deal about the importance of emotion in early childhood may for solid psychological reasons be quite challenged to keep these channels of communication open with their infants, whereas parents to whom this whole proposition might seem quite far-fetched may readily register and respond to their infants' emotional communications without thinking about it in these terms.

Also, as with all PCRCs, this one is bidirectional. What the child brings to the equation is the full palate in potentia—the capacity for joy, fury, sorrow, pride, shame, delight, and all imaginable subtle nuances of emotion. All these treasures of human feeling are invested in the ever-changing family story, offering parents the opportunity to experience (either in direct resonance with the child or via complementary pairings, such as helplessness paired with protectiveness) emotions that may be rarely visited, to sustain feelings they may have little allowed themselves, and to embody states they thought were the purview of others.

Vignette 4.1

Madelaine, a 39-year-old White woman, seeks therapy when her infant, Marcel, is 4 months old. During the initial telephone call, she explains that she is concerned that she is doing "something wrong" because she had anticipated enjoying motherhood but so far has found it very challenging. Madelaine is a college professor, and she and her husband Zack timed the pregnancy very carefully to coincide both with her securing tenure and with her teaching schedule so that the baby would be born at the end of a spring semester. This plan worked, but Madelaine has found it much harder than she anticipated to resume her teaching responsibilities a few weeks ago, despite having a full-time, in-home nanny. She reports feeling exhausted and not being able to get organized or be productive. The IMH worker proposes that Madelaine and Zack come in together for an initial session or two and then incorporate Marcel into two meetings after that, and then they can assess together from there how she might be helpful. Madelaine responds that Zack is out of the country on business, and so instead she comes in twice on her own and then together with Marcel two times. During these meetings, the IMH worker learns that Madelaine worries about almost all aspects of child rearing. Although she has read extensively about early childhood development and what she refers to as "the science of parenting," she feels that what she tries with Marcel does not work. She explains guiltily that she would like to believe that there was something wrong with Marcel that could be treated, but she sees that the nanny, who is very experienced with babies, has no difficulty managing him. The IMH worker learns that anxiety is not new to Madelaine, who states, "I hoped that motherhood would ground me." Instead, she has had the opposite experience. During sessions with Marcel, Madelaine is observed to be very active in making adjustments to his blanket and clothing, offering high-stimulation interaction, and trying multiple strategies in rapid succession to soothe him when he cries. She is very concerned that his crying may be disturbing people in the adjoining offices.

DSM−5 diagnosis: Generalized Anxiety Disorder

ICD−10−CM code: F41.1

Relational Clinical Formulation

The identified client is a 39-year-old White woman who is struggling to meet the demands of new motherhood and to balance this with work responsibilities; she feels ineffective in both realms. She meets criteria for a diagnosis of Generalized Anxiety Disorder as evidenced by preoccupying worries about perceived inadequacies and anticipated catastrophes (e.g., public shaming at work resulting from falling behind in her duties, disturbance in the child resulting from parenting failures), which long predate the baby's birth and plague her on a daily basis. She reports being both chronically fatigued and unable to rest, even when the baby is in the care of her nanny. The client's anxiety is preventing her from settling into a flow of back-and-forth communication with her infant, which does appear to contribute to agitation on the part of the baby. Opportunities for mutual pleasure and shared experience are missed, which could over time introduce complications for the child's social−emotional development. The client and infant will benefit from dyadic intervention focusing on strengthening

PCRC 4. It is also recommended that the client's husband participate in treatment as soon as possible to support progress toward decreasing the client's anxiety, facilitating infant development, and improving family functioning.

Goal: Decrease the client's worry and anxiety via strengthening PCRC 4.

Sample collaboratively generated objectives include the following:

1. At present, the client finds it challenging to work for any length of time, exacerbating her anxiety. Within the next week, the client will report identifying a length of time during which she can concentrate on her work while the baby is in the care of the nanny and implementing this routine on a daily basis without expecting herself to work for a longer period.

2. Constant worry interferes with the client's capacity to attune to her infant emotionally, producing a cycle of distressing emotional mismatch between them. During each weekly IMH session over the next 2 months, the client will describe what she observes in her baby in the moment and what she imagines this behavior might suggest regarding the child's experience.

3. The client reports having no effective strategies for calming her anxiety when caring for her baby, which leads to mutual agitation. The client will practice matching her breathing to her infant's and describe how this practice affects her during at least two out of the next four IMH sessions.

4. The client's anxiety is exacerbated by struggles with caregiving collaboration with her husband. The client and her husband will discuss which states of arousal in their infant they each find most rewarding and most challenging and will report feeling supported by one another in parenting on a daily basis accordingly by [date].

Vignette 4.2

Pedro is a 3-year-old boy of Mexican descent who is referred for IMH services by a public health nurse who visits his family following the birth of his infant sister. The nurse is concerned because Pedro's household—which includes his mother, father, and maternal grandmother—appears to be so preoccupied with the care of Pedro that they have little room for considering the needs of the new baby, Paulina. The family reports that things go best when they organize the household around Pedro because, although he maintains a sweet demeanor most of the time at home, he becomes highly distressed when the family deviates in any way from the daily routines to which he is accustomed. The family has stopped participating in church-related events because Pedro does not play with age-mates or take part in activities, and it is socially awkward for them to make excuses to other parents. The nurse attempted to engage Pedro, but he did not respond to her overtures, instead fingering and peering closely at his grandmother's rosary, which he fished himself out of her pocket. "Don't take it personally!" was Pedro's father's advice when the nurse's greeting of Pedro was ignored.

The Latina home visiting IMH worker who responds to the referral meets with almost exactly the same behavior from Pedro. She recognizes that the family has low expectations for Pedro's enjoyment of or participation in family activities, instead organizing themselves around trying to keep him on as even a keel as possible. When he expresses emotion other than contentment at being provided with familiar experiences, it is generally agitation and distress. His caregivers complain that there are very few foods he will eat or environments he is comfortable in and that they are beginning to share the nurse's concern that Paulina's life will be restricted to the confines of Pedro's comfort zone. In the course of a 2-month long assessment period that includes (with Pedro's parents' approval) collateral contact with Pedro's pediatrician as well as with the public health nurse, the IMH worker discusses with the family her sense that Pedro's difficulties are consistent with Autism Spectrum Disorder, which means that they face challenges as caregivers that are outside of the ordinary and that Pedro, through no fault of his own, needs a great deal of help in upholding his side of PCRC 4.

DC:0–5 diagnosis: Autism Spectrum Disorder

DSM–5 diagnosis: Autism Spectrum Disorder

ICD–10–CM code: F84.0

Relational Clinical Formulation

The identified client is a 3-year-old boy of Mexican descent whose family struggles to respond to his needs and to simultaneously integrate a new baby into the family. The client meets criteria for a diagnosis of Autism Spectrum Disorder, as evidenced by his lack of openness to interacting with anyone outside of his immediate family, the paucity of reciprocity in those relationships, his limited range of affect, his inflexibility about routines and daily activities, and his narrow range of interests (e.g., focus on his grandmother's rosary to the exclusion of toys or social games). The client's family is very dedicated to the client, but these difficulties strain his relationships with family members, and the caregivers are very worried about his future. He is also missing out on opportunities for learning because of the family's accommodation to his discomfort with leaving the home. The client and family will likely benefit from home-based IMH services aimed at strengthening PCRC 4 toward expanding the client's affective repertoire and capacity for reciprocal social interaction. It is recommended that all caregivers—father, mother, and grandmother—take part in the treatment on a regular (though perhaps rotating, as need be) basis so that they will all be coordinated and collaborative on a daily basis in developing approaches to support his development toward a more promising trajectory.

Goal: Expand repertoire of reciprocal emotional experience and expressiveness by strengthening PCRC 4.

Sample collaboratively generated objectives include the following:

1. At present, the family is overwhelmed with the client's care and reports struggling to balance care for him and his sister. Within 2 weeks, the client's caregivers will identify a plan for dividing care of the client and the client's sister between them so that her developmental needs are not neglected while the family meets the client's needs for intensive daily intervention.

2. At present, the client's repertoire of interest is extremely limited, resulting in lost opportunities for learning. During each home-based IMH session, the caregivers will experiment with ways of playing with the client based on his interest in his grandmother's rosary, gradually increasing his flexibility around this object and supporting him in engaging others while interacting with it.

3. At present, the client's self-isolation leads to missed opportunities for learning social interaction, resulting in his rapidly losing ground with social–emotional development. The client's caregivers will, during each home-based IMH session in the course of the next 3 months, take turns successfully drawing the client into play by being persistently "goofy" with him.

4. The client's repertoire of emotional expressiveness is extremely limited, exacerbating his social isolation. The client's caregivers will verbally identify emotional experiences that the client appears to be having during each IMH session over the next 3 months and show him facial expressions that convey what they believe he is feeling.

5. The family's accommodation to the client's social aversion leads to isolation that is straining family well-being. The client will tolerate attending a church function with the family by [date].

CHAPTER 6

PCRC 5—Interpersonal Neurobiology and the Dynamics of Regulation

Snuggle-Me-Up Song

I know the feel that I like best,
It's soft and warm and tight,
And when I'm cuddled up in it
My tummy feels just right.
I like the place I put my head,
I like to bump my nose,
I like to straighten out my back,
And spread my little toes.

—Frances Shaw, *Songs of a Baby's Day* (1928, p. 7)

PCRC 5: Parent has the capacity to self-regulate and to engage in **mutual regulation** with child AND child is able to participate in mutual regulation with the parent and is developing the capacity to self-regulate.

Parent–Child Relationship Competency (PCRC) 5 is closely associated with PCRC 4, which focuses on the link between empathy, attunement, and emotion that takes place at the level of communication between an infant and a parent or caregiver occurring largely outside of conscious awareness. Similarly, the processes described by PCRC 5 happen largely outside of conscious awareness, although they may be learned and enhanced via conscious reflection. Dan Siegel (2001) wrote that

> *From the beginning of life, "self-regulation" is actually*
> *determined in part by an interactive "dyadic" process of*

mutual coregulation...A child uses the state of mind of the parent to help organize her own mental processes. This alignment of states of mind permits the child to regulate her own state by direct connection with that of her parent. (p. 81)

What Siegel is articulating in this article is a vision of human experience that respects powerful mind-to-mind influences. This perspective challenges us to recognize the degree to which human beings who are connected to each other by close affective ties are actually systems rather than discreet individuals.

Regulation involves many aspects of experience. Neonates require the attentive intervention of caregivers to regulate their temperature, hunger and satiation, and other physio-logic processes. Accurate caregiver reading of the infant's sleep and wake states and states of arousal more broadly support responsive care. Mutual gazing and face-to-face interactions, such as sticking out the tongue, are among the astonishing relational delights available to caregivers of new-borns, and these myriad interactions facilitate the attentional regulation necessary for learning and relating (DeGangi, 2000; T. Greenspan & Lewis, 1999). The empathic emotional responsiveness described in the previous chapter supports infants in developing the capacity to self-soothe and, as they develop, to experience and express an increasingly differentiated range of emotions. The capacity to regulate emotion and mood has its roots in the capacity for physio-logic regulation and self-soothing, which an infant cannot accomplish without human partners.

As any parent of more than one child will attest, each infant is unique with respect to coregulation patterns. Whereas vigorous rocking may be soothing and organizing for one baby, the same technique may be overstimulating and disorganizing for another. Louise Erdrich (1995) reflected,

I know from the first that the babyhood of our youngest will be surprising. Her dance has entered my body—a soul rumba, slow, committed, with a

hiccup on the fourth step. She is acutely sensitive, a mine of emotions, an easily saturated sponge for the most minute sensations....Her roots into this life are dartlike, fine hairs. She isn't sure that she wants to be here. Unlike her older sisters, who always seemed absolutely positive, she is still making up her mind.
(p. 55)

Poetic license notwithstanding, there is a fine line between perception and attribution, but PCRC 5 is fueled by a process of minute experimentation, wherein a parent is able to imagine or feel their way into the experience of the child even as it is quite different from their own. Such a parent may find himself undertaking in tender earnestness rather outlandish things, such as making a slow jog around the block with the baby clutched to his chest, head carefully supported, at 3 a.m. Such efforts are registered at the level of implicit memory on the part of the child and rewarded handsomely in trust and love down the line.

Tenet # 4: Recognize and Respect Non-Dominant Bodies of Knowledge

What infants bring to this process is their capacity for fine-tuned, cross-modal organization around the people who care for them. A neonate who does not yet have volitional control of the movement of her limbs will nevertheless move them in synchrony with the rhythm of her parent's voice. Infants are generally equipped to make excellent use of their caregivers' ministrations, which is almost always immediately gratifying to adults. Beebe et al. (2016) have described infants as "contingency decoders," meaning that when an adult interacts with an infant in a way that is responsive to the infant, the infant registers and responds in turn, millisecond by millisecond, resulting in a coherent, connected relational exchange. This process is central to the sense of inherent reward experienced by many parents in the ordinary day-to-day of early parenting. It also fuels parental pride commonly experienced in being the ones who know the baby better than anyone else does.

When infants experience challenges around regulation and have a hard time accepting the offerings of their would-be coregulating partners, the job of parenting becomes exponentially more difficult. There is often a role for the infant mental health (IMH) worker in supporting parents in recognizing a difficulty, tolerating the frustration, healing their wounded pride, bolstering their sense of efficacy, strategizing about work-arounds, and so forth. Conversely, when parents have difficulties around self-regulation, such as when an adult is prone to defensive numbing, angry outbursts, anxious intrusion, or other behaviors that impede coregulation, it is critical that they have access to IMH treatment so that their struggles do not interfere with the child's developing regulatory capacities.

As with all PCRCs, it is important to recognize the wide range and variety of healthy embodiment of regulatory and coregulatory capacities. In one family, community, or sociocultural context, adults might delight in children's high-spirited antics, not expecting them to settle down readily, for example, in response to adult "shushing." In another family or sociocultural context, it might be expected that a child's responsiveness to adult signals regarding modulation be quite fine-tuned and immediate. The IMH worker is not the arbiter of what is correct among this range, but instead is a partner with the parent in determining to what degree this PCRC is functioning in a way that promotes the child's development, the parent's role satisfaction, and the family's well-being.

Vignette 5.1

Claudia was referred for IMH intervention by her 75-day-old infant's pediatrician following the diagnosis of a congenital oral irregularity requiring surgery. The pediatrician reported that the infant, Milo, had had difficulties latching in the first days of life and that a lactation consultant had been assigned to the family; however, breastfeeding support had been unsuccessful, and Milo was now bottle fed. He had continued to cry an inordinate amount and rarely calmed for periods of more than 15 minutes. He had been prescribed medication for reflux, and it was only when this was ineffective that it was finally discovered that he suffered from a mild malformation of the tongue that prevented effective latching and complicated swallowing. "The corrective surgery is quite simple, and the prognosis is excellent," the pediatrician stated, "but the mother has taken this pretty hard."

The IMH worker learned in an initial home visit that Claudia was very disappointed not to be breastfeeding. "Aside from all the benefits to Milo," she said tearfully, "I just wanted that for myself—that closeness with him and that quintessential mother thing." She reports not being able to enjoy even the good moments with Milo and being overcome with grief whenever she gives him a bottle. She expresses guilt and self-reproach for not having insisted on a more thorough evaluation of Milo's condition sooner; she also worries that their rough start will harm their relationship in a lasting way, and she has anxiety about the upcoming surgery.

DSM–5 diagnosis: Adjustment Disorder with mixed anxiety and depressed mood

ICD–10–CM code: F43.23

Relational Clinical Formulation

The identified client is a 34-year-old White woman who is struggling with mood disturbance and role functioning as a new mother secondary to her infant's medical issues. The infant is to undergo a surgery that is reportedly low risk, but the client is extremely worried about it. The dyad was unable to breastfeed, which is a source of great disappointment for the client to the degree that she finds feeding her baby aversive. She meets criteria for a diagnosis of Adjustment Disorder with mixed anxiety and depressed mood, as evidenced by her despondency and pervasive worry. As infant functioning and development may be put at risk by caregiver mood disturbance, it is recommended that the client engage in dyadic treatment together with her infant. Dyad will benefit from IMH treatment aimed at strengthening PCRC 5, with a specific focus on supporting emotional regulation in the client and state regulation in the infant.

Goal: Strengthen PCRC 5 as a means of decreasing the client's symptoms of depression and anxiety and mitigating potential adverse developmental effects of these symptoms on the infant.

Sample collaboratively generated objectives include the following:

1. Client has ceased to lactate and is despondent about this. With the support of the IMH worker, the client will engage a new lactation consultant within the week to explore the possibility of resuming breastfeeding after the surgery.

2. At present, client becomes sorrowful every time she feeds her baby. [In the event that breastfeeding cannot be resumed] The client will identify three things (e.g., music, tea, the company of someone she is comfortable with) that make bottle-feeding episodes more tolerable to her, and she will report putting some of these in place for herself at every feeding over the course of the next 3 weeks.

3. At present, client reports feeling globally ineffective with her baby. Over the course of the next 2 months, the client will identify during each weekly IMH session at least one thing she does that effectively supports her baby around a state transition (e.g., settling or arousing and attending).

4. The client will report perceiving mutual pleasure and satisfaction during feeding exchanges with her baby by [date].

Vignette 5.2

Ginger is a 30-month-old girl who was orphaned in China and adopted at 11 months old by White American parents. Ginger and her parents are referred for IMH treatment by the mental health consultant at her child care because of concerns about behavioral difficulties. Ginger reportedly refuses to stay with the group during circle time, instead retreating to the cozy corner of the classroom on her own; rejects physical holding or cuddling by child care staff even when struggling with separation from parents at drop-off; and appears to have a phobia of the bathroom that adjoins the classroom. During initial meetings with the IMH worker, Ginger's parents disclose painful fears about ways that Ginger's months in an orphanage may have harmed her, and they express hurt and disappointment regarding the lack of cuddliness that they had hoped to enjoy with a child. Strangers have asked them whether Ginger is autistic, and while this made them indignant, they have been reading about autism on the Internet and fear that this may be the case.

During initial home visits, the IMH worker observes Ginger to become silly and giddy when exposed to loud sounds, such as a noisy truck passing by or a flushing toilet. She is observed to engage in affectionate exchanges with her parents, such as a game in which she kisses a toy bunny and passes it to them and then receives it back from them after they kiss it. When first presented to the IMH worker, she stayed close to her parents and studied her from behind their backs, but after a time she engaged with her with curiosity and reciprocated playful overtures. During the assessment period the IMH worker meets with the family at home several times, speaks with Ginger's pediatrician, observes her at school, and speaks with her teachers and the mental health consultant.

DC:0–5 diagnosis: Sensory Over-Responsivity Disorder, tactile (people) and auditory (mid-loud, especially toilet)

DSM–5 diagnosis: Other Specified Neurodevelopmental Disorder

ICD–10–CM code: F88

Relational Clinical Formulation

The identified client is a 30-month-old girl of Chinese descent who has formed well-functioning attachments with her adoptive parents but who is having some difficulties in child care and at home that lead adults to misunderstand her behavior and put her at risk for punitive behavioral intervention or caregiver emotional withdrawal. Ginger meets criteria for a diagnosis of Sensory Over-Responsivity Disorder, as evidenced by her high sensitivity to both touch and sound. She finds physical touch aversive, and she will avoid situations in which physical contact with others is expected. She reacts in a disorganized and anxious way to sudden loud sounds and avoids exposure to predictable loud sounds such as flushing toilets. Because the client's symptoms compound her parents' preexisting worries connected to adoption, triadic IMH treatment is recommended to bolster parental confidence, reduce their anxiety and fears, and build the parents' capacity to advocate for the client with child care professionals and others. A focus on strengthening PCRC 5 will likely embolden the parents to provide the auxiliary support and environmental accommodations that the client needs to manage her sensory sensitivities and to benefit maximally from relationships and learning opportunities.

Goal: Strengthen PCRC 5 to enhance coping with—and prevent negative interactions in response to—the client's sensory sensitivities.

Sample collaboratively generated objectives include the following:

1. Client's parents accommodate client's aversion to physical interaction by withdrawing, leading to missed

opportunities to expand client's window of tolerance for contact. The client's parents will experiment with forms of physical contact that are tolerable for the client during each weekly home-based IMH session over the course of the next 2 months.

2. A meeting will take place before [date] between the client's parents, IMH worker, mental health consultant, and classroom teachers to collaboratively develop a plan to support the client around circle time, bathroom time, and other situations that are sensorially aversive to the client.

3. With accommodations, the client will be able to participate in circle time 5 days per week by [date] (current baseline: zero).

4. The client will, with the help of her parents, be able to identify when she is overstimulated and signal distress directly (e.g., by saying "too loud") rather than becoming dysregulated by [date].

CHAPTER 7

PCRC 6—Impulse Control: The Paradox of Action and Restraint

Degradation of anger. Anger at a child. How shall I learn to absorb the violence and make explicit only the caring? Exhaustion of anger. Victory of will, too dearly bought...far too dearly!...I remember being uprooted from already far to meager sleep to answer a childish nightmare, pull up a blanket, warm a consoling bottle, lead a half-sleeping child to the toilet. I remember going back to bed starkly awake, brittle with anger, knowing that my broken sleep would make next day a hell, that there would be more nightmares, more need for consolation, because out of my weariness I would rage at those children for no reason they could understand. I remember thinking I would never dream again (the unconscious of the young mother—where does it entrust its messages, when dream-sleep is denied her for years?)

—Adrienne Rich (1986, pp. 22–32)

PCRC 6: Parent has the capacity to identify, act on, and also control **impulses** sufficiently to have rewarding relationships and life experiences and can foster these abilities in child AND child demonstrates an age-expectable capacity to identify, act on, and also control impulses.

All the Parent–Child Relationship Competencies (PCRCs) are interconnected, and many are interdependent. This con-nectedness is the case with PCRC 6 and PCRC 5; impulse control is impossible without some capacity for self-regulation. One does not expect an infant to use the toilet because the infant is not yet in possession of the physiologic regulatory capacity—the bowel and bladder musculature development—needed to make the impulse control associated with toilet use viable. This discussion of impulse control is not an account of all the complex, orchestrated maturational processes that make it developmentally possible but rather a consideration of some of the associated psychological and relational issues.

Perhaps more vividly than any other PCRC, this one demonstrates the fact that a PCRC cannot be said to be functioning well unless both sides of the equation are present. A child may demonstrate precocious impulse control—for example, sitting still without making any demands on adults for longer than would be developmentally expected—but if this capacity was constellated in response to a parent who is prone to angry outbursts (an impulse control failure), then this PCRC needs strengthening. When this PCRC is functioning well for a dyad, a child is not motivated to control impulses by fear but rather by a powerful combination of other things, and the parent's capacities for impulse control provides the firm foundation of basic safety necessary for the child's personal exploration of the dynamic play of inhibition and action.

Engaging in rewarding activities—for example, successfully changing a car tire so that one can get back on the road, making tamales, or playing soccer—requires the capacity to identify (both within and outside of conscious awareness) thousands of impulses and to make thousands of instantaneous decisions (largely outside of conscious awareness) regarding which impulses to inhibit and which to act on. The result—the resumed road trip, supper on the table, the winning goal—would not be attained if things had played out differently at the many impulse-related switch points along the way. If alternate action and inhibition pathways had been taken, one might have abandoned the car by the side of the road, had potato chips for supper, or stormed off the soccer field.

Supporting children in developing these capacities for action and inhibition toward a rewarding experience is a large

P-5 1

part of the socialization component of parenting. It takes time for a child to learn and participate in social conventions such as not throwing sand at other children in the sandbox. Children are very much aided in this process when their caregivers think not only in terms of impulse inhibition but also identification and action. That is, it is helpful when a parent recognizes without negative judgment the child's impulse to throw and is able to support the child toward action as well as inhibition (e.g., "Hey strong girl, it hurts kids when you throw sand at them; throw the ball to Papa instead"). Of course, it would be impossible and unduly solicitous if parents spoke to children in such a way constantly. Furthermore, it is not actually necessary—or necessarily culturally appropriate—for such things to be stated at all. However, it is universally supportive of children's developing the capacity to successfully engage in rewarding activities when their caregivers recognize, welcome, and help them to express as well as to inhibit their impulses.

The action side of this equation is frequently neglected in discussions of limit-setting. As Tandon, Cardeli, and Luby (2009) noted, "acting out" children are more likely to be identified as needing intervention than those who internalize or "act in." This occurrence has resulted in more parenting advice and intervention protocols developed to promote impulse inhibition than to guide adults in facilitating children's impulse expression. Both sets of children—"externalizers" and "internalizers"—need help with recognizing and expressing impulses in ways that will lead to pleasure, connection with others, and positive gain. To the tremendous detriment of all, a great deal more social resource is regularly devoted to orchestrating the control of children's impulses (and punishing children for the fact that this is ultimately ineffective) than to investing in opportunities for truly rewarding impulse expression and active endeavor for children. (The subject of limit setting is P-5 4 discussed more fully in Chapter 14.)

Entire bodies of psychological and psychoanalytic literature are dedicated to defining and discussing human impulses.

With respect to PCRC 6, what is critical is the recognition that impulses that may be seen as negative—for example, aggressive impulses—are not only inevitable but also just as vital to psychological health as impulses that may be seen as positive, such as affiliative impulses. Aggression is part of the palate of human existence, and it is necessary in raw form to accomplish such things as fire fighting and in various degrees to win court cases or kick that soccer ball right past the goalie. Chapter 15 postulates a healthy continuum from aggression to assertiveness and suggests that it is well-modulated aggressive impulses that we are marshaling when we engage in such banal experiences as chewing our food or merging onto the highway. The point here is that PCRC 6 functions best when parents are relatively open to and unoffended by their own and their children's impulses.

Such openness is always uneven; personal and sociocultural history limit what impulse-level experience we each find acceptable or unacceptable. Reflecting on one's internal experience with the goal of identifying impulses—both aggressive and affiliative—can be an illuminating and enriching process throughout life—a "royal road" to understanding convictions, desires, and motivations that may otherwise be inaccessible to consciousness. Such a process can shed light on actions one takes that may be self-defeating or injurious to others. Moreover, it can open up possibilities for accomplishment and connection that might otherwise go unrealized. It is imperative that IMH workers undertake such reflection so that they can flexibly and responsively support families. When parents undertake such reflective processes on their own behalf, their children benefit implicitly.

Tenet # 1: Self-Awareness Leads to Better Services for Families

Vignette 6.1

Prince, a 2-year-old biracial child, is referred to an infant mental health (IMH) clinic together with his parents by his pediatrician because of concerns about his eating difficulties and low weight. Medical explanations have been ruled out, and the family has been assigned a nutritionist who states that she is unable to help them. During an initial assessment period, the IMH worker learns that Prince's mother, Angelica, who is Filipina, has struggled with long-standing mental illness and carries a diagnosis of Bipolar Disorder. Prince's father, Mack, is White. Mack is employed as a dock worker, and Angelica has not been employed since Prince was born, although she and Mack had met when she worked as a waitress at a bar he frequented. Prince spends his days with his mother. She is in the care of a psychiatrist but periodically ceases to take her medication, at which times she becomes despondent, extremely jealous, and paranoid, and she threatens to leave Mack. On several occasions, she has in fact left the family and stayed away for several days. Mack has, on each occasion, persuaded her to return home and resume treatment "for the boy's sake." Mack believes that feeding and caring for Prince are Angelica's responsibilities.

The IMH worker observes that during the early assessment sessions, Mack is quite removed, joining in play with Prince only when prompted by the IMH worker and then with a good deal of stiffness and embarrassment. Angelica, by contrast, is fully given over to the play in an almost childlike way, but she is directive and intrusive with Prince, making multiple suggestions about what to play with and how to play, taking toys out of his hands and thrusting others toward him. Prince does not overtly protest, but he repeatedly repositions himself so that his back is toward his mother. When asked about Prince's eating difficulties, Angelica laments, "The doctors think I don't feed him, but I try to feed him all the time! He won't eat. Do you think he doesn't love me?" The IMH worker meets with the parents over the course of several weeks, eliciting their thoughts and discussing with them her observations and speculations regarding some of the family patterns that may be contributing to the difficulty. Both parents are committed to helping Prince and are open to making adjustments in family roles and routines.

DC:0–5 diagnosis: Undereating Disorder

DSM–5 diagnosis: Unspecified Feeding or Eating Disorder

ICD–10–CM code: F50.8

Relational Clinical Formulation

The identified client is a 2-year-old biracial (Filipino–White) boy who is underweight for his age. He meets criteria for a diagnosis of Undereating Disorder, as evidenced by his frequent food refusal, picky eating patterns, and avoidance of situations associated with food (e.g., refusing to join his parents at the table). His relationships with his parents are sorely strained in relation to this issue. Family patterns are counterproductive because the client's father tends to withdraw, and the client's mother attempts constantly and ineffectually to persuade the client to eat. The client appears to refuse food as a way of warding off his mother's intrusive behaviors and perhaps attempting to solicit his father's care. Both parents are dedicated to the client and are worried about his weight; they also feel negatively judged by pediatric providers. Triadic IMH treatment is recommended to interrupt patterns that are not working and to develop approaches to interaction and eating that support the client's weight gain and healthy social–emotional development. A focus on strengthening PCRC 6 will be important so that the client and his father may increase their capacities to act on growth-promoting impulses and the client's mother may be supported to inhibit impulses that impede the client's development.

Goal: Strengthen PCRC 6 such that the client is able to identify and act on impulses to eat.

Sample collaboratively generated objectives include the following:

1. The client's mother will practice "waiting, watching, and wondering" during play sessions for periods of 5 minutes at a time by [date] (current baseline: zero minutes).

2. At present, the client's mother assumes sole responsibility for feeding and engages with the client many times each day in struggles around eating, which contributes to the client's difficulty gaining weight. Within the next 2 weeks, the client's parents will develop a plan that transfers some responsibility for meal preparation from the client's mother to the client's father.

3. At present, the client is encouraged to eat incessantly throughout the day, which exacerbates his resistance to eating. The client's parents will report during weekly IMH sessions over the next 4 weeks inhibiting their impulses to encourage the client to eat other than on five occasions each day (three mealtimes plus two snack times).

4. At present, the client appears never to identify an impulse to eat because he never requests food. The parents will report that the client spontaneously requests food by [date].

Vignette 6.2

Chad, a 52-year-old White man, calls the IMH worker to request therapy at the suggestion of his Alcoholics Anonymous (AA) sponsor. The IMH worker, who is White, uses a wheelchair due to a disability. Chad has a 3-month-old baby, Ruby, with his second wife, Lila, who is 35 and is likewise White. He also has older children who reside in another state with his ex-wife. He pays child support and alimony and has little contact with them. He explains that he has only recently entered recovery. He and Lila used to argue frequently about his drinking, but he had maintained that because he met the bills and had never been convicted of driving under the influence that he could not be an alcoholic. Then when Ruby was born the arguments stopped, but Chad saw that "as soon as I poured myself a drink after work, Lila would gather up the baby and just go in the other room." He continued, "I see the writing on the wall. I don't want to mess up another family."

DSM–5 diagnosis: Alcohol Use Disorder, moderate

ICD–10–CM code: F10.20

Relational Clinical Formulation

The identified client is a 52-year-old man in early recovery from alcoholism. He has a history of drinking to manage painful emotions and to avoid interpersonal intimacy, which has resulted in relationship rupture, loss, and isolation over the years, including alienation from his children. His new recovery is motivated in part by the birth of his daughter, with whom he hopes to have a better relationship than has been possible for him with his older children. The client meets criteria for a diagnosis of Alcohol Use Disorder, moderate, as evidenced by his persistent drinking despite harmful effects on relationships, having difficulty refraining from drinking or cutting down on drinking, and missing out on valued life experiences due to drinking., These patterns have negatively affected the client's relationships and role functioning. As the client's parental functioning has historically been impaired as a result of this alcoholism, the client's infant's social–emotional development may be at risk. Family treatment focused in part on strengthening PCRC 6 in support of the client's inhibition of his impulses to drink is recommended.

Goal: PCRC 6 will be strengthened, as evidenced by the client's refraining from drinking.

Sample collaboratively generated objectives include the following:

1. The client states not being clear about what triggers his tendency to isolate from his family. During each weekly IMH session over the course of the next 2 months, the client will identify interpersonal experiences with the

infant and his partner that prompt in him the impulse to withdraw.

2. Alcoholism has historically prevented the client from attending to the emotional experiences of loved ones. During each weekly IMH session over the course of the next 2 months, the client will, with his partner's support, describe impulses he perceives or imagines that his daughter may be experiencing.

3. The client states that attending AA meetings is helpful in supporting his recovery, and thus promoting family well-being, but getting himself to meetings can be challenging. The client will report in each weekly IMH session over the course of the next 2 months having participated in a minimum of three AA meetings during the intervening week.

CHAPTER 8

PCRC 7—The Joys of Joint Attention

One stormy autumn night when my nephew Roger was about twenty months old I wrapped him in a blanket and carried him down to the beach in rainy darkness. Out there, just at the edge of where-we-couldn't-see, big waves were thundering in, dimly seen white shapes that boomed and shouted and threw great handfuls of froth at us. Together we laughed for pure joy—he a baby meeting for the first time the wild tumult of Oceanus, I with the salt of half a lifetime of sea love in me. But I think we felt the same spine-tingling response to the vast, roaring ocean and the wild night around us.

—Rachel Carson (1956, p. 1)

PCRC 7: Parent is able to pay attention and focus as needed and to engage child in attending and focusing AND child demonstrates a developmentally expectable capacity for **shared focus/mutual attention** and is on a path toward being able to focus and attend on his or her own.

The capacity to focus and pay attention is critical to well-being in all realms of human experience. It is a key ingredient of mutually respectful and satisfying relationships, and it is a necessary component of performing well and attaining goals. When people struggle with this capacity, many difficulties and sometimes hazards follow. Driving safely, for example, requires the capacity to focus and attend. Learning is exponentially more difficult for students who struggle to focus and attend. Work productivity is undermined and the satisfactions of working are diminished when one is prevented from becoming absorbed in the tasks. Furthermore, relationships suffer when partners feel neglected or are misunderstood. Although opportunities exist to build our capacities for focus and attention throughout life, the early weeks, months, and years are the time when the stage is set for how readily these capacities will come.

S. I. Greenspan and Greenspan (2003) proposed four functional–emotional organizational levels of development, of which the first, initially established in the first 3 months of life, involves a child's capacity to attend and engage. The two primary (and indivisible) characteristics of this level are (1) "Affective interest in sights, sound, touch, movement, and other sensory experiences. Also, initial experiences of modulating affects (i.e., calming down)," and (2) "Pleasurable affects characterize relationships. Growing feelings of intimacy" (S. I. Greenspan & Greenspan, 2003, p. 8). In a book addressing an audience of parents, T. Greenspan and Lewis (1999) emphasized the fact that infants find the motivation and wherewithal to pay attention to the world around them on the basis of their passionate interest in their caregivers. "As your love," they wrote,

> magnetically pulls her into the world, your baby becomes more excited about the sights, sounds, touches, and tastes that surround her crib. You'll be literally enticing her into an awareness of things outside of her own body. Obviously, the more sensations your baby can tune into, the richer her understanding of the world will be. (T. Greenspan & Lewis, 1999, p. 56)

Toward this end, T. Greenspan and Lewis (1999) have encouraged parents during the first 3 months of a baby's life to pay close attention to and gently expand the range of the child's interest: "When you offer your baby various sights and sounds and patterns of touch and movement that intrigue him…this will often lead to even a split second more of shared looking and shared listening" (p. 36).

From a Parent–Child Relationship Competency (PCRC) perspective, it is important to celebrate not only parents' tremendous ingenuity and dedication in bringing the world to the baby in manageable bits (Winnicott, 1965c) but also the pleasure and wonder that the baby brings to the parent by bringing the parent's attention to otherwise overlooked details of their own person and the environment. A baby's appetite for gazing at a parent's face and movements is, under ordinary circumstances, nearly insatiable, although it is the extraordinary adult who is otherwise accustomed to being the object of such rapt attention while she goes about her mundane business. Without the tutelage of infants, adults can easily overlook the fairy dust that shimmers in a shaft of light through the blind, or they may register the tear in the upholstery of the sofa, underneath which a small piece of a silky underlayer is palpable, with irritation rather than fascination.

It can be frustrating for parents that infants and toddlers are so specifically focused on their personal effects. The quintessential example is keys. Despite the efforts of toy-production industries to capitalize on infants' interest in keys, the plastic ones rarely get traction. Even an old set of real keys unearthed for the toddler's delight will not likely garner the level of interest enjoyed by exactly those keys that the child sees so often in the hands of his parent—the set that must not be dropped from the stroller through the grate and into the sewer! This fascination occurs because the keys (or purse or coffee cup or cigarettes or cell phone) are saturated with a kind of essence-of-parent through a network of associations reinforced via hundreds of cumulative experiences. Babies pay extremely close attention to parents and intuitively do the math of what is important to them—and they are motivated to partake.

When PCRC 7 is functioning well, parents know (consciously or not) that, taxing or humbling as it may feel at times, their child's routing of interest in the world through their person is tantamount to gold in their hands. On the basis of this circuitry, they guide the child's attention toward opportunities for learning and interacting. A bus ride for a parent and toddler who are enjoying this PCRC may be characterized by looking together out the window and pointing to high-interest sights (e.g., perhaps, garbage trucks) with shared excitement. A bus ride for a parent and toddler struggling with PCRC 7, by contrast, might be characterized by discord around sitting safely in the seat, remaining calm and occupied, and so forth.

Parents themselves have varying levels of challenge around the capacity for absorbed, focused attention. Some research points to a general phenomenon of decreased capacity for focused attention when correlated with increased amounts of time spent interacting with electronic devices such as cell phones (Zheng et al., 2014) and other digital media (Ra, Cho, & Stone, 2018). Many other things, of course, may interfere with parents' capacities in this area. Often, there is a role for the infant mental health (IMH) worker in helping parents to appreciate the power of this relational capacity, to identify and work to address interferences, and to protect and promote opportunities for parent–child experiences of shared focus and mutual attention. Moments of this shared experience with their first intimate partners accumulate for children and undergird their capacity to focus and pay attention on their own as they grow.

P-5 2

Vignette 7.1

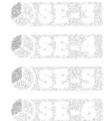

The mental health consultant from Upsy Daisy Preschool refers Luke, a 3½-year-old White boy, and his family to an IMH worker when her attempts to support the school in meeting his needs have not been successful. She reports that the preschool director is close to asking the family to find another school for Luke because staff find it too taxing to manage his behaviors. Luke has an extremely difficult time settling into activities—such as circle time, listening to stories, or even active play—that require collaboration and turn-taking. The parents of other children in the classroom have become alarmed because he can be physically rough with children (e.g., crashing into them on trikes) and also with objects—for example, tearing other children's drawings and toppling their block constructions. Teachers are frustrated because he "doesn't listen" and has difficulty following through when given verbal direction. They have tried assigning a "floater" teacher to him, which does help, but feel they cannot afford to provide as much one-on-one support as he requires. In parent–teacher conferences, the parents, Jack and Jill, have been dismissive of the concerns raised by teachers, suggesting that the school may be too focused on rules, whereas they favor "letting kids be kids." In a recent meeting with the director, Jack and Jill were defensive, blaming the school for not having staff with sufficient skill to manage children with a range of temperaments.

In meeting with Jack and Jill, the IMH worker learns that Luke has a sister, Leslie, who is 1 year old and that the parents have actually experienced a good deal of stress in child rearing because Luke has the same difficulties at home that he displays at school. A great deal of vigilance is necessary in supervising the siblings because Luke can be rough with Leslie and cannot settle into activities on his own while the baby is being attended to, instead requiring constant monitoring and engagement. The parents are completely overwhelmed and disheartened at the thought that they may lose the respite of Luke's time at school. They give the IMH worker permission to meet with the school director and teachers to gather more information and are open to meeting all together in the hopes of salvaging the situation.

DC:0–5 diagnosis: Attention Deficit Hyperactivity Disorder

DSM–5 diagnosis: Attention Deficit Hyperactivity Disorder

ICD–10–CM code: Disturbance of Activity and Attention (F90.1)

Relational Clinical Formulation

The identified client, a 3½-year-old White boy, meets criteria for a diagnosis of Attention Deficit Hyperactivity Disorder as evidenced by extreme difficulty attending and focusing both at home and at school. He is rarely able to settle into a calm activity for more than a few minutes, and in active play he cannot easily wait his turn or collaborate. He is rough and disruptive with his baby sister (e.g., knocking her over, taking her bottle away from her, waking her from sleep by picking her up from her bassinet and carrying her to the next room). He engages in group activities in ways that frustrate children and adults (e.g., throwing a ball over the fence deliberately, dumping out the bubble mixture, grabbing toys from other children, crashing trikes). These symptoms strain his relationships with family, peers, and teachers, and they lead to missed opportunities for learning and connecting with others. At present, his school placement is at risk as a result of his behavioral difficulties. IMH intervention involving the client's parents so that they may develop strategies for intervening on a daily basis and also including collaboration with school personnel is recommended. The client will benefit from treatment aimed at strengthening PCRC 7.

Goal: The client will increase his capacity for focused attention through the strengthening of PCRC 7.

Sample objectives developed collaboratively with the client's parents include the following:

1. The client's parents and the IMH worker will meet with school personnel within 2 weeks to strategize collaboratively about how to maintain the client in the classroom.

2. The parents are presently at a loss as to how to support the client in calming down enough to focus and learn when he is dysregulated. Within the next month, the client's parents will, with the support of the IMH worker, identify three calming strategies (e.g., putting his hand on his heart to feel his heartbeat, blowing a pinwheel, using

a squishy ball) that can help the client listen to adults when they are giving him direction.

3. The parents will report during weekly IMH meetings supervising the client and his sister closely so that there are zero incidents of the client endangering his sister (current baseline: 1–2 incidents per week).

4. As observed by the IMH worker, the client's capacity to settle into and enjoy a calm activity, such as listening to a story, will increase from several minutes to 15 minutes within 3 months.

5. The parents will report in weekly IMH meetings taking the client one time per day to a park or other appropriate environment where his high energy level and need for physical stimulation will not conflict with social– environmental expectations.

Vignette 7.2

Shea is referred to an IMH clinic by the public health nurse who has been visiting her since the birth of her daughter, Nya, 6 months ago. "Nya is overfed, but other than that I haven't really had any medical concerns," the nurse explains, "so I need to close their case, but I think Shea is depressed, and I know they are really isolated. I hate to stop visiting."

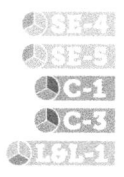

The IMH worker visits and learns that Shea, a 27-year-old African American woman, is indeed quite isolated socially and rarely leaves her apartment. Her extended family lives nearby, but she keeps her distance from them because she reports that many family members struggle with substance abuse, and she wants to "stay out of that drama." She reports that Nya's father has been incarcerated since before Nya was born and that she had not known him well and has not tried to inform him about Nya's birth. She does not want to pursue a relationship with him, but she suffers from worry and guilt at the idea of Nya not having a father. Shea states readily that she suffers from depression, adding "I've been depressed as long as I can remember." She saw a counselor in high school and found this helpful but has not engaged in therapy since then.

Nya is a quiet, solemn baby. She appears comfortable in her mother's arms, but she will also lie for long periods in the infant seat without demanding interaction. Shea is adept at diapering and feeding Nya, but she does not play with her or provide her with regular opportunities for being on the floor, resulting in Nya being a bit delayed with respect to gross motor development (i.e., sitting). Nya is bottle fed, and Shea has not yet introduced solids, despite the public health nurse's encouragement. "I'm just not ready for that," Shea tells the IMH worker. When asked what "all that" refers to, she replies "going out and getting food, dealing with people—and her growing up."

DSM–5 diagnosis: Persistent Depressive Disorder (Dysthymia)

ICD–10–CM code: F34.1

Relational Clinical Formulation

The identified client is a 27-year-old African American woman who is a single parent to a 6-month-old baby. She has struggled with symptoms of depression for as long as she can remember and meets criteria for a diagnosis of Persistent Depressive Disorder (Dysthymia). Her symptoms include staying very socially isolated; persistent feelings of sadness, guilt, and worry; not being able to identify or engage in pleasurable activities; and persistent low energy. These troubles are negatively affecting her sense of herself as a mother and are interfering with her infant's development because opportunities for growth-promoting exploration and interaction are restricted. Aside from feeding-related interactions, the dyad engages in very few activities involving shared focus and mutual attention that would be mutually pleasurable and would support the infant's development. These difficulties are best addressed in the context of the infant–parent relationship so that both the client and the infant may participate in and benefit from intervention. The dyad will benefit from IMH intervention aimed at strengthening PCRC 7.

Goal: Reduce symptoms of depression as reflected in increased capacity to enjoy shared focus and engage in mutual attention with the infant.

Sample objectives developed collaboratively with the client include the following:

1. Within 1 month, the client will begin working with a psychiatrist to see whether medication may reduce symptoms of depression.

2. Client reports not being able to identify any joint activities aside from feeding that she and her baby enjoy engaging in together. During weekly infant–parent psychotherapy meetings over the course of the next 2 months, the client will develop alternatives to feeding that the baby enjoys, such as experimenting with the textures and sounds of various household objects, looking at picture books together, or watching passers-by together from the front steps.

3. At present, the client only leaves her apartment to accomplish necessary tasks once or twice a week, and her isolation likely compounds her depression. In each weekly meeting with the IMH worker over the next 2 months, the client will report having taken the baby for daily walks in the stroller and noticing together sensations, landmarks, or objects of interest.

CHAPTER 9

PCRC 8—The Little Engine That Could: Problem-Solving as a Mindset

"I think I can. I think I can. I think I can. I think I can."
Up, up, up. Faster and faster and faster and faster the
little engine climbed, until at last they reached the top
of the mountain.

—*The Little Engine That Could*, retold by Watty Piper
(1930/2009, pp. 34–35)

PCRC 8: Parent possesses and conveys to child reasonable confidence that many things can be figured out/worked out successfully AND child demonstrates age expectable confident **problem-solving** capacities.

The capacity to stick with and solve problems has at least as much to do with one's experience and attitude when confronted with challenge as with their discrete cognitive capacities. When we are agitated or distraught, simple difficulties may feel insurmountable. The very same difficulties will likely feel less daunting when we are calmer or feel optimistic. As Zadra and Clore (2011) established through empirical research, hills look steeper when we are sad.

Although they are variable in attitude moment-to-moment, general attitudes toward encountering challenges are developed over time and in a relational context. A typically calm woman with the capacity to respond forthrightly to difficult situations tended to panic if her toddler suffered minor illnesses or injuries. She was both irritated and embarrassed by her own tendency to startle and gasp loudly, for example, if the toddler bumped his head on the kitchen table. Upon reflection, she realized that this tendency to react with alarm to minor physical ailments was a pattern of her own mother's. She had clearly absorbed it and was repeating this behavior in her relationship with her child. She was determined not to continue this pattern. She dedicated herself to be calm and suppress her impulse to gasp in such moments so as to convey to her child a greater sense of physical sturdiness than she herself had inherited. She wanted to instill in him a sense that he could persist rather than panicking at a physical challenge.

Young children can be excellent problem solvers, sometimes seeing possibilities that elude adults. A 4-year-old student at the Reggio Emilia School in Italy reflected that you can learn by listening (Reggio Children, 2008). He explained, "You can listen to the noise of a place; a tree, for example, tells us about the wind." His 5-year-old peer reported that "You can listen to the future, too…if you close your eyes and open your mind." Even newborn infants have remarkable capacities such as the ability to track caregivers in their visual field, which can develop later into recognizable problem-solving capabilities such as searching for hidden objects when the cognitive capacity (object permanence) emerges.

The problems of the world are boundless and can crush us in an instant. Psychological health involves developing a relationship to the problems of the world that is neither too disengaged and cut off from them nor so engaged as to be engulfed, but instead establishing the highly personal zone and mode of engagement that is "just right" for the individual: morally and ethically bearable, personally meaningful, and psychologically sustainable. In a similar fashion, relational health involves taking the problems of loved others seriously and joining in solving them to the degree that works. We are each challenged to attend to the problems of loved others without losing sight of the "otherness" of the other person and their problems and without ceasing to do what one can to attend to one's own problems (perhaps relying on others for help) and to shared problems. Working toward this differentiated balance in parent–child relationships is a gradual, dynamic process occurring across the lifespan, as parents and children are psychologically intertwined in perpetuity.

Parent–Child Relationship Competency (PCRC) 8 describes the dynamics in the parent–child relationship around encountering challenges and solving problems. The basic premise is that all human beings are presented with both large and small challenges in life, and parents can help their children to be equipped to meet challenges with a sense that they bring their own reliable internal resources to this effort. When this PCRC is functioning well, the parent is one who is able to face adult challenges and work toward solving them. In addition, the parent interacts with the child in ways that promote this capacity in the child. Returning to the earlier example, this mother wished to foster in her son a capacity to "get up, shake it off, and carry on" if he were to stumble and fall in the playground, and she hoped and believed that this capacity would generalize to her son's ability to recover from failures or disappointments down the line. She did not want him to be dissuaded from trying physically challenging gross motor activities or, later in life, to shy away from experiences that might seem daunting because of a misperception of himself as fragile.

Many things contribute to how individuals, families, and cultures construe the meaning of life's challenges, including history, religion, cosmology, and ideology. Also, as the *Diversity-Informed Tenets for Work With Infants, Children, and Families* (© Irving Harris Foundation; see www.diversityinformedtenets.org/) remind us, different societies are not level playing fields. Individuals and families are variably affected by intersecting systems of oppression. Qualities such as optimism and determination are developed not in a vacuum but in a sociopolitical and relational context. In a given family or cultural context, optimism or determination may be encouraged or absent, and they may be experienced or deemed inappropriate. Problem-solving strategies may be individualistic or collectivistic. Whereas striving to be

Tenet # 3: Work to Acknowledge Privilege and Combat Discrimination

P-5 5
"problem free" may be seen as a virtue by some, others may hold the opposite value, associating struggle with virtue, for example. Acceptance may be valued more than rebellion, and either may constitute problem-solving effort.

P-5 2

There is often a role for infant mental health (IMH) workers in helping families identify and tackle their challenges, supporting the processes of differentiation and balance, and helping parents to nurture in their children the approach to problem solving that is personally and culturally appropriate for them. It is critical, however, that IMH workers understand and respect the varied expression of this PCRC so that it is families, rather than IMH workers, who determine what constitutes a problem for them and what solving it will look like.

Tenet # 4:
Recognize
and Respect
Non-Dominant
Bodies of
Knowledge

Vignette 8.1

SE-2
SE-4
SE-5
SE-6
C-1
L-1

Three-year-old Terrence, an African American boy, has been referred to an early childhood mental health program by the teacher at the Head Start program where he is newly enrolled because of concerns about his aggressive behavior with other children and difficulty engaging in group activities. The teacher reports that Terrence has "been through a lot." He and his mother, Akira, had lived in another city together with his father, Leroy, but the parents had had a high-conflict marriage with a lot of arguing (although no physical violence). The parents separated, and Terrence and Akira now reside with Akira's mother, Ms. Stanton.

The IMH worker, who is biracial (African American and White) meets with Akira to gather more history and find out what her concerns are. With Akira's permission, she observes Terrence once in the classroom and then begins to make home visits to work with Terrence and Akira together. Ms. Stanton also joins these visits from time to time.

During the classroom observation, Terrence refuses to join in an art project that a teacher is facilitating and throws a truck at a child who makes an overture to play with him. In early home visits, the IMH worker notes that Terrence gets easily frustrated, for example, knocking over a stool when he tries unsuccessfully to balance a ball on top of it. While at school, Terrence's presentation is defiant; at home, he collapses into tears when he becomes frustrated. The IMH worker and Akira agree that Terrence is struggling to adjust to many changes and that he seems to lack confidence in his ability to take effective action or solve problems.

DC:0–5 diagnosis: Adjustment Disorder with mixed anxiety and depression

Relational Clinical Formulation

The identified client is a 3-year-old boy who meets criteria for a diagnosis of Adjustment Disorder with mixed anxiety and depression, as evidenced by his apparent worry that he will not succeed at tasks and social interactions, his proneness to disintegrating into tears when met with frustration, and his aggressive acting out with peers. These symptoms and behaviors strain his relationships with family, peers, and teachers. He has suffered a significant relationship loss because his parents have recently separated, and he now resides at a considerable distance from his father. The client's mother is distressed herself as a result of the separation and is preoccupied with efforts to forge a new life for herself and the child; hence, her patience with the client is limited. The client seems to be struggling with a sense of his lack of control over life circumstances and concern that problems are insurmountable. These difficulties are best addressed in the context of the parent–child relationship so that the client's mother can participate as a collateral partner to increase her patience and to restore the client's sense that problems may be solved, which will likely help restore the client to a healthy trajectory of social–emotional development. This dyad would benefit from services aimed at strengthening PCRC 8.

Goal: Reduce depressive and anxious symptoms by strengthening PCRC 8.

Sample collaboratively generated objectives include the following:

1. At present, the client's emotional difficulties lead to his easily giving up when he experiences challenges, thus missing out on learning opportunities. The client's mother will arrange a meeting within 2 weeks to include the IMH worker and the client's teachers to collaboratively generate a plan to increase the client's sense of success in the classroom.

2. Due to high levels of marital conflict, client's mother often ignores calls from client's father, exacerbating client's sense of loss and lack of predictability and control. Within 2 weeks client's mother will arrange with client's father a regular time for a phone call with client in order to increase client's sense of connectedness and predictability.

3. At present, the client's mother reports rarely offering client verbal affirmation. During weekly home-based IMH visits over the next 3 months, the client and the mother will engage in child-directed play, with the mother noting and affirming verbally the client's actions (e.g., "You are driving that truck FAST!").

4. Stress has recently prevented the client's mother from responding to the client's need for relaxing, playful interactions with her, which exacerbates his depressive symptoms. The client's mother will report providing opportunities at least once each morning and once each evening for a period of 30 minutes or more for the client to select and direct pleasurable activities for the family (e.g., reading stories, playing).

5. At present, the client remains socially isolated at school. The client's teachers will report that the client is able to engage with peers in collaborative play and projects on a

daily basis by the parent–teacher conference scheduled for [date].

Vignette 8.2

Lorna enters therapy in the wake of a divorce. Her husband of 13 years, Wallace, has left her and has entered a relationship with a much younger colleague. Lorna and Wallace have three children who are 11 years, 8 years, and 20 months old. Although they had been in graduate school together when they met, Lorna did not complete her degree. For the past 11 years, she has dedicated herself full time to child rearing, whereas Wallace was the sole breadwinner. Lorna is enraged and indignant that the determination in court was that she and Wallace will have joint custody and that although she will receive child support, she must seek employment and the children will be in the care of their father half time. She is especially upset in relation to the 20-month-old, Angie, who is still breastfeeding. She reports that this child had been "conceived in love" and that she and Wallace had explicitly recommitted to their marriage in anticipation of her birth, only to find themselves increasingly alienated after Angie was born. Lorna feels that both Wallace and the court system have treated her cruelly and unfairly, and she feels the custody arrangement will be injurious to the children, especially Angie. She reports constant worry (intensifying when she attempts to sleep) about her and the children's future and a sense of dread at the thought of looking for work. She feels it is a bitter irony that she must find employment now, when her sense of well-being and confidence are so shaken.

During an assessment phase, the Chinese American IMH worker holds weekly individual sessions with Lorna to provide consistent opportunities for Lorna to freely express and address her distress, as well as weekly dyadic sessions with Lorna and Angie together to assess how the changes in the family are affecting Angie. During the dyadic sessions, Lorna frequently weeps. Angie is very attentive to Lorna's states, bringing her tissues and patting her knee. Lorna sometimes invites Angie to nurse at such moments. On several occasions when Angie is exploring manipulative toys in the office such as building blocks with interest independently, Lorna redirects her to interactive doll play. The IMH worker shares with Lorna her impression that the current anxiety-based collapse of Lorna's problem-solving capacities prevents her from promoting these in Angie.

DSM–5 diagnosis: Generalized Anxiety Disorder

ICD–10–CM code: F41.1

Relational Clinical Formulation

The client has recently undergone a divorce and is contending with significant life changes as a result. The client meets criteria for a diagnosis of Generalized Anxiety Disorder, as evidenced by her near-constant state of worry about family and work, her catastrophic thinking, her disturbed sleep, her difficulty focusing on anything other than the court proceedings, and her chronically inflamed emotional state. These symptoms undermine her capacity to seek employment and are negatively affecting her relationship with her child, who is aware of and concerned about her mother's distress, engaging in role-reversal behaviors. The client's anxiety prevents her from supporting her daughter's developmentally important autonomy and exploratory impulses. These difficulties are best addressed by a treatment format including both individual and dyadic sessions so that the client can be supported in reducing her anxiety and tackling her adult life challenges, while concurrently practicing developmentally attuned, growth-promoting interactions with her daughter during this critical time of family transition. The client and her daughter will likely benefit from intervention aimed at strengthening PCRC 8.

Goal: Reduce symptoms of anxiety by strengthening PCRC 8.

Sample collaboratively generated objectives include the following:

1. At present, the client states that her constant worry about her children makes it hard for her to tell whether they are emotionally okay in any given moment, which, in turn, exacerbates her anxiety. During weekly dyadic sessions over the next 2 months, the client will identify signs in her daughter that breastfeeding and other nurturing interactions are emotionally responsive in the moment.

2. During weekly dyadic sessions over the next 2 months, the client will identify signs in her daughter that interactions supporting her autonomy and exploratory impulses are emotionally responsive in the moment.

3. At present, the client is at a loss as to how to support her daughter in transitioning to her father's house as per the custody arrangement. In individual sessions over the next 2 weeks, the client will develop with the IMH worker specific language to use with the daughter around transitions to and from the ex-husband's home to build and support a sense in the daughter that these transitions will be manageable.

4. Symptoms of anxiety, including global and catastrophic thinking, currently prevent the client from seeking employment. During each individual session over the next 2 months, the client will counter her sense of being overwhelmed by breaking down the life tasks that she faces into component parts that are accomplishable day by day.

5. At present, the client finds it difficult to refrain from criticizing her ex-husband in the children's presence, which puts their social–emotional development at risk. The client will report ceasing to discuss her distress about her ex-husband within earshot of her children by [date], instead using treatment to work through her feelings.

CHAPTER 10

PCRC 9—The Birth of the Speaking Subject

I marched on over the next few miles, my pace quickened by my rage, but soon I slowed and stopped to sit on a boulder. A gathering of low flowers grew at my feet, their barely pink petals edging the rocks. Crocus, I thought, the name coming into my mind because my mother had given it to me. These same flowers grew in the dirt where I'd spread her ashes. I reached out and touched the petals of one, feeling my anger drain out of my body. By the time I rose and started walking again, I didn't begrudge my mother a thing.

—Cheryl Strayed (2012, p. 267)

PCRC 9: Parent talks to child and otherwise facilitates child's entry into **language and literacy** (including multilingualism as appropriate) and confidence in communication AND child is developing at age level the capacity for two-way gestural and/or verbal communication.

Language links people. Interpersonal connections are often forged and framed through language. Cultures are delineated and reproduced largely through language. Moreover, the human capacity for language is widely recognized as our primary distinguishing feature as a species.

Infants are typically bathed in a language environment even before they are born, as is reflected in the neonate turning her head to the sound of the already familiar voice of her mother the first time they meet face to face. Infants are primed to organize themselves around parents' and caregivers' voices (as well as our faces), such that even before they have volitional control of the movements of their limbs, they will move involuntarily in rhythm with our voices. As the early months unfold and they do gain motor control, they make use of this development to participate in and further exchanges around words even though they cannot yet reciprocate verbally, positioning themselves to better hear the parent, for example, or to be able to read the parent's facial expression together with hearing the voice. They come into the world capable of learning and speaking any language, and their brains are literally shaped in response to the languages they are exposed to. They spend the first months of life immersed in language that they do not yet understand and cannot reproduce but that gradually (and often in sudden bursts) captures their attention. Language is meaningful to them as an experience even as the precise meaning eludes them.

P-5 5
P-5 1

There are several important precursors to a toddler's learning to talk. Being spoken to is a major experience. When a baby is addressed directly, they are being invited into language. When we say "Hello little one in your striped pajamas!" we are both playing and offering a part, saying, "I recognize you as a person, and I offer you a place in this language event between you and me, and in our language-linked community." This experience of being addressed gives the baby a sense of belonging in the world of those who speak that precedes and paves the way for being able to speak.

When we speak and the baby wiggles and makes a sound, we might ask, "Is that so? I never thought of it just that way!" When infants are invited into an exchange of this sort, rich with affect and with plenty of interesting vocabulary and inflection, they pay attention with their whole selves. They show us with their facial expressions, their heart rates, the pace of their breath, the sounds they emit, and their physical movements that they are taking in a great deal of information from the communication even though they cannot yet understand our words. They can also show us that they know the difference between verbal communications that are mild or urgent, informational or playful, light-hearted or grave. Furthermore, they show us that they recognize that they are doing things to further the exchange.

Speaking to a baby establishes a sense of expectation—the baby is expected to speak one day as well as to comprehend what is said. This sense of expectation is part of what pulls the toddler into speech. This sense of expectation is conveyed in a wide range of individually and culturally meaningful ways, including in environments where children may be socialized to be quiet under certain circumstances—in church, for example, or when there are guests. Offering a developing child a place in the world of speaking subjects is not limited to cultures that groom children to be garrulous.

Tenet # 5:
Honor Diverse Family Structures

A shared sense of meaning around an exchange of words precedes verbal comprehension. The baby in the striped pajamas probably gathers not only that he is the addressee— the "there, there" who is being spoken to—but also that he is quite fetching. People often underestimate what infants can notice and make use of. It is easy not to be aware of the amount of emotion children pick up on from those around them and how nuance is not lost on them. Imagine, for example, a baby whose mother is experiencing grief and is crying. The baby is likely alerted to his mother's distress, although the source of the problem eludes him. It is possible to comfort a baby in such a moment by responding with a calm narrative that may include "Your mommy is crying, and she is sad, but she will be all right." The older the child, the more detailed information one might layer in. It is quite remarkable to note how a "preverbal" infant responds when something very important is said to him when it is delivered in an emotionally resonant manner.

Tenet # 6:
Understand That Language Can Hurt or Heal

The reciprocal language relationship is a duet. The adult who knows how to talk plays a part, and the baby coming along toward being a person who can talk plays the other part. The baby's part fills out as the child develops. A baby shows her developing awareness that she can use her voice to get her parents' attention and perhaps to initiate a chain of back-and-forth interactions. Her voice changes and comes increasingly under her control as the baby is able to produce and experiment with a broadening range of sounds, patterned more and more after the sounds of the languages spoken around her. She comes to recognize names and words and can signal this recognition through gestures and by producing sounds containing elements of the words. Eventually, she imitates words, and ultimately she uses them spontaneously. When we lump infants and toddlers into categories labeled "preverbal" and "verbal," we lose sight of all of the intricate processes whereby language populates, animates, and connects people.

Literacies are developed hand-in-hand with language development. Developing a pleasurable relationship with books can be an immeasurably rich and rewarding experience for infants and toddlers, laying the groundwork for a lifelong positive relationship with reading. Parents can promote such positive reading experiences by joining in the pleasure with infants and toddlers, celebrating books as interesting objects and making reading-together time cozy and playful (Pawl, 1991). This outcome is more easily achieved when parents' own relationships to reading have been likewise supported in positive ways. Often, this experience is not the case, and indeed in many instances reading is associated with painful or traumatic experiences of exclusion, frustration, or shame (Kozol, 2005).

There can be an important role for the infant mental health (IMH) worker in unearthing such painful histories with parents and paving the way for a new reading experience for the parent together with the baby. This process often entails examining with the parent interpersonal dynamics or the forces of oppression that conspired to block pleasurable pathways and access to rewarding reading experiences for them in the past. Sometimes, finding the right books for each family—books that reflect their lives, capture their imagination, speak to matters of importance to them—is a critical element of promoting family literacy. IMH workers can access diversity-informed, library-building resources from organizations such as Welcoming Schools (www.welcomingschools.org) and the National Association for the Education of Young Children (www.NAEYC.org).

Tenet # 3: Work to Acknowledge Privilege and Combat Discrimination

Bilingual and multilingual families offer an amazing wealth of language and literature to their children, potentially providing a sense of belonging in not just one global language community but in two or more, with access to the multiple cultures that each language delineates. Bilingualism may also be fraught with conflict for parents—bound up, for example, with immigration experiences that may have been painful or traumatic, with experiences of discrimination and oppression, or with separation from homeland and loved ones. The birth of a baby often presents opportunities for parents to identify and address some of the emotional complexities with which language may be saturated, which can help them to bestow with less conflict the gift of bilingualism that is their child's birthright. Learning two languages simultaneously is not in and of itself an impediment to language development; on the contrary, it is an enhancement.

Tenet # 7: Support Families in Their Preferred Language

P-5 5

There are many kinds of literacy, and we need to be cognizant of literacies beyond word-based reading and writing. Oral traditions, musical traditions, and traditions of visual representation are all examples. Culture is preserved, shared, and innovated through these pathways, and literacy in such traditions varies from one person to the next. It is easy but injurious to overlook these non-dominant forms of literacy.

Tenet # 4: Recognize and Respect Non-Dominant Bodies of Knowledge

Aside from reading print material, people also have more and less well-developed capacities to decipher online and virtual spaces; urban, rural, and wilderness environments; or specific cultural contexts. One person may feel quite oriented and able to readily pick up subtle pieces of information in an emergency room but be oblivious to significant signals at a social gathering. The ability to read such cues is important in managing a variety of environments.

Promoting racial literacy in children is a parenting task that some parents execute competently as a matter of basic protection, whereas others falter. Howard C. Stevenson (2014) defined *racial literacy* as "the ability to read, recast, and resolve racially stressful social interactions" (p. 4). He argued that children benefit from being actively taught how to read the racialized meanings in the social world, and indeed that if adults fail to teach them in considered ways, we will be teaching them lessons inadvertently that may be injurious. Stevenson wrote, "The teaching of racial literacy skills protects [children of color] from the threat of internalizing negative stereotypes" (p. 4).

PS①

White children, too, are injured when their parents fail to cultivate their racial literacy. White supremacy is the commonly held fantasy that perceived "Whiteness" is better than racially marked "otherness." This fantasy naturalizes racial inequity, suggesting that the privileges that accrue to Whiteness are a measure of its superiority. White supremacy is not innate; children are socialized into it. Racial illiteracy for White children can manifest in White fragility (DiAngelo, 2011), xenophobia, the entitlement of unexamined privilege, and alienation connected with conscious or nonconscious White supremacism. There is often a role for the IMH worker in helping parents to reflect on how race has influenced them in their lives so that they can promote racial literacy in their children.

Tenet # 3: Work to Acknowledge Privilege and Combat Discrimination

The question of agency is a key issue when considering adults' relationships to literacies of various sorts, and this, in turn, influences how they promote literacies in their children. When parents see themselves as valuable and competent participants in linguistic and cultural exchanges, they can usher their children into such exchanges, providing a sense of access and value. Conversely, when parents feel disempowered and excluded, it can be very challenging for them to pave the way for their children to have an experience different from their own, however much they might wish for this outcome.

In a discussion of an effort to promote literacy skills in adults, Paolo Freire (1974/2007) argued that it is important first to help people understand that literature and other cultural artifacts belong to and issue from them, not exclusively from some official realm of art or scholarship outside of them. "By discovering himself to be a maker of the world of culture," Freire wrote,

> by discovering that he, as well as the literate person, has a creative and re-creative impulse...he would discover that culture is just as much a clay doll made by artists who are his peers as it is the work of a great sculptor, a great painter, a great mystic, or a great philosopher; that culture is the poetry of lettered poets and also the poetry of his own popular songs—that culture is all human creation. (p. 41)

IMH workers can likewise ground efforts to support family literacy of all sorts in bringing attention to family culture and to the special literacies that each parent holds and offers.

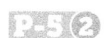

Vignette 9.1

A 30-year-old El Salvadorian woman, Elana, is referred to an IMH clinic by her 20-month-old son Raphael's pediatrician. The pediatrician is concerned about Raphael's possible language delay but also notes that Elana brings him in frequently with health concerns that seem to be unfounded. The IMH worker, who is a bilingual/bicultural clinician and an immigrant from Argentina, meets with Elana and Raphael to begin the assessment. Elana carries Raphael in a shawl that is wrapped around her and tied snugly and keeps him on her lap during the initial meetings, which he does not protest. Raphael is passive and quiet during these meetings, exploring the treatment room (which is set up with many brightly colored developmental toys) only with his eyes. The IMH worker is surprised initially that although Elana struggles with English, having immigrated just 5 years prior, she declines to speak Spanish with the IMH worker, stating that she wants Raphael exposed only to English. She alludes to "bad things" that happened to her in El Salvador and in the process of immigrating to the United States. The IMH worker suggests that it may be important to be able to think about some of those things together and notes that it seems Elana does not want to talk about them in Raphael's presence. She wonders whether Elana might be able to come in for a couple of individual meetings. Elana reports that Raphael is never cared for by anyone other than his parents, and his father works long hours. They develop a plan to meet in the evening several times so that Elana's husband, Mark, can join in the appointments during after-work hours. This arrangement will allow the IMH worker to get to know the whole family and to spend some time conversing privately with Elana while Raphael is in the care of his father.

DSM–5 diagnosis: Posttraumatic Stress Disorder (PTSD)

Relational Clinical Formulation

The identified client, a 30-year-old woman, is experiencing stress related to parenting in a new country. The client suffered a series of traumatic experiences in her home country that led to her decision to emigrate. She then encountered traumatic experiences in the process of immigration. She meets criteria for a diagnosis of PTSD, as evidenced by her feeling as though she is in acute danger nearly all the time, fearing that if she lets her son out of her sight something terrible will happen to him, and oscillating between emotional numbing and being overwhelmed with fear. These symptoms are negatively affecting her functioning as a parent because she frequently presents at urgent care when her son is in fact healthy, and both she and the toddler are quite isolated because there are so few places that the client feels are safe for them to go. The client's son's opportunities for learning and exploration are quite restricted as a result of the client's fear. Finally, because of the client's PTSD-related emotional distancing from her native language, Spanish, and her belief that it will be protective for her son to learn only English, she does not speak with him in Spanish. This decision results in his being exposed to very little language, because the client's English is limited, and they are alone together most of the time. The client's husband is mono-lingual English-speaking, but he spends little time with the client and his son because of long work hours. The client will benefit from services aimed at increasing her sense of safety and her functioning as a parent via strengthening Parent–Child Relationship Competency (PCRC) 9. It will be important to include the client's son as a collateral partner in the treatment on a regular weekly basis to prevent adverse developmental outcomes secondary to the client's PTSD and to also include the husband as a collateral partner as his schedule permits.

Goal: Reduce symptoms of PTSD as reflected in strengthening PCRC 9.

Sample collaboratively generated objectives include the following:

1. The client will consider during weekly IMH meetings research findings shared by the IMH worker related to children raised bilingually and will develop a plan for supporting her son's language development by [date].

2. At present, the client describes having no strategies for calming herself when suffering from traumatic re-experiencing. The client will practice during weekly IMH meetings over the next 3 months engaging in "up-regulating" and "down-regulating" games and songs with her son to develop awareness of internal states and to expand capacities for calming herself while also promoting his language development.

3. At present, the client describes being too afraid to explore her neighborhood, resulting in extreme isolation. The client, son, and IMH worker will take walks together on a monthly basis in the neighborhood of the clinic to increase the client's and the son's comfort with exploration and sense of safety moving about in the world.

4. The client will report that her son's language development is deemed to be within expectable range by the 24-month pediatric appointment.

Vignette 9.2

The IMH consultant at a preschool refers Benita, a 3½-year-old girl, and her mother, Isabel, to the IMH clinic because of concerns about recent changes in Benita's behavior. "Her mom has a lot of challenges, but she is very devoted to Benita, and Benita's a great kid," the consultant explains. "But the family has recently gone through some big transitions, and I think it is taking a real toll on Benita. She seems sad all the time and has virtually stopped talking."

The IMH worker contacts Isabel and arranges a meeting during a time when Benita will be in school. She learns that Isabel, who is Puerto Rican, grew up in New York, and moved many times in her early adulthood, is in early recovery. She and Benita recently moved into an apartment together after having spent the past 18 months living at Phoenix House, a residential substance abuse treatment program for families. With Isabel's permission, the IMH worker observes Benita at the preschool and meets with Benita's teachers. She then conducts a home-based assessment, meeting with Benita and Isabel together for a few weeks. An aftercare case worker from Phoenix House who has known Isabel and Benita for a long time joins two of these visits to share her impressions and thoughts. It is clear that Benita can talk, and does some, but Isabel, the Phoenix House case worker, and Benita's teachers all concur that she has been much quieter, more subdued, and less vibrant than usual since the move. Isabel reports that Benita is also having a hard time falling asleep in her new bed, and she does not have the appetite she usually does. Isabel says, "We finally have our own kitchen, and she won't eat anything I make!"

During an individual meeting with Isabel at the end of this assessment period, the IMH worker talks with Isabel about her sense that moving out of Phoenix House has been hard on Benita, and she seems to be struggling with depression. She had relationships with many staff people and other children and mothers, and all of that changed very suddenly for her. Things are much quieter in the apartment with just the two of them than they were at Phoenix House, where there were always so many people everywhere and so much happening. The IMH worker explains that young children sometimes show their sadness by seeming to go backward in their development, and Benita's new silence at school might be an example of that. The IMH worker suggests that she continue to visit Isabel and Benita in their apartment on a weekly basis so they can think together about how to support Benita with the transition and make their new life together as much the way they want it to be as possible. Isabel is amenable to this.

DC:0–5 diagnosis: Depressive Disorder of Early Childhood

DSM–5 diagnosis: Major Depressive Disorder

ICD–10–CM code: F32 Depressive Episode

Relational Clinical Formulation

The identified client, a 3½-year-old girl, was referred because of recent cessation of previous expressive language. The client's reduced talking is part of a larger pattern of subdued behavior, somber mood, and loss of previously established developmental accomplishments, such as falling asleep readily at bedtime. She also demonstrates loss of appetite. In general, she presents with low mood and lack of capacity to take pleasure in previously enjoyable activities. Taken together, these behaviors meet criteria for a diagnosis of Depressive Disorder of Early Childhood. These difficulties reflect distress, are impeding the client's capacity to benefit from learning opportunities, and cause worry for her mother and other caregivers. The client's depression is likely secondary to relationship loss related to her family's recent move. Weekly home-based IMH services including the client's mother as collateral partner are recommended so that the mother can implement strategies on a daily basis to reduce the client's symptoms of depression and help her restore her previously acquired capacities for talking, playing, and enjoying life.

Goal: Reduce symptoms of depression via strengthening PCRC 9.

Sample collaboratively generated objectives include the following:

1. At present, teachers report that the client produces few verbal utterances during the school day, limiting her capacity to benefit maximally from learning opportunities. The client will engage in conversation with peers or teachers once per hour of each school day, as reported by teachers by [date].

2. The client's mother describes that she has been focused on setting up the apartment, and she has not prioritized interacting with the client when the two of them are home together, which may exacerbate the client's sense of loneliness. The client's mother will report engaging with the client in at least 30 minutes of focused play, reading, or other language-based interaction before and after each school day over the course of the next 3 months.

3. The client appears confused and at a loss to understand and process recent changes in her life related to her family's move, undermining her social–emotional development. During weekly home-based IMH sessions,

the client and her mother will engage in talking and playing directed at putting themes of moving and saying goodbye into words.

4. The client's mother has been puzzled by the client's depressive symptoms, thinking that the client would be excited about the family's move and imagining that a child of the client's age would be too little to experience depression, leaving the client feeling alone and misunderstood. During each weekly home-based IMH meeting over the course of the next 6 months, the client's mother will verbally identify plausible emotional meanings signaled by the client's behaviors.

CHAPTER 11

PCRC 10—Play and Meaning-Making: Symbolic Networks

Block City

What are you able to build with your blocks?
Castles and palaces, temples and docks.
Rain may keep raining, and others go roam,
But I can be happy and building at home.
Let the sofa be mountains, the carpet be sea,
There I'll establish a city for me:
A kirk and a mill and a palace beside,
And a harbor as well where my vessels may ride.

—Robert Louis Stevenson (1885)

PCRC 10: Parent is able to take satisfaction from **symbolic activities** and may use conversation, narration, play, and/or other practices to promote these capacities in child AND child is able to use symbols in developmentally expectable ways to play, process, and partake in meaning-making.

Parent–Child Relationship Competencies (PCRCs) 9 and 10 are intertwined, but whereas PCRC 9 focuses on language and literacy specifically, PCRC 10 is broader. It has to do not only with language but with all the forms of symbolic activity that human beings can engage in: visual and performing arts, crafts, cooking, sports, religion, media, and so forth. All these activities are potentially meaning-making. For most people, when all is going well enough, engaging in symbolic activity is inherently meaningful, a route to pleasure or satisfaction. Listening to music on the radio while driving to the grocery store is an example. Driving to the grocery store is a goal-oriented activity bound up with accomplishing something.

The yield is material: procuring groceries. Listening to the radio is a separate endeavor, incidental to grocery shopping, which provides its own satisfactions—symbolic ones. (This contrast is simply illustrative. In fact, grocery shopping, too, is bound up with many symbolic systems—e.g., exchange, currency, advertising, culinary arts, food politics, and consumption.) In situations of ordinary psychological health, symbolic experiences enrich human existence and can provide pleasure, inspiration, comfort, connectedness, and solace. Most fundamentally, they provide meaning.

Symbolic networks surround and organize us in ways both visible and invisible. Lacan (1977) described the abiding and influential presence of symbolic networks such as language and other systems of representation. From this perspective, individual agency is exercised within the context of systems that color and delimit what might be imagined, conceived, desired, or willed by an individual. From an infant mental health (IMH) perspective, it is important also to consider the power of early relationships in shaping an individual's experience of being ushered into the world of symbolic networks. PCRC 10 describes these dynamics.

Tenet # 6:
Understand That
Language Can
Hurt or Heal

When people contend with certain psychological difficulties, their capacities to engage in or draw pleasure or satisfaction from symbolic activities can be constricted. When someone suffers from severe depression, for example, symbolic activities that would otherwise be rewarding to them are likely to be experienced as empty and meaningless, or perhaps even aversive. In certain states of psychosis, symbolic systems fail entirely as organizing forces, resulting, for example, in the extreme phenomenon of "word salad," when an individual can produce words from their language but cannot apply the rules of syntax that make language intelligible and meaningful. One of the defining characteristics of Autism Spectrum Disorder for some people is a restricted capacity to engage in symbolic activity. Experiencing a trauma can leave a person preoccupied with the horror that the concrete world sometimes presents. This experience can arrest their capacity to derive pleasure from our usual symbolic activity. All these extreme examples illustrate psychological difficulties with symbolic activity and meaning-making. Most people encounter milder challenges around these processes at times of personal crisis.

For children, the primary mode of active engagement with symbolic activity is play. In situations of ordinary develop- **P-S 1** mental and psychological health, infants and children learn and process their experience through play. They perform this behavior spontaneously and with incredible ingenuity; play behavior will emerge without toys or any adult prompting or organizing. Although the form play takes is widely varied across communities, cultures, and individuals, its importance is universal. A child's play is the forerunner of the adult's capacity to work and engage in cultural activities of all kinds.

These symbolic networks surround children in ways that are both perceptible and imperceptible. They are absorbed by children through osmosis regardless of a parent's actions. Nonetheless, this PCRC posits a link between a parent's relationship to symbolic activity and that of the child. As with all PCRCs, its expression is individually and culturally varied. In one cultural and family context, it might be that a parent provides a child with toys saturated with cultural significance particular to the parent and actively facilitates the child's engagement with the toys. (Toy industries are fond of this avenue of expression.) In another cultural and family context, it might be that a parent does not provide toys or facilitate a child's play but has his own routes to symbolic pleasure and meaning-making—for example, watching sports or attending church services. He allows for the child's developmental need for play by monitoring for safety while the child manipulates household objects, rolling cans on the floor, stacking empty boxes, or repeating rounds of fill-up-the-bucket-with-clothespins and dump-the-clothespins-out. It is highly likely that, as the child develops, the symbolic themes that are important to the parent and present in the household will find their

> **Tenet # 4:** Recognize and Respect Non-Dominant Bodies of Knowledge

way into the child's play. It is equally true that the capacity will vary greatly.

It is enormously helpful for children when they know that their parents and the adults in their surroundings welcome and appreciate their play, and they will readily accept adults' offers to join them in play when all is going well enough relationally. Adults, with their wealth of knowledge and experience, can support and expand children's play if they are so inclined, and this act can be enriching and delightful for both child and adult. Still, children's capacity to play is not dependent on adult solicitation or facilitation. It is critical when IMH workers assess the functioning of this PCRC that they suspend their own personal and imported ideas regarding how parents "ought to" interact with children around play. If a child's capacity to play is developing

Tenet # 1:
Self-Awareness
Leads to Better
Services for
Families

well, this PCRC is likely functioning well, regardless of whether the parent plays actively or in obvious ways with the child. What is important is that the child be able to count on the parent as a partner in meaning-making exchanges. There is a role for the IMH worker to intervene around this PCRC if the parent is interacting with the child in ways that undermine the child's developing capacities for meaning-making or inhibit the development of play—that is, if the child is experiencing difficulties that make play or meaning-making inaccessible or fraught. When this problem occurs, the parent needs help in learning to support the child in play behavior; the parent will also need help when she is experiencing her own difficulties in her own relationship with symbolic activity

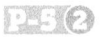

such that the child's relationship to the symbolic world is put at risk.

Vignette 10.1

A child welfare worker refers 2-year-old Lulu and her 20-year-old mother, Talia, to an IMH clinic as part of a plan to support their recent reunification. The worker explains that Lulu was placed in foster care following her exposure to an incident of mutual interpersonal violence between Talia and a man she had been dating that led to police involvement. Lulu and Talia had been living together with Talia's sister during Lulu's first year of life, but this sister had moved out of state subsequent to a falling out with Talia. In her sister's absence, Talia seems to have struggled to provide safety and stability for Lulu. At this point, however, Talia has met all benchmarks for reunification, and the dyad is living together with consistent child care in place and 6 more months of services available to them. "It is hard to pinpoint what's wrong now," the worker reports. "Talia loves Lulu and dotes on her in some ways, but they get into it constantly. Lulu is really challenging with her, disobeying her and provoking her all the time. And she's not like that in foster care or child care."

During an assessment period, the IMH worker, who is biracial (Japanese American and White), meets with Talia individually several times, observes Lulu at child care several times, and then makes weekly home visits over the course of a month to meet with the dyad together. She learns that Talia is of Samoan descent. Talia identifies as a single mother, stating that she "never tried to figure out" who Lulu's biological father might be. "It was me and her at the beginning and it's me and her now," Talia stated, "we are two peas in a pod."

The IMH worker's observations are consistent with the child welfare worker's description. Lulu looks very different at home and at child care. At child care, she is calm and cooperative. She interacts competently with peers and teachers and seems to enjoy a range of activities: active play outdoors, collaborative play with blocks and vehicles indoors, circle time with a story read aloud, a congenial snack with eight toddlers and two adults around a low table, and settling down for naptime. At home with Talia, by contrast, Lulu is very keyed up and contrary, saying "no" indiscriminately and engaging in risky behaviors such as climbing up the back of the sofa and lowering herself to the floor by hanging onto the drapes. The play skills she is in possession of at child care seem to elude her at home. She is provocative with her mother; on one occasion, she poured her mother's coffee on the floor while looking at her defiantly. Talia describes feeling constantly frustrated and overwhelmed to the point that she dreads taking Lulu out in public and also dreads being home with her for long stretches.

Talia's behavior with Lulu is likewise concerning. She alternates between pleading with the child to behave and yelling at her angrily. She is also preoccupied with Lulu's appearance. She often dresses Lulu in outfits that match her own, and many of their struggles center around Talia's near-constant attempts to fix Lulu's hair or adjust her clothing. When Lulu does, on occasion, settle into solo play, Talia frequently interrupts this play with grooming behaviors. When the IMH worker suggests that Talia join Lulu in play, Talia commandeers the play, dictating what should happen, and Lulu disengages. On one particularly disturbing occasion, the IMH worker finds Lulu asleep on the couch when she arrives for a home visit. Talia awakens the child and insists on dressing her, despite Lulu's sleepy protests. When Talia persists in her efforts to dress her and brush her hair, Lulu spits at her mother, runs to the edge of the room, and pulls a rug up over her head, thereby toppling a table and chair with a crash.

Clearly, Talia and Lulu are struggling in relation to many PCRCs. They could benefit from support around limit-setting, for example. However, the IMH worker determines that the highest priority initially is to help the dyad move away from these chaotic exchanges toward exchanges characterized by a sense of shared meaning, and away from the constant conflict toward play and pleasure. The IMH worker proposes this approach to Talia, explaining that her hope and expectation would be that as the two learn to play and learn to understand each other better, Lulu's oppositional behavior will diminish. Talia is receptive to this idea, if not wholly convinced, and they work collaboratively to describe what markers of progress would look like as they begin this work.

DC:0–5 diagnosis: Relationship Specific Disorder of Infancy/ Early Childhood

DSM–5 diagnosis: Parent–Child Relational Problem

ICD–10–CM code: Other Specified Problems Related to Upbringing (Z62.820)

Note: In some contexts, this diagnosis would not meet criteria for establishing medical or service necessity. This child could also legitimately be assigned a diagnosis of Oppositional Defiant Disorder, which would be more likely to be included in a list of qualifying diagnoses but is less comprehensive or developmentally appropriate in this instance because it does not account for the relational component.

Relational Clinical Formulation

The identified client is a 2-year-old girl who meets criteria for a diagnosis of Relationship Specific Disorder of Infancy/ Early Childhood by virtue of her exhibiting a pattern of problematic behaviors exclusively in her relationship with her mother. Although she is able to interact with other adults such as child care providers in developmentally expectable and cooperative ways such that she is able to benefit from learning opportunities, when she is in the care of her mother, she engages in near-constant oppositional behavior. The client's mother contributes to this problematic dynamic by frequently interacting with the client in an intrusive manner and not being able to set limits effectively. The two have no reliable routes to mutual pleasurable interactions at this time, and they are not able to enjoy conflict-free meaningful interactions. Although some of these problematic dynamics most likely took shape during the client's infancy, they may have been exacerbated by the loss of the client's maternal aunt, who resided with the dyad and aided the client's mother with caregiving until she moved out of state when the client was 1 year old. These problematic dynamics could also have been compounded by the intimate partner violence–related trauma that the client witnessed and by the dyad's recent child welfare–related separation and reunification. The struggles that the dyad engages in cause both of them significant distress and restrict their capacity to enjoy growth-promoting activities. The client's social–emotional development is at risk, and it is possible that without intervention, the relational patterns that are currently restricted to her relationship with her mother might become generalized to the client's other relationships. Child–parent psychotherapy aimed at strengthening PCRC 10 is recommended to reduce the level of chaos in the home environment, increase the sense of shared meaning and purpose, and build the dyad's capacity to interact in ways that support the client's social–emotional development.

Goal: Strengthen PCRC 10 to improve problematic patterns of relating.

Sample collaboratively generated objectives include the following:

1. The client's mother will allow the client to take the lead in play sequences of 10 minutes' duration as observed by the IMH worker during weekly home visits by [date].

2. The client's mother will verbally describe to the IMH worker a possible emotional antecedent when the client engages in oppositional behavior one time during each home visit in the next [specify number] weeks.

3. The client will reduce incidents of oppositional acting out from several per hour to several per day as reported by the mother by [date].

4. The client will engage with the mother in a mutually pleasurable and meaningful activity at least one time per day per the mother's report by [date] (current baseline: zero).

5. Over the course of the next [specify number] weeks, the client's mother will develop and relay to the client a developmentally meaningful family narrative describing the challenges (including traumas and losses) that they have encountered.

Vignette 10.2

Andre, 23 years old, and his 1-year-old son, Demarea, are referred to an IMH clinic by Andre's 30-year-old sister Tanesha, with whom they reside, She explains that Andre and Demarea lived with the baby's mother's family at first, but they were asked to leave 3 months ago due to conflict between Demarea's parents. Tanesha states, "I'm glad to have them here, but Andre needs to learn some parenting skills. He is addicted to video games, and all he wants to do is stay in his room and play. He needs to learn to teach Demarea things. Plus the games are violent. I don't know if a baby should be seeing all that shooting." Tanesha confirms that Andre is open to having the IMH worker visit him.

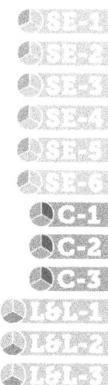

The IMH worker, who is a Latino man, meets with Andre and Demarea several times. The first time he visits, Tanesha joins them and describes to Andre her concerns about the video games, saying "I don't think they are appropriate for babies, but this is a baby expert—he can tell you." The IMH worker proposes that they take a few weeks to get to know one another and think about the video games together as part of that. In the course of their subsequent conversations, he learns that Andre values the video games for many reasons, not the least of which is his sense that they keep him and his son safe as male African Americans in a racist world. "They can't shoot me or arrest me for gaming in my room," he states. He is also proud of his skill level and knowledge about the video games he plays, and he feels connected with others who play, many of whom he is acquainted with only virtually. He discloses that he is grateful to Tanesha for housing him and Demarea but resents her "acting like she's my mother." He keeps to his room partly to keep the peace. "I know it's good for Demarea to have the roof over his head," he states, "so I'm in here for him, but I'm not used to this." Andre stays in the apartment to stay off of the streets and stays in his room to avoid stressful interactions with his sister.

Demarea is a somber infant. He does not smile or otherwise respond to overtures by the IMH worker, although he does smile when addressed and handled by his father. The IMH worker observes Demarea to be cooperative and comfortable with his father around diaper changing and feeding. However, he is not observed to initiate interactions, and he spends what strikes the IMH worker as a remarkable amount of time sitting passively in his stroller during visits.

The IMH worker tells Andre, in the course of the assessment period, that he shares Tanesha's concerns about the video games. He describes research findings regarding what helps and what hinders infants' and toddlers' learning and the developmental significance of play. He thinks that Demarea is too young to enjoy the video games and that he is ready for other kinds of play—play that involves direct interaction with his father. He proposes that they identify together the valuable skills one can develop playing video games (e.g., manual dexterity, motor planning and agility) and find activities that Demarea can engage in that will help him build these skills. He also says that he believes Andre's concerns regarding his and his son's safety as Black men are extremely important. He proposes that they work together on reducing the time Demarea is exposed to video games and replacing those hours with activities geared toward building a sense of safety and comfort for both of them and expanding Demarea's play skills.

DSM–5 diagnosis: Adjustment Disorder with Anxiety

ICD–10–CM code: F43.22

Relational Clinical Formulation

The identified client is a 23-year-old African American man who, as of 3 months ago, is a single father to a 1-year-old boy. He is experiencing stress in the transition to single parenthood and to residing with his sister, which he manages by remaining isolated with his son in their room for large amounts of time. He also relies heavily on video games for self-regulation and anxiety management. These patterns negatively affect the client's functioning in his parenting role and restrict his son's opportunities to engage in activities that promote his development. The client identifies the dangers of racist targeting of Black men and boys as an exacerbating condition leading to his isolation, and he reports experiencing anxiety as a parent in relation to this discrimination. These difficulties are best addressed in the context of the infant–parent relationship so that the client may develop growth-promoting parenting skills with the direct participation of his son. Infant–parent services aimed at strengthening PCRC 10 are recommended. Collateral engagement with community resources and other service providers may be useful in increasing the client's sense of confidence in navigating a racist world and protecting his son.

Goal: Reduce isolation by strengthening PCRC 10.

Sample collaboratively generated objectives include the following:

1. The client and his son will visit the neighborhood library together with the IMH worker by [date] to explore infant books representing Black people.

2. During each weekly visit with the IMH worker over the course of the next [specify number] weeks, the client will engage his son with a range of play activities and will verbally identify his son's emerging abilities and interests.

3. By [date], the client will identify three trustworthy support people he could call immediately in the event that he feels unsafe when in public.

4. By [date], the client will identify 10 destinations (e.g., parks, community resource centers, sports facilities) that are enjoyable for him and his son to visit.

5. The client will report taking his son on daily excursions by [date].

6. The client will report that incidents of experiencing anxiety are reduced from [specify number] times per day to [specify number] times per day by [specify date].

CHAPTER 12

PCRC 11—Water, Water Everywhere: Accessing Resources

¡Mamá...Cuéntame Por Qué Viniste!

Mommy...Tell me, why did you come here?...

¡Mama, ya se cómo viniste! ¡Viniste usando todo tu amor y todo tu valor! ¡Ahorita quiero saber por qué viniste! ¡Por favor cuéntame!

Mommy, I know how you came here! You came using all your love and all your courage! Now, I want to know why! Please tell me!

¡Ya sé! ¡Mamá, viniste porque sabés que aquí yo podría viajar donde quisiera cuando sea grande como vos!

I know! Mommy, you came because you knew that I would be able to travel anywhere I wanted when I am a grown-up like you!

—Silvia Juarez-Marazzo (2016, pp. 17–20)

PCRC 11: Parent is able to **access resources** on behalf of child and family AND child is able to make use of resources accessed by parent and is on a path toward accessing resources as developmentally expectable.

Resources are things we can draw on and make use of to further particular aims, beginning with staying alive. The question of access to resources is always political, with groups of people often divided against one another as the interests of some are safeguarded at the expense of others. Access to resources such as food, water, and medicine is a human rights issue that clearly affects infants, children, and families around the globe and is a matter of life and death.

Tenet # 2:
Champion Children's Rights Globally

Tenet # 3:
Work to Acknowledge Privilege and Combat Discrimination

Tenet # 8:
Allocate Resources to Systems Change

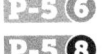

Tenet # 9:
Make Space and Open Pathways

Tenet # 6:
Understand That Language Can Hurt or Heal

Although it is important to be aware of global politics affecting resource allocation, it is also critical not to lose sight of the prevalence of access disparities, including food scarcity, within the United States, which is one of the resource-richest countries in the world.

Within the infant and early childhood field, "accessing resources" often refers to securing not only such things as food and shelter but also services, such as early intervention, early care and education, parenting support, and so forth. Infant mental health (IMH) workers are often well positioned to support parents and families in accessing needed resources of this sort. This work can be difficult to undertake. It can be time consuming to investigate options, navigate systems, and advocate on behalf of families, and it can be profoundly dispiriting when what is available is inadequate. It can be easy to believe that such efforts must be someone else's job! However, it is important for programs and systems to think critically about who is responsible for undertaking this part of the work. The more one is in a position to make resource allocation decisions within a program or a system, the more important it may be for that person to have current, on-the-ground experience with the challenges of connecting families with resources outside of the program or system, otherwise programs and systems can drift far from understanding families' lived realities.

Interlocking systems of oppression conspire to erect barriers to access. Service settings may be hostile or unwelcoming to certain families—for example, those who do not speak English, those who are not heteronormative, or those with members who have disabilities. It can be difficult from a dominant perspective to perceive the access barriers that are erected—the things that send a message to such families that they do not belong. Often, IMH workers can serve as brokers and advocates, identifying and addressing such barriers on behalf of families so that the burden does not fall to families to expose and challenge exclusionary institutional practices.

Although such external factors frequently block access to resources for vulnerable families, there can be internal impediments as well. Depression saps energy, and anxiety squanders it. Either can impede a parent's capacity to access available resources. A parent's self-judgment that they ought to be self-reliant could prevent that person from availing themselves of needed support—so could a conviction that one is undeserving or that nothing "out there" is trustworthy or holds promise. As a result, sometimes parents automatically interact with would-be helping professionals and other resource gatekeepers—such as landlords, doctors, teachers, benefits administrators, clerks, and receptionists—in ways that backfire on them, and then their children suffer as well.

When adults clearly have entrenched patterns of relating that lead to interpersonal embattlement, alienation, or hostility, such patterns often have their roots in early relational experiences that were painful. These patterns can be hard to change and can complicate and undermine parents' capacities to secure or hold on to resources on behalf of their families. When a parent has difficulty taking up or making use of available resources or successfully navigating relationships with resource gatekeepers, this can be a clear sign that an IMH worker (rather than another kind of practitioner) is the appropriate person to help the family. That is, it sometimes requires mental health expertise to understand and address the internal impediments parents struggle with to accessing and making use of resources, especially in the context of the many systems of oppression that regularly target and exclude particular groups.

Resources are not always "things" in the sense of material goods or services. It is equally important to attend to internal resources. A person may have very few material resources but be rich from the perspective of their internal resources.

They may be favored with great courage, for example, or with creativity, generosity, ingenuity, wisdom, spirituality, or humor. Internal resources include myriad capacities for peace of mind, pleasure, cognition, self-regulation, organization, sensory integration, perceptual experience, and interpersonal relating. States of arousal, mood, emotion, and powers of imagination are all realms of experience by which we can be painfully afflicted or, conversely, nourished and enriched. All these questions are of internal resource. In taking the measure of a person's well-being, it is ultimately internal resources that win the day. Moreover, early relationships powerfully influence a child's capacity to build and marshal internal resources.

P-5 3

Parent–Child Relationship Competency (PCRC) 11 can be said to be functioning well when a parent is able to access both internal and external resources on behalf of themselves, the child, and family, and when the child is able to make use of both the internal and external resources. The child is thus supported by the parent in building and benefiting from their own internal resources. There is a role for the IMH worker when difficulties arise at any of these levels. That is, the IMH worker may need to focus on external barriers and clear the path so that families can access the needed resources. Alternatively, they may need to help a parent strengthen their own internal resources or diminish barriers to accessing resources. The worker may also need to directly help the child to build internal resources or benefit from the resources the parent accesses. Efforts are often directed at helping the parent learn to support the child's internal resource-building processes.

As is true of all PCRCs, this one is fueled bidirectionally: The parent is motivated to access resources on behalf of the child, and the child is motivated to accept the resources not only because of their inherent properties but also because this action pleases the parent. Imagine the classic scene of a parent offering the baby a spoonful of oatmeal, saying "one bite for Mommy," or the toddler eagerly presenting the parent with a "treasure" they have found or created, or demonstrating a skill they have mastered. The toddler's pleasure is derived both from the treasure or skill and also from the parent's approval and appreciation. Without the parent's enthusiasm, the treasure almost always loses luster for the child. The parent–child relationship is the motivator for both parties to avail themselves of and enjoy what the world has to offer.

Vignette 11.1

Tom, a 37-year-old White man, calls the IMH clinic because he is worried about his wife, Suzette, and their 5-month-old baby, James. Suzette is a 33-year-old White woman with a physical disability resulting from cerebral palsy. She uses a wheelchair because of limited functioning of her legs. Tom reports that Suzette has managed the transition to parenthood "like a champ" but that she is increasingly worn out and distressed. He says James is "as sweet as they come...except that he cries constantly."

The IMH worker conducts a home-based assessment. She learns that Suzette and Tom are well connected to local and national disabilities communities and have appropriate material resources for parenting, including adaptive baby equipment that lets Suzette readily bathe and diaper James as well as get him in and out of his crib. Both parents are loving and completely competent in caring for James, yet the worker does see what Tom described—James cries a great deal and is difficult to console. The parents report that mornings are okay, but afternoons are often hard, and they are completely exhausted from nighttime episodes. Typically, they both get up with him and try together to soothe him because the effort is so frustrating and dispiriting. They report that James has been through "every imaginable medical assessment," and the doctors have concluded that he has "colic."

Suzette reports tearfully that everyone assumes James's crying signals her failure as a parent with a disability—that somehow he is unhappy because she is in a wheelchair. Although she knows this is preposterous, she does not have the same thick skin for able-ist discrimination that she usually does. "What if they are right?" she asks, "What if I just can't do this?" Because of her exhaustion and James's proneness to crying, Suzette has not been participating in the social and activist commitments that she engaged in prior to James's birth, and the family has become increasingly isolated.

DC:0–5 diagnosis: Excessive Crying Disorder

ICD–10–CM code: Nonspecific Symptoms Peculiar to Infancy (Excessive Crying in Infants): R68.11

Relational Clinical Formulation

The identified client is a 5-month-old White boy who meets criteria for a diagnosis of Excessive Crying Disorder, as evidenced by his pattern of crying many hours of most afternoons and evenings, with little capacity to be soothed by his parents. This pattern has persisted since birth, with several periods of abatement lasting approximately 10 days. Pediatric assessments have ruled out identifiable medical conditions. The client's crying causes distress for his parents, especially his mother, who worries that she is to blame for his discomfort and dysregulation. These difficulties are exacerbated by the able-ist discrimination that the family encounters because the mother has a physical disability and contends with stigma related to this disability. These patterns are leading to isolation and undermining parental confidence and stamina. The client will benefit from weekly home-based IMH sessions with the parents as collateral partners geared to strengthening PCRC 11.

Goal: Strengthen PCRC 11 to counter family exhaustion and isolation.

Sample collaboratively generated objectives include the following:

1. The client's parents become frustrated and despondent multiple times on a daily basis when efforts to soothe the client are unsuccessful. In the course of the next 3 months, the client's parents will practice implementing mindful self-regulation strategies when the client cries during weekly home-based IMH sessions.

2. At present, the client's parents rely solely on each other to manage their frustration with the client's crying, which puts strain on the marital relationship. The client's parents will access the hotline for infant crying three times per week as needed over the next 3 months.

3. At present, both of the client's parents are exhausted because they both stay up with him during nighttime crying episodes, resulting in neither sleeping longer than 4 hours at a stretch. Over the course of the next 3 months, the client's parents will implement a nighttime schedule and take turns caring for the client when he cries so that each parent gets adequate sleep.

4. The client's mother's distress related to his crying has led her to discontinue social contact and activist work, exacerbating family isolation. The client's mother will report reconnecting with friends and coworkers by [date].

5. The client will be able to be soothed by his parents' ministrations such that crying episodes diminish from seven per day to two per day by [date].

Vignette 11.2

Mindy, a 29-year-old White woman, is referred to the IMH clinic by her son's pediatrician. The pediatrician is clearly exasperated. He reports that the child, Danny, who is now 23 months old, was born with congenital heart disease that required surgery immediately following his birth and has necessitated consistent monitoring and intervention by several different specialists. Mindy has moved her son from one medical group to another three times in less than 2 years, each time beginning by expressing tremendous appreciation for the care her son is receiving and then suddenly leaving in great anger, stating that her son has been failed by the providers. "I was sympathetic when she brought him to us," the pediatrician explains, "because I know how hard heart disease is on parents, and it's true, doctors do mess up sometimes. She was so grateful to us at first. Now she is threatening to sue. I can assure you that her accusations are unfounded. My concern really is for the kid. He really does need consistent monitoring, and I'm worried about where she'll take him now."

The IMH worker meets with Mindy and Danny several times to understand who they are and what their struggles are. She is careful to request from the start that Mindy let her know whether something that she says or does fails to sit right with Mindy. She says, "I understand that you have been disappointed by the care you and Danny have received from others. I am sure that I will make mistakes too, and I hope that when I do you will tell me. That way, we can have a chance to work things out." The IMH worker also inquires regularly throughout these early meetings about how Mindy is experiencing her words and actions.

The IMH worker learns in these early meetings that Mindy's sensitivity to injury and betrayal has roots in her own early history. Mindy was molested by her stepfather during her childhood, and her mother first refused to believe her when she told her it was happening, and then her mother shifted to blaming her. Mindy has had a difficult time sustaining relationships with men, moving from intense and passionate beginnings to sudden, angry endings. She broke up with Danny's father early in her pregnancy with Danny, never telling him she was pregnant. When asked about her feelings for Danny, Mindy says tearfully, "He is the light of my life. He's all I live for now. If he doesn't make it, I won't either."

Danny is a charming little boy with a sunny disposition. He expresses delight in the toys in the therapy room, and he moves back and forth between exploring toys and playing on his own with absorption and bringing things to his mother's knee to show her. During these moments of connection, they engage in slightly stylized, affectionate games that are clearly repetitions. Danny also brings Mindy pretend tea when she cries, and he pats her arm.

DSM–5 diagnosis: Borderline Personality Disorder

ICD–10–CM code: F60.3

Relational Clinical Formulation

The identified client is a 29-year-old White woman with characteristically limited modes of relating, negatively affecting her functioning. The client meets criteria for a diagnosis of Borderline Personality Disorder. This disorder is evidenced by her history of relationship intensity and instability and her self-reported long-standing feeling of emptiness, which her son intermittently relieves. She is vulnerable to experiencing and acting on intense anger, precipitated by feeling that she has been betrayed or intentionally injured. She has a pattern of taking impulsive actions when feeling unsafe. The client's interpersonal difficulties likely issue in part from her history of childhood sexual abuse.

These patterns (instability, impulsivity, inability to trust, and heightened sensitivity to the perceived poor treatment by others) prevent the client from establishing consistent care on behalf of herself or her child. It is characteristic of her to lose faith, mistrust, and refuse to rely on others. If she had a physically healthy child, this condition would be difficult enough; however, with a child who is medically vulnerable, it is dangerous—he is put at medical risk by the disruptions in his care.

These patterns of relating leave the client isolated, strain the parent–child relationship, and impede the child's social–emotional development. He appears to organize himself around the client's moods in an effort to calm, please, and enliven her and to avoid triggering her anger. Treatment involving her son as a collateral partner is recommended so that the client can learn to engage in modes of relating that promote the child's well-being and build family stability and security. Individual sessions are also recommended to address her childhood sexual abuse. Collateral contact with pediatric providers will likely be important to support and coordinate family services and to address communication challenges that may arise.

Goal: Bolster internal resources and secure consistent care via strengthening PCRC 11.

Sample collaboratively generated objectives include the following:

1. At present, the client's son's medical care is suspended. Within 2 weeks, the client will be able to agree to an appointment with a pediatric provider to resume monitoring of her son's condition.

2. At present, the client alternates between interacting excitedly with her son and becoming preoccupied and directing her attention elsewhere, leaving her son at a loss emotionally. In each weekly dyadic meeting over the next 3 months, the client will practice interacting with her son in a sustained, calm state through activities such as play and reading to bolster internal regulatory resources.

3. The client reports not being aware that she is beginning to feel unsafe until it feels "like an emergency," resulting in her taking extreme actions. In each weekly meeting with the IMH worker over the course of the next 3 months, the client will identify experiences throughout the week that have increased or decreased her sense of interpersonal safety.

4. The client avoids reflecting on her own childhood because it was so painful, which puts her at risk of re-enacting aspects of it. During each regularly scheduled individual meeting with the IMH worker over the

course of the next 6 months, the client will develop an understanding of how her adverse childhood experiences affect her relationship with her son.

5. The client will report addressing any concerns with providers as they arise and working to understand and resolve these issues to support consistent medical care for her son over the course of the next year.

CHAPTER 13

PCRC 12—Peopled World/ Nested Child

For dinner we had turkey and blazing pudding, and after dinner the Uncles sat in front of the fire, loosened all buttons, put their large moist hands over their watch chains, groaned a little and slept. Mothers, aunts and sisters scuttled to and from bearing tureens. Auntie Bessie, who had already been frightened, twice, by a clock-work mouse, whimpered at the sideboard and had some elderberry wine. The dog was sick. Auntie Dosie had to have three aspirins, but Auntie Hannah, who liked port, stood in the middle of the snowbound back yard, singing like a big-bosomed thrush. I would blow up balloons to see how big they would blow up to; and, when they burst, which they all did, the Uncles jumped and rumbled. In the rich and heavy afternoon, the Uncles breathing like dolphins and the snow descending, I would sit among festoons and Chinese lanterns and nibble dates and try to make a model man-o'-war, following the Instructions for Little Engineers, and produce what might be mistaken for a sea-going tramcar.

—Dylan Thomas (1954/1978, pp. 31–33)

PCRC 12: Parent is able to maintain and enjoy a **network of family and/or friends**, that may include a co-parent, and to support child's relationships with this circle AND child is able to enjoy developing relationships with this network of people.

As the frequently quoted adage goes, "it takes a village to raise a child." Children respond positively to being nested in a community of people who know and value them, enriching their lives with a sense of belonging that extends beyond their immediate family. Very young infants track familiar faces closely, recognize the difference between new and known figures in their milieu, and make meaning from routines involving people whose lives are interconnected with their own. When raised in circumstances in which contact with people outside of the family occurs infrequently, young children nonetheless orient themselves to this sense of a peopled world that comes to them via their parents' and caregivers' sense of connectedness with others. Moreover, children can make excellent assessments of who in their environment is good for what—who can be counted on for a high-spirited bounce on the knee, whose silky tie feels good on the cheek, who tends to carry licorice in his pocket. Infants and young children also apprehend how other people affect their parents: They will often be glad to see someone in whose presence their parent tends to be relaxed, and they will be apprehensive when someone comes around whose presence is associated with stress or discord.

Parents also benefit from being "villagers." Parenting is a tremendous undertaking that affects all other relationships for good or ill. Babies can be magnets that draw people into their sphere—curious neighbors, other new parents, and long-lost relatives. Becoming a parent can feel like a sort of passport to humanity, linking new parents with a world community of parents and with parents across the generations. However, the opposite can also occur. Many people experience losing friendships that cannot adapt to the presence of the baby in the mix, being forced to leave jobs that cannot accommodate caregiving demands, and needing to set boundaries with family members who persist in interacting in problematic ways. Couple relationships commonly encounter developmental crises around new parenting, and many couples part ways in the early years of their children's lives. People often experience painful isolation from others and from the baby.

When interviewed, Toni Morrison said this regarding parenting:

I believe that suggesting that a one-parent family is crippled in some way is somebody else's notion. I do know that no one parent can raise a child completely. But it is also true that two parents can't do it either. You need everybody. You need the whole community to raise a child. And one parent can get that community. You have to work at it. You have to decide....You have to collect around you the people who can serve that function for you, and provide multiple kinds of resources for your children. I have women friends who raise their children alone and are working, whose children relate to her friends like family members. They call on one another in times of crisis and duress. They really use each other as a kind of life-support system....You need a tribe. I don't care what you call it, extended family, large family. That's what one needs. (Denard, 2008, p. 36)

Tenet # 5:
Honor Diverse Family Structures

Feeling supported by the "village" can have a powerful buoying effect for parents, even in very difficult moments with children. For example, when an infant is crying at the grocery store, a parent is likely to feel calmed and understood if the clerk expresses understanding and sympathy. The parent's sense of calm could be a critical aid in calming the baby. Unfortunately, parents often feel unsupported by the people around them. A survey conducted by ZERO TO THREE (Lerner, 2017) revealed that almost all parents feel judged almost all of the time. A staggering number of parents—nine out of 10 surveyed—reported feeling judged or criticized by others in relation to their parenting almost constantly. Therefore, it is more likely that the parent described earlier would feel judged by the clerk and the other shoppers at the grocery store, leaving him feeling helpless and ashamed. This judgment would likely exacerbate the parent's distress and make it harder for him to calm his infant via coregulation.

Many forces mitigate against parents having access to support from their communities. The interests of various groups of parents are often pitted against one another, resulting in divisions and alienation where people might otherwise experience interconnectedness. Family-leave policies in

Tenet # 10:
Advance Policy
That Supports
All Families

the United States are so meager that few parents of infants and young children who are in the workforce have sufficient time away from work to cultivate relationships with other families during the intense months and years of early parenting. Families excluded from the mainstream workforce by structural racism, xenophobia, and other forces of oppression face economic hardship often associated with frequent relocation, interrupted phone service, and other experiences that undermine community-building efforts. Regardless of how parents are located socially, they are vulnerable to isolation.

Parent–Child Relationship Competency (PCRC) 12 describes the capacity of parents to create and maintain relationships with people other than their child, despite these formidable challenges, as well as young children's capacity to benefit from being part of this circle of connectedness. Parents' tending of their relationships with friends, neighbors, extended family, and the communities of which they are a part is important for their own well-being, separate of their parenting roles. Furthermore, it is important for children, including infants and toddlers, to understand that although they may be the center of their parents' world in very real ways, there exists a wide human world that does not revolve around them, although they are a special part of it. Depending on a child's social location, they may be more at risk regarding one half of this equation than the other. That is, young children whose social location places them on the upside of privilege along multiple axes may be deprived of opportunities to experience their noncentrality, and thus,

Tenet # 3:
Work to
Acknowledge
Privilege
and Combat
Discrimination

they may have difficulty being part of groups without being central and may grow to mistake their privilege for their own self-worth. Conversely, young children whose social location places them on the downside of privilege along multiple axes may be deprived of opportunities to experience their rightful claim to the world and may be at risk of internalizing the devaluation to which they are exposed.

Regardless of social location, parents have opportunities to help children understand that the world holds promise for them and to facilitate their feeling a part of it. Children, for their part, can take pleasure and pride from having relationships with people other than their parents, but they will calibrate their experiences of others on the basis of the messages they receive from their parents about these other people. An infant who is just a few months old will register conflict between adults and be apprehensive about interacting with someone with whom his parent is antagonistic. With an emotional "green light" from his parent, by contrast, he is likely to be open to at least shy, tentative interaction regardless of the stranger's temperament, provided the stranger is able to interact in reasonably contingent ways.

These issues can be especially complex when there is conflict between parents. An 18-month-old toddler picked up the telephone and repeated in distress "Mama–Dada–Baby!" when her parents were arguing, which signaled both the crisis she experienced at the unity of the family being threatened and her sense that there was someone out there to call to the family's aid. Research has demonstrated that, contrary to parents' common belief that their infants and young children are unaffected by parental conflict, in fact babies whose parents argue frequently demonstrate greater reactivity in brain regions associated with emotion regulation when exposed to angry tones of voice—even while they are asleep (Graham, Fisher, & Pfeifer, 2013). When anger and hostility permeate a parental relationship, children are placed in terrible binds. They may sense that they are at risk of losing one parent, imagine or accurately perceive that their closeness with one parent constitutes an injury for the other, or conclude that relationships are fraught with pain and irreconcilable conflict. Given the developmentally expectable egocentrism of childhood, they are likely to harbor the belief that they are responsible for the distress in the family. This complex early egocentrism is a healthy and desirable state under ordinary developmental circumstances. When all goes well enough, reality gradually diminishes its power without stripping it away brutally—reality takes a reasonable pace. However, this egocentrism becomes a liability in conditions of undue stress, because the child is likely to hold herself responsible.

P-5 1

Difficult though it can be, forging a functional co-parenting relationship—what James P. McHale (2007) termed the *co-parenting alliance*—on behalf of infants and young children is the best way to shield them from unnecessary adverse effects of parental relationship conflict or dissolution and to secure their unencumbered access to each parent. McHale's research has suggested that all parenting figures substantially responsible for a child's rearing should be thought of as co-parents, whether they are raising the child in the context of being together as a couple or outside of a marriage or partnership, such as in the case of separation or divorce, birth parents who were never a couple but are both engaged parents, or when a grandparent and parent are raising a child together. Stepparents in many instances are also active partners in child rearing, which can open up multiple axes of co-parenting alliances. Additional co-parenting constellations exist, and it is incumbent on infant mental health (IMH) workers to cultivate eyes and ears for less conventional arrangements, otherwise critical co-parenting figures may remain unrecognized.

Tenet # 5:
Honor Diverse Family Structures

Focusing on PCRC 12 helps the IMH worker to see the child in the context of a network of potentially enriching relationships and to see the work that the parent does to provide this network. It also helps the IMH worker to identify impediments to the full functioning of the competency. A family may be very isolated in ways that negatively affect them. Sometimes, a child needs support in forging, navigating, and enjoying their relationships with co-parents or people other than their parents. Sometimes, parents need support in recognizing or accessing the people who are available to them and their child. This need may result from a parent's emotional vulnerability, interpersonal challenges or relational tendencies, or from extrinsic barriers, as in the case of forced separations related to incarceration, deportation, or child welfare intervention. In any of these instances, the IMH worker's efforts always need to be directed toward eliminating barriers to the family's connectedness and strengthening PCRC 12.

P-5 ②

Tenet # 8:
Allocate Resources to Systems Change

Vignette 12.1

A 26-month-old Afghan boy, Zemar, has been assigned a diagnosis of Early Atypical Autism Spectrum Disorder by a clinic specializing in the assessment of Autism Spectrum Disorder. His parents, Mateen and Taara, (who are both bilingual) and his pediatrician had become alarmed when he stopped using some of the words he had previously acquired in both Farsi and English. He also stopped reliably responding when addressed by his name, became more focused on objects and less responsive to people, and became increasingly inflexible around moving through daily life. Zemar's father, Mateen, works long hours outside of the home, and Zemar is cared for by his mother, Taara, who has become increasingly isolated as his condition has developed. Taara reports avoiding going out in public with her son because transitions are difficult and interactions with others cause him distress and her embarrassment. For example, she reported that at the playground, "He will walk right over a little baby in the sand, knocking her over without even noticing, and take what she was playing with and fall apart when I take it away from him. Needless to say, we are not popular!" The parents are ashamed of Zemar's condition and have not informed anyone in their extended family. The family has been referred for IMH treatment by the assessment clinic.

SE-1
SE-2
SE-3
SE-4
SE-5
SE-6
C-1
C-2
C-3
LG-1
LG-2

A bilingual/bicultural Farsi-speaking Iranian American IMH worker conducts a follow-up assessment to determine together with Mateen and Taara what services might be helpful to the family in light of this recent diagnosis. This assessment begins with some discussion of language and culture, including exchanging some information about the family and the IMH worker's immigration experiences and the prospect of their working together. It becomes clear that the family's stress is exacerbated by the xenophobia they frequently encounter in moving through life in the US. Together they decide that the IMH worker will visit twice a week to address Zemar's symptoms in the context of his relationship with his parents. They generate a plan of care together that includes both professional services and attending to their co-parenting relationship and their network of family and friends.

DC:0–5 diagnosis: Early Atypical Autism Spectrum Disorder

DSM–5 diagnosis: Other Specified Neurodevelopmental Disorder

ICD–10–CM code: Pervasive Developmental Disorder, Unspecified (F84.9)

Relational Clinical Formulation

The client, a 26-month-old Afghan boy, meets criteria for a diagnosis of Early Atypical Autism Spectrum Disorder, as evidenced by a lack of expectable capacity to interact with others, lack of responsiveness when called by name, and inflexibility regarding routines and difficulty with transitions. These symptoms significantly strain his relationship with his mother, who is his primary caregiver. The client's mother is overwhelmed by her caregiving responsibilities, grieved by her son's challenges, and increasingly isolated because of her sense of embarrassment regarding her son's behavior. These conditions result in an unfortunate cycle wherein the client's opportunities for learning prosocial, communicative, and interactive skills are increasingly restricted. The family's isolation is compounded by the parents' sense of shame and stigma surrounding their son's diagnosis and by the xenophobia they frequently encounter as immigrants from

Afghanistan. These difficulties are best addressed in the context of the parent–child relationships. The family will benefit from intensive services aimed at strengthening PCRC 12.

Goal: The client will expand capacities for reciprocal interaction with others via strengthening PCRC 12.

Sample collaboratively generated objectives include the following:

1. At present, parents have no child care and are depleted and alienated as a result of parenting stress, which makes it hard for them to engage energetically with client. The client's parents will, within 2 weeks, arrange for at least 3 hours of weekly child care so that they can spend restorative time together.

2. The client's parents will, with the support of the IMH worker, develop a way of describing their son's condition that they are comfortable with, and the parents will notify at least one extended family member within 1 month.

3. Stigma-based family isolation restricts client's opportunities for engaging in reciprocal interaction with others. The client's parents will, within 1 month, identify a family through the local Afghan community center who they are comfortable disclosing their son's status to and request weekly play visits.

4. Client's parents will access additional early intervention resources provided by IMH worker by [date].

5. The client will respond when the parent or the IMH worker calls his name two times per session (current baseline: zero times) within 2 months.

6. The client will complete 10 loops of reciprocal interaction (e.g., turn-taking, creative elaboration, question–answer, or joint decision making in play) with the parents or the IMH worker per session (current baseline: 1–2) within 2 months.

Vignette 12.2

A 41-year-old African American woman, Sydney, has been referred by her individual therapist for dyadic treatment together with her 19-month-old toddler, Chloe, and possible co-parenting counseling with her ex-husband, Cameron. Sydney is an accomplished professional who has struggled with long-standing low-grade anxiety that has been managed in individual therapy for several years. She and Cameron had challenges conceiving, which had exacerbated tensions in their relationship. They had imagined that the birth of the long wished-for child would solidify their relationship, but they found the opposite to be true; their conflict and alienation escalated during the first year of Chloe's life, resulting in their decision to separate.

As the parents have now established separate residences and the divorce becomes finalized, Sydney has moved out of a hyper-competent mode of coping, and symptoms of anxiety are coming to the fore. She has difficulty sleeping and is consumed with worry that Chloe will suffer lasting harm as a result of the divorce; moreover, despite the fact that Cameron has been a competent caregiver and has a warm relationship with Chloe, she experiences agitation verging on panic when Chloe is in his care.

The court-mediated custody arrangement involves Chloe spending alternate overnights with each parent in light of the fact that she had been cared for jointly by both parents prior to the divorce. The parents communicate primarily by text or e-mail, and exchanges are very tense. The therapist feels that these issues require direct relationship-focused intervention to ensure that Chloe's developmental needs are being addressed. The IMH worker, a White woman, meets with Chloe in the context of both of her homes during an assessment phase and then discusses with Sydney her impression that Chloe needs more help from her parents adjusting to her two households and being protected from parental conflict. Together, the IMH worker and Sydney develop objectives that will ease Sydney's anxiety and support Chloe.

DSM–5 diagnosis: Adjustment Disorder with Anxiety

ICD–10–CM code: F43.22

Relational Clinical Formulation

The client is a 41-year-old recently divorced African American woman who meets criteria for a diagnosis of Adjustment Disorder with Anxiety, as evidenced by insomnia, worry about the future, and agitation at separating from her daughter—symptoms that have emerged and intensified since her divorce. The client's parental functioning is adversely affected by this condition. The client has a court-mediated shared custody arrangement with her ex-husband. The client's daughter is 19 months old and spends alternating overnights with her two parents, who cared for her jointly prior to their separation. The client's caregiving system is sorely challenged when her child is out of her care, exacerbating her symptoms of anxiety. The child has strong relationships with both parents but becomes solemn at exchanges and has been more clingy and less playful since the separation. When she is at the home of one parent, she asks repeatedly for the other. The client's anxiety limits her ability to soothe her daughter or engage in effective co-parenting collaboration with her ex-husband, which negatively affects the child's capacity to adjust to the divorce and places the child's social–emotional development at risk. Dyadic infant–parent treatment with collateral co-parenting sessions is indicated to strengthen PCRC 12.

Goal: The client will strengthen PCRC 12, as evidenced by relief from anxiety around separations from her daughter, improvement in the co-parenting alliance, and expanded capacity to support the child's relationship with her father.

Sample collaboratively generated objectives include the following:

1. Client's exclusive focus on her daughter's vulnerability heightens her anxiety, which she cannot help but

convey to her daughter. The client will identify during each infant–parent meeting one sign of her daughter's emotional sturdiness and capacity for resilience. (current baseline: zero)

2. The client will report, within 3 months, practicing calming techniques such as deep breathing to reduce her anxiety during pick-up/drop-off exchanges of child with ex-husband 50% of the time (current baseline: zero).

3. The client will articulate during each co-parenting meeting over the course of the next 3 months one concrete request of her ex-husband that will ease her worry about the time her daughter spends with him.

4. The client's daughter's mood during exchanges will be lighter three out of four times within 1 month per the client's report, as reflected in increased playfulness and decreased clinginess (current baseline: clinginess and somber mood at all exchanges).

CHAPTER 14

PCRC 13—Fire: The Gift of Aggression

The night Max wore his wolf suit and made mischief of one kind and another his mother called him "WILD THING!" and Max said "I'LL EAT YOU UP!" so he was sent to bed without eating anything.

—Maurice Sendak (1963, pp. 1–5)

PCRC 13: Parent is able to manage frustration and channel **aggression** in appropriate directions, and to promote these capacities in child AND child is developing these capacities at age level.

The very well-known words that begin the story *Where the Wild Things Are* (Sendak, 1963) are accompanied by equally well-known pictures. The first page depicts little Max dressed in his wolf suit creating a fort by hammering a nail into a wall, presumably in the family living room. The second page renders him chasing a frightened pet dog down a set of stairs while wielding a fork with glee. The third page shows Max in the bedroom to which he has been banished, wolf-hand resting on his wolf-hip and an angry scowl on his be-whiskered face. From here, interesting things begin to happen! The story continues, "That very night in Max's room a forest grew and grew—and grew..." (Sendak, 1963, pp. 7–11), and Max is transported a few pages later to the land where the wild things are.

This story captures the generative power of aggression. The wild things Max encounters on his imaginary journey are larger than life. They "roar their terrible roars," and "gnash their terrible teeth," and "roll their terrible eyes," and "show their terrible claws" (Sendak, 1963, pp. 17–18). They may be understood as embodiments of the wild, larger-than-life aggressive impulses that, when unbridled, get Max (and all of us) into trouble in polite society. These same impulses animate us and afford us an inner sense of being mighty, audacious, unstoppable—awesome, in the old-fashioned sense of the word. Their potency is depicted in the fecundity of the foliage that overtakes Max's sparsely furnished bedroom and the raucous sea onto which he sets sail. We can find reflections of the primal force of aggression in such natural phenomena as lightning bolts, lava flows, earthquakes, and avalanches. We marshal these impulses and, sometimes, such images when aspiring to take powerful actions.

Max's mother is apparently animated by her own aggressive impulses in response to Max's provocations. She shouts at her son and shuts him in his room without any supper, exercising her power to punish, deprive, contain, and condemn. Selma Fraiberg has written about the powerful aggressive impulses that parents routinely experience in relation to children, even when childish mischief is absent. Fraiberg suggested that nursery rhymes and baby games often both reveal and bind such universal aggressive parental impulses. Consider, for example, the lyrics to the lullaby "Rock-a-Bye Baby": "Rock-a-bye Baby; In the tree tops; When the wind blows, the cradle will rock; When the bough breaks, the cradle will fall; and down will come Baby, cradle and all." Although the cadence of this song may be soothing, the words certainly are not. (See Winnicott, 1949.) Fraiberg (1974) wrote that

> games and play have another function: they regulate, through ritual and through the conventional disguises of play, the discharge of forbidden impulses. In the case of parent and baby there is a biological contract... which normally guarantees that the love bonds will protect the baby against harmful or potentially harmful parental impulses, that aggressive impulses will not be discharged in physical acts against the body of the baby and must find pathways away from

the body and the person of the baby. Normally, the game circumstance permits discharge in ways that are harmless to the baby, and the game conventions afford regulation and inhibition of hostile motives. (p. 202)

It is in this way that the essence and personhood of the baby is protected. Fraiberg (1974) contended that all parents face the challenge of finding ways of discharging the aggressive impulses they feel toward children while protecting and nurturing their children and that the capacity to do so is a sign of psychological health. From this perspective, banishing aggressive impulses is neither desirable nor possible. Rather, aggressive impulses are to be expected, respected, and recognized as they seek and find nonharmful forms of expression. At best, they may be tapped and channeled in constructive and growth-promoting directions.

Parent–Child Relationship Competency (PCRC) 13 is rooted in this respect for aggression as a primal expression of life force. From this perspective, aggressive and loving impulses are natural, universal, and inextricable; they both fuel us in fundamental ways, and these impulses are often intermixed and not dangerous. When PCRC 13 is functioning well, the parent–child relationship is animated by big, ferocious feelings that are mutual. Both parties can experience the fierce "I'll eat you up!" feelings articulated by Max in the story. Both can experience and benefit from their own aggressive energy with the confidence that it will not harm the other and can perhaps even experience enough security to be able to enjoy at times being the special object of the other's aggressive attention. Each is warmed by the other's inner fire and knows that they are the special experience that the other desires—but will not, in fact, devour. A parent–child relationship tempered in the fire of mutual controlled aggression withstands life's tumult and supports both partners in meeting life's challenges with mettle.

Frequently, however, parents and children encounter difficulties in the realm of aggression. Parents may be uncomfortable with or unaware of their own aggressive impulses and may have difficulties supporting children in recognizing, accepting, and channeling theirs. Parents may act out aggressively in ways that put the family in harm's way. They may direct aggressive impulses at the child in action in obvious or subtle ways. It is not unusual for parents to feel controlled and persecuted by the relentless needs of infants and young children and, thus, to feel when they lash out at their children that they are merely retaliating and protecting themselves. (Spanking and other forms of corporal punishment often serve this function for parents, allowing them to discharge rage under the guise of socializing the child.) Alternatively, a parent may direct aggression inward, harming themselves and depriving the child of this vital relational force.

P.5.1 Children need help learning to manage frustration and channel aggression. Achieving the capacity to express aggression in words is extremely useful. When a parent can help a child recognize their aggressive impulses and articulate them, this is tremendously relieving and empowering for the child. Fraiberg (1959) described the dilemma for children who do not yet have the verbal capacities to discharge aggression in this manner. She recounted the story of a 28-month-old boy who experiences aggression toward a new baby sister and expresses this anger at first by hitting her. A more verbally advanced child, Fraiberg wrote, would be encouraged to put his feelings of jealously and anger toward the baby into words. "Through expressing his feelings in words he diminishes the need for jealous and destructive acts towards the baby; the words are substitutes for the acts, and verbal expression will usually afford the child enough relief so that he can inhibit the hostile actions toward the baby" (Fraiberg, 1959, p. 153). However, when a toddler is not yet developmentally capable of expressing aggression verbally, parents must help them find other acceptable outlets. Symbolic or presymbolic play involving themes of aggression can offer a fruitful avenue of expression, as can vigorous physical activity. The key is to refrain from socializing children to express only "nice" or "gentle" impulses and instead to demonstrate that fierce, angry impulses are expected, respected, and even celebrated.

Forbidding expression of aggression altogether, Fraiberg cautioned, leads to more complex difficulties. Fraiberg (1959) wrote, "A little girl who was spanked repeatedly for attacks against a baby brother became a model child who showed no signs of aggression at all after a while, but she developed a serious sleep disturbance and a number of fears which caused her to cling to her mother all day" (p. 155). Another little girl "who was taught to substitute loving acts for hostile acts against her little sister developed a pattern of displaying exaggerated love for anyone toward whom she felt hostile, and acquired a symptom through which the suppressed anger could be discharged: bedwetting" (Fraiberg, 1959, p. 155). Rather than forbidding aggression, then, parents are encouraged to help children find constructive avenues for its expression.

The same is true of parents. When they believe that their aggressive impulses toward children are monstrous and unacceptable, these impulses do not evaporate, but they may be suppressed or repressed, and complex difficulties ensue. Parents may become depressed as a result of directing aggressive impulses inward. Alternatively, they may direct aggressive impulses toward children in directly harmful ways, perhaps rationalizing such harm by justifying their actions as a form of instruction or socialization. Without constructive avenues for the expression of aggressive impulses, parents might also act out aggressively in other realms of their life in ways that negatively affect the family— for example, through parental job loss or involvement with the criminal justice system.

It is critical to note in relation to legal systems involvement that perceptions of aggression are often filtered through racism such that people of color are grossly dispropor- tionately represented in the child welfare and criminal justice systems. Such disparities begin in early childhood. In groundbreaking research, Walter Gilliam (2005, 2008)

Tenet # 3: Work to Acknowledge Privilege and Combat Discrimination	revealed the alarming fact that preschool-age children face expulsion at rates more than 3 times greater than their K–12 counterparts, with African American boys being disproportionately targeted. In her 2014 report, *Black Girls Matter: Pushed Out, Overpoliced, and Underprotected*, Kimberlé W. Crenshaw demonstrated that African American girls are also "on the receiving end of punitive, zero-tolerance policies that [subject] them to arrest, suspension, and/or expulsion" (p. 7). Attributions of aggression constitute a risk factor to which children and families of color are chronically exposed.
Tenet # 10: Advance Policy That Supports All Families	

Sexism, misogyny, and heteronormativity also lead to distortions in perceptions of aggression. Dominant patterns of socialization often lead to girls and women being discouraged from avowing and constructively discharging aggressive impulses, whereas boys and men are encouraged to discharge aggression in unconstructive and injurious ways, and they are thus deprived of opportunities to find constructive and connective pathways.

Infant mental health (IMH) workers can make positive contributions in all these areas: countering systems of oppression leading to the distorted perception and expression of aggression, supporting recognition of and respect for universal aggressive impulses, and helping parents find constructive pathways for the discharge of their own and their children's aggression.

P-5 6

Vignette 13.1

SE-3
SE-5
SE-6
C-1
C-3
LSL-1

Brian and PJ seek consultation from an IMH worker because they have newly adopted 16-month-old Jimmy and are worried about his weight and patterns around eating. The pediatrician has told them that Jimmy is overweight for his age and height. They were referred to a nutritionist, but they feel conflicted about implementing her recommendations. "He has been through so much,"

Brian explains. "He gets so upset when we try to limit his food. We don't want to say no to him about anything!"

The male, Filipino American IMH worker meets initially with Brian (who is African American) and PJ (who is native Hawaiian) for several sessions and then with the three of them together. He learns that Jimmy, a biracial Black/Latino child, was removed from his birth mother at 3 months old following a finding of nonaccidental injury. His mother was struggling with substance abuse, and after a brief period in a substance abuse treatment facility, she relapsed and failed in reunification efforts. His birth father could not be identified. Jimmy spent time in three different foster homes before being placed with Brian and PJ for adoption.

Jimmy is vigilant around transitions into and out of the IMH worker's office, ceasing play, for example, when PJ leaves the room to go to the bathroom and not being able to re-engage until PJ returns. Instead, while PJ is gone, Jimmy stands near his stroller and drinks from his bottle, ignoring Brian's attempts to re-engage him in play. Throughout the session, Jimmy is preoccupied with the bottle and the snacks that Brian and PJ have brought with them, and he is also interested in the toy food and play kitchen equipment in the office. At several moments when protest might have been expectable—for example, when Brian initiated a diaper change somewhat abruptly—Jimmy whimpered for his bottle. Brian and PJ report that whimpering for the bottle or food is Jimmy's way of responding to almost all unwelcome experiences. They also describe that Jimmy is preoccupied with food, opening the cupboards and attempting repeatedly to open the refrigerator at home. He likes to hold food in his hands and will keep food in his mouth for long periods.

Brian and PJ had planned to have Jimmy enter child care right away so they could both resume work, but they are worried that the snack and meal routines at child care might be too hard for Jimmy. They are wondering whether they should keep him at home longer in hopes that the feeding issues will resolve. They are also avoiding taking him to social gatherings, because they report being "sick of hearing everyone's negative judgments and cheap advice."

DC:0–5 diagnosis: Overeating Disorder

DSM–5 diagnosis: Unspecified Eating Disorder

ICD–10–CM code: F50.4: Overeating Associated with Other Psychological Disturbance

Relational Clinical Formulation

The identified client is a 16-month-old boy who has spent the majority of his life in multiple foster homes and who was recently adopted. The client meets criteria for a diagnosis of Overeating Disorder, as evidenced by his overconsumption of and preoccupation with food: locating food initially when entering any new space, insisting on having food or a bottle in response to a broad range of anxious experiences, and using food and the bottle as his exclusive route to comfort and self-regulation. These patterns are leading to social isolation for the family and prevent the client from engaging in growth-promoting experiences. The client appears convinced that his overall needs will not be met by people and that they constitute relational liabilities. Because it appears that the client uses food and the bottle to stifle aggressive impulses as well as for many other anxious purposes, the client and his family will benefit from services aimed at strengthening PCRC 13. It will be critical that the adoptive parents be engaged as collateral partners in the treatment so that they can implement strategies on a daily basis to open growth-promoting pathways to expression of aggressive and other impulses, reducing the client's reliance on food to stifle impulses and to cope with stress. (Note that in children younger than 2 years old, Overeating Disorder is less common than Overfeeding Disorder, but the client appears to have suffered deficits in caregiving that have led him to seek out food in a precociously self-reliant manner.)

Goal: Relieve reliance on food for self-soothing by strengthening PCRC 13.

Sample collaboratively generated objectives include the following:

1. At present, the client never actively protests unwelcome experiences, instead whimpering for a bottle. Per the parents' report, the client will actively protest unwelcome experiences at least three times per day within 3 months.

2. The client will direct aggressive impulses outward via shouting, aggressive symbolic or presymbolic play, or physical actions such as stomping or banging a pillow three times per day per the parents' report (current baseline: zero).

3. As observed by the IMH worker, the client's parents will state out loud to the client the healthy aggressive impulses they perceive may underlie food-seeking behaviors at least one time per session (current baseline: zero).

4. The parents will report engaging with the client in highly physical activity several times each day (current baseline: 1–2 times per week).

5. The client's weight will be trending toward expectable range by the next pediatric visit scheduled for [date].

Vignette 13.2

Rachel contacts the IMH worker because she is worried about the impact of her husband, John's, "anger issues" on their family. She initially meets with the IMH worker individually and reports tearfully that she feels ashamed for putting up with John's behavior for as long as she has, but she feels stuck in the marriage. They are at a crisis point now because John was recently fired "again" as a result of being belligerent with his boss. Rachel is seeking help at this time because she has come to realize that she is not able to protect her 3-year-old daughter, Sara, from the effects of John's temper.

The IMH worker conducts an assessment that involves meeting with each parent individually, with the two parents together, with Sara with each parent alone, and with the whole family together. Among other things, she learns that John has a history of having received harsh discipline bordering on physical abuse as a child. He is vehement about not using corporal punishment with Sara; however, it is clear to the IMH worker that Sara fears her father's frequent angry verbal outbursts and that the family is organized around his anger, with Sara and Rachel both "walking on eggshells" in a futile attempt to avoid provoking him. After this lengthy assessment process, she meets with the two parents together again to share her impressions and proposes a treatment structure alternating between co-parenting and family sessions, with John as the identified client. Both parents agree to this, and together they identify treatment objectives.

DSM–5 diagnosis: Intermittent Explosive Disorder

ICD–10–CM code: F63.81

Relational Clinical Formulation

The identified client is a 35-year-old White man who meets criteria for a diagnosis of Intermittent Explosive Disorder, as evidenced by having frequent angry outbursts at home and at work; engaging in "road rage" behaviors when feeling offended by other drivers; going on loud, angry verbal tirades with his spouse and occasionally with his 3-year-old daughter; and pounding furniture and slamming doors when angry. Although the client and spouse report a period of reprieve during their engagement, this pattern was present beginning in the client's adolescence and resumed when client's wife became pregnant. The client's explosive behavior has led to job loss on several occasions, has caused significant marital discord, and has negatively affected the client's daughter's social–emotional development, placing her at risk of developing an internalizing disorder.

Family intervention is recommended to change the client's behavioral patterns so that the child may be redirected to a healthy developmental trajectory and family well-being may be achieved. Treatment focused on strengthening PCRC 13 is recommended to interrupt problematic patterns of relating and to help all family members establish healthy patterns in relation to aggressive impulses.

Goal: Strengthen PCRC 13 as a means of curbing the client's damaging aggressive acting out and opening pathways for the client's daughter's growth-promoting experience and expression of aggression.

Sample collaboratively generated objectives include the following:

1. Per the client's and the spouse's reports, incidents of physical aggression (e.g., hitting furniture and slamming doors) in the daughter's presence will cease (current baseline: 1–10 times per month).

2. As observed by the IMH worker during weekly co-parenting sessions, the client will use deep breathing and other self-regulating strategies to stay engaged and refrain from retaliating one time per session when his spouse expresses hurt or criticism (current baseline: zero).

3. At present, the client's daughter always curbs aggressive impulses. The client's daughter will experiment with expressing aggression through play one time per weekly family session, as observed by the clinician.

4. The client will report increasing incidents of taking a walk around the block when feeling provoked rather than yelling at family members from zero to seven times per week.

CHAPTER 15

PCRC 14—No Means No

*Among the trees I achieved absolute vacancy of mind.
I had no thought of being hurt or of hurting anyone
else, not even as I notched my arrow and pulled it back
intent on some movement in the shadows ahead. I
was doing just that one afternoon, drawing my bow,
ready to fire as soon as my target showed himself...
when I heard a rustling behind me. I spun around.
Sister James had been about to say something. Her
mouth was open. She looked at the arrow I was
aiming at her, then looked at me. In her presence, my
thoughtlessness forsook me. I knew exactly what I
had been doing. We stood like that for a time. Finally
I pointed the arrow at the ground.... "Practice is over,"
she said. Then she turned and left me there.*

Tobias Wolff (1989, p. 11)

PCRC 14: Parent is able to set limits with child in
ways that promote development AND child is able
to make good use of **limit-setting** interactions
in working toward internalizing the ability to
avoid danger, consider others, follow rules, defer
gratification, etc.

Parent—Child Relationship Competency (PCRC) 14, which
has to do with limit setting, follows PCRC 13 because
although aggression is to be expected, respected, and
celebrated, it must be bridled. The same is true of sexuality
and the many other impulses that animate human beings.
Although cultures, communities, and families vary widely
with respect to specific ideas about how children are to
be socialized, all cultures, communities, and families have
a stake in this process, and limit-setting must be grappled

with. Often, parents reproduce without much reflection patterns that were passed on to them in childhood or that they observe around them. Sometimes, these inherited or absorbed patterns are productive and growth promoting. Often, however, they are not, although they may be quite widespread.

As they develop, infants gradually become capable of beginning to comply with and internalize the limits set by adults. It is convenient (and perhaps not a coincidence from an evolutionary perspective) that an infant who is developmentally capable of crawling is usually also developmentally capable of registering that her mother does not want her to put her little finger in the electrical outlet at the baseboard. This understanding does not mean, however, that she is capable of stopping herself from doing so. Learning to inhibit the impulse to explore in this way—to accept and internalize the limit set by the adult—is a complex process that unfolds in the context of relationships and generally with many iterations and approximations before it is firmly established.

The 2010 documentary film *Babies* (Chabat & Balmés) illustrates the wide sociocultural variance with respect to limit-setting conventions. Four infants in four different countries—Japan, Mongolia, Namibia, and the United States—are tracked from their first moments of life to their first birthday. There are many fascinating differences between the worlds that the four babies are born into. Prime among these differences is the variance from one family and sociocultural context to the next regarding the degree to which the child is allowed room to navigate the physical environment on their own versus being managed and handled by an adult or allowed access only to a "childproofed" physical environment. One does not need to search so far to find variability along these lines; such differences exist within countries, from one household to the next, and sometimes within a single household when different caregivers have different approaches.

When PCRC 14 is functioning well, the parent is comfortable with limit setting as part of what the Circle of Security model describes as the parent being "bigger, stronger, wiser, and kind" (Powell et al., 2014), and heeding these limits is on the whole developmentally possible for the child. In one household, this expectation may mean that a child does not leave the family home except in the company of an adult until they are old enough to have a child themselves, whereas in the next family, a 3-year-old is welcome to run around the corner to so-and-so's house—but it is understood that they are not to cross the street. There is also a healthy range with respect to the degree of limit testing a child may engage in, with differences often evident among siblings despite parental efforts at consistency. Challenge around limit setting, limit testing, and limit heeding is to be expected and is not an indication that this PCRC is in need of strengthening. On the contrary, when a parent–child dyad can resolve and benefit from limit-related tussles, this occurrence may be a sign that this PCRC is a source of strength.

However, it is not uncommon for families to struggle in this area. It is critical that infant mental health (IMH) workers learn from parents about what kind of limit setting is in keeping with family, community, and sociocultural expectations and about any areas of confusion or conflict. Parents may be attempting to set limits that are developmentally unrealistic or, conversely, may have difficulty setting limits that would be developmentally supportive. It is crucial that within the parent–IMH worker relationship the parent has opportunities to reflect deeply on their own historical and contemporary experiences around limits, as complex and contradictory feelings often lodge in this arena and find expression in action if they do not find their way into words. The IMH worker can be helpful to a parent in this way only if they have had their own opportunities to become aware of any biases or unresolved conflicts they themselves have around limits.

Tenet # 1:
Self-Awareness Leads to Better Services for Families

Any emotional or psychological difficulty with which a parent struggles can make limit setting hard for them. A history of trauma can make it difficult for a parent to distinguish between safety and danger, leading them either to impose unnecessary or inappropriate limits because the historical danger they were exposed to is still present for them, or to fail to register the need for limit setting because their alert system has been disabled. When parents suffered harsh or abusive treatment from caregivers, they may find themselves interacting in this way with their children, perhaps inflicting suffering under the socially sanctioned auspices of limit setting (Fraiberg, 1980). Depression may erode a parent's energy and sense of efficacy, leading them to feel that they cannot muster the wherewithal to set a limit or that they do not know how to set boundaries effectively.

For many parents, children offer a reflection of their inner experience of the world. They may experience their child as being out of control, unreasonable, or unrelentingly demanding not because such traits are inherent in the child but because this view is consistent with their experience of life. For better and for worse, children are sensitive to their parents' perceptions of them, and sometimes patterns become established such that children take on the characteristics and behaviors that their parents are ready to find in them (Silverman & Lieberman, 1999).

When PCRC 14 is strained, impaired, or absent, it is important not to jump to child-focused problem solving without developing an understanding with the parent of what they bring to the table. What was the parent's early experience of limit-setting interactions? What does the idea of "limits" evoke for them? What degree of child trial-and-error versus adult orchestration do they deem optimal? It can also be very useful to wonder with the parent about how they imagine the child feels or what the child may be experiencing or exploring with the unwelcome behavior.

Several principles can be helpful when supporting parents in finding and implementing limit-setting interactions to promote child and family well-being:

No limits—no safety. Unlike other species in which neonates are ready to fend for themselves, human infants and young children require a tremendous amount of adult ministration and protection to survive. Raising a human infant means setting limits to ensure physical safety. When adults set limits confidently with children, it also helps children develop a sense of emotional safety, because it conveys to them that they are not alone and exposed to danger but are adequately protected.

Pick your battles. Most infants, toddlers, and young children will present parents with infinite decision points around limit setting. Conflict can be minimized when parents are clear about the zones and issues in which limits do not need to be imposed, those that are negotiable, and those that are nonnegotiable. How these principles are established can always usefully be examined and discussed.

Safeguard the potency of "no." Sometimes, parents find themselves saying "no" so much that their child has become inured to the word. From the child's perspective, if it is impossible to avoid eliciting "no" on a regular basis, and if "no" frequently gives way to "oh, well, alright," then "no" ceases to be an impressive or coherent word. By the same token, the parent is finding the word useless, leading to frustration and discord.

Limits are not punishment. Often, parents are confused about this principle, feeling that to set a limit is to punish or deprive a child. Parents frequently set limits intentionally as a form of punishment (e.g., limiting screen time as a method of discipline for another infraction), which complicates matters tremendously. Also, parents often engage in limit-setting behaviors in moments of anger, which is very understandable, but it makes things much more difficult. Parents will usually find that calming themselves before entering into limit-setting interactions will produce better results.

Bankrupt the problem zone. Often, when parents and children struggle around particular issues, these issues become saturated with conflict-ridden memories and meaning for both people. For both parent and child, every time the conflict plays out in that arena, more lifeblood is invested there, more parts of themselves are associated with the drama, the stakes get higher, and the potency mounts. Sometimes, the zone of conflict increases, seeming never to end. It can be helpful to explore when the limit is actually necessary and when it is irrelevant. That is, if the parent can treat the issue as low stakes and uninteresting while holding firm around any truly necessary limit, the intensity and scope will often dissipate.

Cooperation versus compliance. Families vary with respect to the amount of deference a child is expected to show an adult. Still, even in the most proudly hierarchical households, parent–child relationships do best when the heeding of limits is based in a spirit of mutually respectful cooperation rather than submissive compliance. Because cooperation is an active and flexible mode of relating, it builds a foundation for successfully negotiating limits at later developmental stages. Bowlby (1969/1982) coined the phrase "goal-corrected partnership" to describe this growth-promoting quality in a parent–child relationship. It is important to anticipate the child's development. An IMH worker can ask a parent to imagine what is likely to work to achieve the desired results when the child is much bigger—when they can no longer be picked up bodily, for instance—and to begin to establish this kind of collaborative partnership while the child still could be physically overridden.

Children are inclined to want to please their parents. This fact is easily lost sight of when parent–child relationships are characterized by frequent struggle and conflict. However, the child's dearly held wish to please a parent is nearly inextinguishable. Often, behaviors that seem designed to elicit parental displeasure and disapproval can be traced to the opposite motivation by following a surprisingly short path. It can be exceedingly helpful if limit-setting interactions are deliberately balanced with clear opportunities for the child to feel their parent's approval and their shared pleasure.

Internalizing limits is a process. It is important to apply a developmental lens when assessing the degree to which a child is capable of heeding limits on their own. Parents must initially take responsibility for imposing limits as needed and as socioculturally appropriate. They can gradually transfer responsibility to the child for recognizing and accepting them on their own. Part of bringing a developmental lens to bear is remembering that development unfolds in fits and starts, with inclines, plateaus, and regular dips.

A for effort. Often, a child will show glimmers or clear evidence of attempting to heed a limit before failing to do so. When a parent is able to focus on recognizing, affirming, and celebrating these efforts rather than focusing exclusively on the failure, this behavior builds the child's confidence in their capacity to succeed. Parents often need help and support in shifting their focus in this way.

Outlast doubt. When conflictual patterns are well established in a parent–child relationship and limits have constituted an area of difficulty, children sometimes need to accumulate substantial evidence that things are actually different now. It can be helpful if parents are supported in remembering that this is playing out over time and adopting the positive attitude that the child is presenting them with lots of opportunities to demonstrate their new limit-setting skills as parents. Perhaps the parent can imagine that the child's limit-testing behavior is a way of asking, "Are you *sure*?" giving the parent a chance to calmly respond, "Very sure." Talking with the child directly about the good reasons why they might wonder can also be helpful. The parent might say, "I know that in the past I wasn't good at helping you to know when enough TV is enough, so it is hard for you to believe me now. But I am getting better at that now, and I am going to help you find something else enjoyable to do."

Vignette 14.1

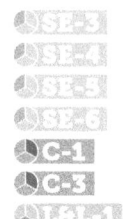

The mental health consultant at an Early Head Start site refers 30-month-old Kevin and his mother, Analyn, to the IMH clinic. "The teachers are working really hard with him in the classroom, but they are pretty maxed out. He is very hard to manage, and we have had a hard time engaging the mom," the mental health consultant explains. She describes that Kevin is very quick to become enraged and regularly hits, kicks, throws objects, and spits at other children and sometimes teachers. Expectedly, he also hurts himself frequently, such as by crashing his tricycle into the fence on purpose. "The teachers get so confused," the consultant goes on, "because he can be really affectionate with them, and he is clearly very distressed about his own behavior, but one minute he will be sobbing in their arms and the next minute purposefully doing the opposite of what they ask him to do."

The White Jewish IMH worker meets with Analyn and Kevin several times at their home to conduct an assessment. She learns that the family is Filipino. Kevin's father, Marlon, works in the construction industry. Analyn is at home with the children: Kevin, his baby brother, Kholo, and two other young children, Kevin's cousins. Analyn expresses anger and resentment at Kevin's school. She feels criticized and blamed by them for Kevin's behavior. At the same time, she is also frustrated with Kevin and overwhelmed by the caregiving demands she contends with. "They ask me how to control him. I don't know! They're the professionals!"

During the initial home visits, the IMH worker observes Kevin engaging in many of the same behaviors described by the mental health consultant, including defiance in the face of his mother's admonitions. For example, he climbs on the sofa, and when she orders him to get down under threat of time out, he climbs higher, balances precariously on the back for a moment, and then jumps to the floor, landing inches from Kholo, who is in an infant seat. When Analyn yells at him to go to his room, he kicks the infant seat, runs to the bedroom, slams the door, and refuses to return to the living room when invited back. "You see?" Analyn demands of the IMH worker, "It is like he is trying to get me mad."

During a parent meeting with Analyn and Marlon at the end of the assessment period, the IMH worker inquires about their family histories. The conversation includes their sharing information about each of their immigration experiences, some reflection about the impact of colonialism in the Philippines, and their perceptions regarding differences between child-rearing practices in the Philippines and the United States. The IMH worker proposes meeting with Kevin and Analyn at home on a regular weekly basis to work together on decreasing the conflict and helping Kevin learn self-control. She suggests that Marlon join in these meetings whenever possible and that they can decide together when it might also be helpful for her to meet with Kevin's teachers and the mental health consultant. Analyn and Marlon agree to this plan.

DC:0–5 diagnosis: Disorder of Dysregulated Anger and Aggression of Early Childhood

DSM–5 diagnosis: Disruptive Mood Dysregulation Disorder

ICD–10–CM code: F34.8: Other Persistent Mood Disorders

Relational Clinical Formulation

The identified client, a 30-month-old Filipino boy, meets criteria for a diagnosis of Disorder of Dysregulated Anger and Aggression of Early Childhood, as evidenced by his daily angry outbursts and states of being extremely upset; defiant acting out in response to limit-setting attempts on the part of caregivers; and kicking, hitting, pushing, and spitting in response to frustration or perceived affronts from peers.

These behaviors seriously strain his relationships with family, peers, and teachers, limiting the client's capacity to benefit maximally from relationships and learning opportunities at home or at school. The client's mother reports feeling ineffectual in her parenting role and worries that younger children in the household may be harmed by the client, and she responds positively to the idea of receiving help in developing new ways of interacting with the client. Home-based IMH treatment with the client's mother as a collateral partner is recommended to strengthen PCRC 14. Also involving the client's father as a collateral partner whenever his work schedule permits will likely benefit the client. Collateral contact with the mental health consultant at the client's Early Head Start program is also indicated to coordinate services and support the client across caregiving environments.

Goal: Strengthen PCRC 14 in order to promote cooperation, decrease conflict, and increase relationship satisfaction.

Sample collaboratively generated objectives include the following:

1. The client's mother reports never having had an opportunity to reflect on the impact of historical or interpersonal trauma in her family. The client's mother will identify during each weekly IMH meeting in the course of the next 3 months at least one connection between historical experiences and present parent–child challenges.

2. The client's mother reports never offering the client a positive alternative to undesirable acting-out behavior. The client's mother will report offering the client a positive alternative to negative acting-out behavior rather than threatening punishment three times per day over the course of the next 2 months.

3. The client's incidents of physical aggression toward other children will decrease from three times per day to three

times per week per the mental health consultant's report by [date].

4. The client's capacity for engaging in interludes of mutually enjoyable play with peers without disintegrating into emotional dysregulation will increase from 10 minutes to 30 minutes per the mental health consultant's report by [date].

5. The client will cooperate with the mother's calm limit-setting intervention four out of five times per session, as observed by the IMH worker during weekly home visits within the next 6 months.

Vignette 14.2

Gina, a 28-year-old White woman, calls the IMH clinic at the urging of her 12-Step sponsor, Sheila, stating "My son is working my last nerve, and Sheila said I better get some help."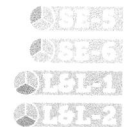

During a home-based assessment process, the IMH worker learns that Gina is in early recovery from methamphetamine addiction. She lives alone with her 22-month-old son, Max. Throughout Max's first 18 months of life, they had resided in another state together with Max's father, who also suffers from addiction. Gina's mother supported Gina to move and enter an 8-week, hospital-based detox program, during which time Max resided with his grandmother. For the past 2 months, Gina has been participating in an outpatient program and attending 12-Step meetings.

In the home visits, the IMH worker sees that Gina and Max engage in near-constant struggles. Max is reckless, impulsive, defiant, and provocative with his mother—for example, excitedly throwing objects out of the window into the courtyard below while Gina screams at him to stop. Gina alternates between ignoring Max's problematic behaviors; pleading with him to stop; yelling at him with global, condemning statements such as "you are impossible"; and threatening punishment.

Gina recounts to the IMH worker painful aspects of her history, including describing the course of her addiction, the decline of her relationship with Max's father, and various dangerous and injurious situations the family experienced as a result of their addiction. Max would become increasingly dysregulated when Gina relayed such things, but Gina appeared not to notice the effect of her words on him. At the end of the assessment period, the IMH worker suggests that she continue to visit Gina and Max once a week to support Gina in learning to "parent clean," as Gina puts it, with an immediate focus on learning to cooperate around limit-setting interactions. Gina agrees, and together they identify objectives that Gina imagines may be possible to achieve that would be a relief to her.

DSM—5 diagnosis: Stimulant Use Disorder, severe, in early remission

ICD—10—CM code: F15.20

Relational Clinical Formulation

The identified client, a 28-year-old White woman, has been assigned a diagnosis of Stimulant Use Disorder by the hospital-based detox center where she was recently treated following a period of substance abuse—related turmoil. She is in early recovery and is struggling to remain abstinent. Her early recovery—related challenges include irritability, distractibility, low frustration tolerance, mood lability, and difficulty with self-regulation. These symptoms negatively affect her functioning as a parent, contributing to a dynamic of constant conflict and struggle with her 22-month-old son, which, in turn, negatively affects his social—emotional development. Without intervention aimed at improving their patterns of interaction, the client is at risk of relapsing, and the client's son is at risk of developing diagnosable behavioral and emotional difficulties. Weekly dyadic home-based intervention is recommended to address mental health and relational challenges to the client's continued recovery, expand her repertoire of parenting skills, and support parent–child interactions that restore the client's son to a path of healthy social–emotional development.

Goal: Support recovery by strengthening PCRC 14.

Sample collaboratively generated objectives include the following:

1. At present, the client engages in power struggles with her son approximately three times per hour when he is awake. Incidents of engaging in power struggles will reduce to three per day per the client's report by [date].

2. The client frequently misses early signals that her son requires assistance or containment, responding only after there has been a mishap. During each weekly home-based IMH session over the next 3 months, the client will proactively identify and respond effectively to a signal that her son needs help or containment at least one time as observed by the IMH worker.

3. At present, the client states that struggles with her son contribute to her having an impulse to use methamphetamines approximately 20 times per day. Within 6 months, the client will report a reduction to once a week of instances of feeling triggered to use by interactions with her son.

CHAPTER 16

PCRC 15—Apart and Together Again: The Promise of Separation

After he turns four, she drops him off and fetches him from the university-run nursery school three mornings a week. For the hours that [he] is at nursery school, finger painting and learning the English alphabet, Ashima is despondent, unaccustomed, all over again, to being on her own. She misses her son's habit of always holding on to the free end of her sari as they walk together....To avoid being alone at home she sits in the reading room of the public library, in a cracked leather armchair, writing letters to her mother, or reading magazines or one of her Bengali books from home.

—Jhumpa Lahiri (2003, p. 50)

PCRC 15: Parent has the capacity to plan for and support the child around **separations** in ways that promote development and well-being AND child displays an age-expectable capacity to manage and benefit from developmentally reasonable separations from parent.

Separation is negatively inflected in the minds of many of us. The word often conjures images of isolation, fear, and sorrow; indeed, for many people, experiences of separation are in fact linked with interpersonal rupture and pain. However, this experience does not need to be the case, and it certainly is not always the case.

Parent–Child Relationship Competency (PCRC) 15 posits that separation is not only unavoidable in the flux and flow of life but potentially growth promoting and an important ingredient of family well-being. Newborn infants require near-constant care and tending, but a healthy toddler will eschew too much close togetherness, thriving instead on many growth-promoting loops of exploration and return-to-base as captured by the *circle of security* framework (Powell et al., 2014). For almost all families, separation is a natural part of participation in society via school, work, or other activities. Even sleep involves separation, as is discussed later. The question is not whether separation is good or bad but rather how it is experienced and navigated in each parent–child relationship.

One of the core challenges of parenting, which persists in ever-evolving spirals well beyond the early years, is finding the right balance between holding on and letting go. In the spirit of D. W. Winnicott's (1956, 1966) useful phrase "good enough," the goal is not to achieve a formula for perfection but rather to strive for a balance between experiences of being together and those of being apart that supports development, honors relationships, and serves the particular family in the context of their community, culture, and society.

The valance that the prospect of separation holds for parents will inform how they read their children's behaviors around separations and how they interact with them both in anticipation of parting and on reunion. As attachment research has demonstrated, for many parent–child dyads, separation is an arena of relating that is prone to powerful intergenerational influence. For example, when parents have had formative painful experiences around separation—for example, having felt abandoned and alone routinely at early ages—they are vulnerable to bringing these experiences into the contemporary relationships with their children and very often in ways they are not aware of (Fraiberg, 1980). This occurrence can shape separation experiences that might otherwise have been nonproblematic for their children, resulting in this pattern being passed from one generation to the next.

This possibility is present when infants and young children spend time in child care. As Jeree Pawl (1990) pointed out,

> understanding the experience of infants in day care does not...primarily involve an understanding of issues of separation. In fact, that focus as a major issue of concern may be far more central to the experience of the parent than it is to the experience of the child. (p. 1)

For infants, many other things come into play in the course of a morning or a day in child care, but certainly the meaning they make of being there will be affected by their parents' attitudes. Often, there is a role for the infant mental health (IMH) worker in helping parents reflect on their own experiences around and attitudes toward separation so that choices around child care may be decided with maximal clarity and freedom, and children can be supported in approaching child care as a place that holds promise.

A baby's days, however, are made up of separations and reunions far less dramatic than being signed in for 8 hours at a center. She may experience separation when she is settled into a rear-facing car seat in the back seat while her father climbs into the driver's seat; when she has been enjoying a back-and-forth babbling "conversation" with her mother, who suddenly takes a call on her cell phone; or when it is time to go to sleep. These ordinary daily separation experiences provide infants and young children with opportunities to develop important coping capacities, including what Winnicott described as a sense of *going-on-being*. This term refers to a basic existential sense of self-security that is not innate, although the potential—perhaps likelihood—for its establishment is. It is a sense that is built up over time as a result of not being too sorely tested. It takes work to build it up—caregiving work on the part of the parent, who engages in striving for the "good enough" balance of holding on and letting go that feels comfortable, and social—emotional work on the part of the child, who brings her developing internal resources to the challenge and opportunities that separations present.

One 2½-year-old boy called to his mother from the bathroom where he was sitting on the potty, "Mama, keep me company! I need some privacy!" His paradoxical request captures the complexity of gradually learning through connectedness to benefit from separateness. IMH workers can support parents in appreciating such paradoxes rather than feeling dismayed, confused, and conflicted that the impossible is being asked of them. They can help parents to develop strategies for making separation predictable and profitable for children as well as themselves, whether this means establishing bedtime routines or learning to sleep through the night, planning for transitions between households when parents live separately, or executing the countless tasks leading to morning drop-off without undue frenzy or conflict on anyone's part.

In addition to conceptualizing growth-promoting experiences of separation, Winnicott also offered a framework for thinking about when separation is injurious to children. Winnicott described an infant's capacity to hold on to an internal mental representation, or "imago," of a parent that is associated with a reassuring felt memory. This imago sustains the infant through ordinary separations. Winnicott postulated what happens when this capacity is overtaxed. He wrote,

> The feeling of the mother's existence lasts for x minutes. If the mother is away more than that x minutes, then the imago fades, and along with this the baby's capacity to use the symbol...ceases. The baby is distressed but this distress is soon mended because the mother returns in x + y minutes. In x + y minutes the baby has not become altered. But in x + y + z minutes the mother's return does not mend the baby's altered state. Trauma implies that the baby has experienced a break in life's continuity....We must assume that the vast majority of babies never experience the x + y + z quantity of deprivation. (Winnicott, 1971, pp. 96–97)

It is important to recognize that z is different for different babies, meaning that how much separation constitutes "too much" separation is not absolute but varies from child to child. Still, $x + y + z$ separation—traumatic separation—harms children. Sometimes—for example, when a parent dies in an accident—traumatic separation may be unavoidable, although it is still harmful. Healing will be required, and even under the best of circumstances, the wound will be carried forward throughout the child's life. What is carried forward is the disruption of a basic sense of trust. Certainly, there is a role for the IMH worker in such instances, mitigating the damaging effects of trauma and loss.

Harder yet to countenance are the $x + y + z$ deprivations that are avoidable and that are matters of social injustice, such as the grossly disproportionate numbers of (a) children of color in the child welfare system (Roberts, 2002), (b) children of color who lose fathers and other family members to the prison industrial complex, (c) African American babies who lose their mothers during childbirth and postpartum (Solomon, 2018), and (d) immigrant children who are forcibly separated from their parents at the U.S. border. Traumatic separations such as these incidents are injurious and unacceptable. There is absolutely a role for the IMH worker not only in mitigating the damage to social–emotional development for afflicted children and families but also in educating society to the moral affront that such systematic practices constitute.

Tenet # 3:
Work to Acknowledge Privilege and Combat Discrimination

Tenet # 10:
Advance Policy That Supports All Families

Vignette 15.1

Keandra, a 46-month-old African American girl, is referred to an early childhood mental health clinic by her pediatrician when her adoptive mother, Tiffany (her maternal aunt), discloses how overwhelmed she feels by Keandra's emotional and behavioral challenges. After Keandra had been with her for 3 years, Tiffany had a birth

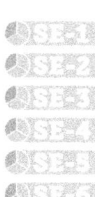

child, Shanice, who is now 1 year old. She is raising the two girls on her own. Keandra was removed from her biological mother's care at birth on the basis of a positive screening for substance exposure combined with interactions her mother had with hospital staff that they found alarming. Keandra's mother struggled with addiction and did not pursue reunification, instead relinquishing Keandra to her sister's care. Keandra's father, Eli, supported this placement. Whereas Keandra's mother now resides in a different state and has little contact with Keandra, Eli lives nearby and visits on occasion. These visits have been sporadic, in part because he has had several periods of incarceration since Keandra was born. Tiffany discourages Eli from coming around because Keandra gets very excited when he appears, but she is extremely distraught when he leaves. Tiffany also fears he may be a "bad influence" because he has had struggles with the criminal justice system.

Tiffany reports that Keandra has always been easily upset but that this behavior became worse when Shanice was born. Tiffany has a hard time managing the two children because Keandra will be rough with the baby, taking toys from her hand and shoving her at times. She also becomes extremely upset at being dropped off at preschool—protesting, clinging, and crying. On a semiregular basis, her teachers call Tiffany to return to school and pick her up because she cannot settle in. Mornings are difficult in part because Keandra resists sleep at night. Tiffany often resorts to letting Keandra fall asleep watching television with her, but this method sometimes backfires if Keandra wakes up when Tiffany tries to transfer her to her own bed.

DC:0–5 diagnosis: Separation Anxiety Disorder

DSM–5 diagnosis: Separation Anxiety Disorder

ICD–10–CM code: F93.0: Separation Anxiety Disorder of Childhood

Relational Clinical Formulation

The identified client is a 46-month-old African American girl who was adopted at birth by her maternal aunt. The client meets criteria for a diagnosis of Separation Anxiety Disorder. Symptoms include her being extremely upset when being dropped off at preschool, which persists on a regular basis such that her mother needs to retrieve her early; her fighting sleep; and her vulnerability to states of being extremely upset around separations from her birth father, who visits her on occasion. The client's symptoms are very hard for her adoptive mother, who is also caring for a 1-year-old infant. The client's symptoms prevent her from benefiting maximally from the preschool environment and strain her relationships with her adoptive mother and her sister. Her relationship with her birth father is also at risk, because the client's vulnerability to being extremely upset leads her mother to question whether contact with her father is in her best interests. These difficulties are best addressed in dyadic work with the client together with her adoptive mother as a collateral partner so that the adoptive mother can implement useful strategies for helping the client on a daily basis. Regular one-on-one collateral meetings with the adoptive mother are also recommended to address her concerns directly without exposing the client to this content. Collateral meetings involving the mother and the preschool teachers are also recommended to engage the early childhood education providers in strengthening Keandra's comfort with separation. Dyadic therapeutic services including the birth father may also be indicated if the adoptive mother is in favor of this strategy.

Goal: Bolster the client's functioning in multiple domains (e.g., school and primary support) via strengthening PCRC 15.

Sample collaboratively generated objectives include the following:

1. Within 6 months, the client will be sent home from school zero times per week per the mother's report (current baseline: two to three times per week).

2. Client's mother, at present, reports feeling perplexed by client's separation-related difficulties. Over the course of the next 3 months, the client's mother will consider during individual collateral meetings with the IMH worker the contributing factors to the client's and family's separation-related experiences using a trauma- and diversity-informed lens (e.g., how systems of oppression have led to criminalization of the client's father and substance abuse struggles for the client's birth mother).

3. The client's mother will use individual collateral meetings with the IMH worker to plan developmentally meaningful language to use with the client to talk about her father's incarceration-related comings and goings from her life by [date].

4. At present, client does not have a bedtime routine, and her separation anxiety is often heightened at night. Within 3 months, the client's mother will develop and implement on a daily basis a bedtime routine for the client that is consistent and predictable.

Vignette 15.2

Yusef and Jamila, an Eritrean couple, enter therapy at Jamila's urging to work through parenting challenges following a family loss. Jamila is 25, and Yusef is 27. Jamila was born in the US and Yusef immigrated from Eritrea as a child together with his mother following his father's death. They have a 16-month-old toddler, Amanuel.

Yusef has been grieving the loss of his own mother who died of cancer just 2 months after Amanuel's birth. Her condition had been diagnosed late-stage, and she had suffered a series of strokes secondary to a brain tumor. Treatment had not been possible, and the time between the diagnosis and the death was a 4-month period just before and just after Amanuel's birth.

Yusef had originally planned to take family leave to care for Amanuel for a couple of months following Jamila's family leave. They had hoped this plan would keep him home for his first few months of life, and they had planned that he would then be in a shared care arrangement with a few other Eritrian families in their neighborhood, with his mother being one of the caregivers. Since his mother's death, however, Yusef has been overwhelmed with sorrow and has not felt able to return to work. He had been close with his mother and had anticipated with pleasure the flowering of a new phase in family life with her as an actively involved grandmother to his child. He misses her terribly and laments her absence from their lives on a daily basis. He feels that Amanuel is his only solace, and in being with Amanuel he sometimes has a sense of his mother's presence, as he remembers and emulates her loving parenting style. He is also haunted by guilt and worry that Amanuel was injured irreparably by being born into a time of such pain and sorrow for the family. He wants to do all he can to make up for this occurrence, and he believes that putting Amanuel in child care would constitute a compounding injury. He points to his mother's death as evidence that "you can lose people in the blink of an eye" and cannot tolerate the thought of letting Amanuel out of his sight. At the same time, however, Yusef feels ashamed of burdening Jamila and failing to support his family.

Jamila is distressed for several reasons. She feels bad about not being able to comfort Yusef, and she is wounded that nothing she does or says seems to ease his grief. The loss of income also scares her, and she resents the long hours she is working because she is now the sole breadwinner for the family. She feels deprived of one-on-one time with Amanuel resulting from the present division of labor. Also, she believes that Amanuel would benefit from having contact with other children and exposure to a wider variety of experiences than characterize his days with his father. She describes that when she arrives home from work Amanuel is eager for her to take him on a walk, and indeed Yusef confirms that some days he feels too down to go out.

During the assessment period, the IMH worker, a Mexican American woman, speaks with Yusef and Jamila about their differing experiences of being part of the Eritrean diaspora, and how these differences affect their respective experiences of loss. They determine that Yusef will be the identified client and that treatment will focus on supporting him in working through his grief so that he can regain his lost sense of strength and purpose as a husband and a father.

DSM–5 diagnosis: Other Specified Trauma- and Stressor-Related Disorder: Persistent Complex Bereavement Disorder

ICD–10–CM code: F43.8

Relational Clinical Formulation

The identified client meets criteria for a diagnosis of Persistent Complex Bereavement Disorder secondary to his mother's untimely death, as evidenced by his preoccupation with his mother's death, persistent yearning for her and lamentation for their lost future as a family, his inability to re-engage with work or activities he previously enjoyed, and his lack of trust that the world may be safe and promising for his son. These symptoms are negatively affecting the family's economic security, the marital relationship, and the parent–child relationship, because the client's perceptions of the child are colored by his grief. The child is at risk of being held back from growth-promoting experiences as a result of the client's sorrow and fear. The client and family will benefit from treatment aimed at strengthening PCRC 15. Regular triadic IMH sessions with concurrent couples sessions and occasional individual sessions are recommended.

Goal: Work through grief, as evidenced by strengthening PCRC 15.

Sample collaboratively generated objectives include the following:

1. Client reports feeling overwhelmed with grief at the prospect of separating from his son for a workday. Client will identify verbally during each weekly IMH visit possible contributing factors to this experience, including immigration-related losses and separations that he may be re-experiencing at this time.

2. At present, client reports never registering his son's desire for exploration or separation, and instead only seeing signs that his son wishes to stay close. During each family session over the next 2 months, the client will practice identifying signs in the child's behavior indicating an impulse and appetite for exploration.

3. Client states that he has fallen out of the habit of engaging in formerly pleasurable activities, instead spending all of his time engaged in child care, which exacerbates his depression. The client will report spending time alone in an activity he finds rewarding (e.g., reading) while his wife has one-on-one time with their son on a regular weekly basis by [date].

4. The client and his partner will collaborate to generate a plan for entering their son in child care by [date].

CHAPTER 17

PCRC 16—All Families Are Traditional

Stories were very important in our family. It was a way of passing down oral tradition, history, and language. Our storytellers were mainly, but not limited to, grandparents. Stories were told while stringing chili, sitting before a fireplace and eating pinons, and so forth.

—Frances Torivio Pino, quoted in Babcock, Monthan, and Monthan (1986, p. 104)

PCRC 16: Parent takes pride and pleasure in his or her (or family) **culture(s)**, respects other cultures, and has the capacity to promote a sense of cultural identity and respect for other cultures in child AND child is able to take pleasure and pride in family culture(s) and demonstrates respect for other cultures.

All families are traditional. When the phrase "traditional family" is used to refer to dominant cultural norms, the rich lineages and meaningful shared practices of families arranged otherwise are discounted. The same is true of the phrase "intact family"; it implies that some families are whole, whereas others are not. In fact, all family units are simultaneously complete systems as they are and also open systems, fragments of larger constellations of people. Infant mental health (IMH) workers are best able to support families around Parent–Child Relationship Competency (PCRC) 16 when they recognize that all families are connected to sociocultural traditions and when they understand culture in the broadest

Tenet # 5:
Honor Diverse Family Structures

and most nuanced sense. The definition offered by the *New World Encyclopedia* is as follows:

> *The word culture, from the Latin root* colere *(to inhabit, to cultivate, or to honor), generally refers to patterns of human activity and the symbolic structures that give such activity significance....Culture is a complex of features held by a social group, which may be as small as a family or a tribe, or as large as a racial or ethnic group, a nation, or in the age of globalization, by people all over the world....Culture is both defined by the social activities of the group and also defines the behavior of the members of the society. Culture...is not fixed or static; rather, it involves a dynamic process as people respond to changing conditions and challenges.* ("Culture," n.d., paras. 1 and 3)

Families make culture, and culture makes families. Members of families link other members to cultural groups and traditions that they might not otherwise be part of, such as when parents become members of a child care community by virtue of the fact that their child is cared for there. Whether deliberately or inadvertently, parents inculcate children into many aspects of the cultures they are part of and convey messages about other cultures. Infants and young children perceive many things regarding culture and cultural differences and can benefit from adult support in making meaning of what they perceive.

PS 1

When PCRC 16 is functioning well, families derive a sense of meaning and connectedness from the culture(s) with which they identify. Parents convey to children that children are part of a shared fabric of human life larger than themselves. This phenomenon—being part of a human community—is inherently pleasurable for children, and parents are often gratified by seeing their children inhabit, cultivate, and honor the cultural traditions they are offered. Culture may be experienced and expressed in terms of race, ethnicity, nationality, religion, language, food, clothing, hair, prayer, songs, games, sports, rituals, routines, iconography, literatures, region, neighborhood, social group, demographic, occupation, craft, political affiliation, and heroes. The ways that culture manifests are infinite. Cultural identification can buoy people in times of challenge; link people across time and space; and fortify people against existential alienation, loneliness, meaninglessness, and despair.

Many things may lead to this PCRC being strained, impaired, or absent. Cutting people off from aspects of cultural experience is an explicit tactic of colonization and domination. Interlocking systems of oppression may produce a sense of stigma or shame for a parent or a child around aspects of their cultural identity. Young children are usually exquisitely sensitive to their parents' pain. They are also ready to identify with their parents, and so the relational stage is set for children to adopt a sense of shame right along with aspects of shared cultural identity. Misogyny is commonly reproduced this way through the generations, with girls forming a sense of gender identity that is laced through with impressions of inferiority, and boys equating masculinity with superiority or internalizing a right to act out aggressively or enjoy more than their fare share (a dollar on a woman's 80 cents, say) via relationally and psychologically costly social and psychic zoning. Internalized racism is likewise highly transmittable, with children of color being at risk of developing a sense of defectiveness that is inextricable from their developing racial identification and White children being at risk of identifying with the White supremacy into which they are indoctrinated.

Trauma can impede parents' capacity to take pleasure and pride in their cultural identities and their ability to promote sustaining cultural identities in their children. For example, Joy DeGruy (2005) has introduced the concept of *Post Traumatic Slave Syndrome*. DeGruy wrote,

> *Post Traumatic Slave Syndrome is a condition that exists when a population has experienced multigenerational trauma resulting from centuries of slavery and continues to experience oppression and institutionalized racism today. Added to this condition*

is a belief (real or imagined) that the benefits of the society in which they live are not accessible to them. (p. 121)

DeGruy (2005) illustrated how the trauma of the history of enslavement in the United States is transmitted intergenerationally. An important ingredient of this phenomenon is the "cognitive dissonance" produced by the obvious present-day sequelae of this history together with a simultaneous disavowal of it. It is a persistent pretense that the national history of enslavement exists only in the distant past, without any present-day reverberations, or that it did not happen at all.

The cognitive dissonance produced by the massive disavowal of historical trauma suffered by many cultural groups—including Native American, Chinese, Japanese, and other peoples as well as by African Americans—affects everyone in the United States. White parents regularly transmit to our children White privilege and White supremacy along with a noncritical cultural identification with Whiteness, which reproduces racism at the level of cultural identity. This kind of White identity is concocted via projection onto and dis-identification from (and often some degree of dehumanization of) people of color, disavowal of the political forces that conspire to disenfranchise them, and obfuscation of investment in perpetuating the unjust status quo. Such processes take place largely outside of conscious awareness but in and through thousands of daily transactions. At the same time, these processes become extremely obvious and can be readily recognized.

"Whiteness" draws its power in part through disembodiment and deracination. According to its logic, "other" groups are particularly socially located, racially marked, and history bound, whereas Whiteness operates outside of such confines. In fact, of course, people who identify as White also have ancestral lineages, ethnic heritages, and migration histories that DNA tracing can shed light on. However, many people are unaware of or disconnected from these parts of their life story because social location has been surrendered across generations in exchange for disembodied Whiteness, with the benefits accruing to it—benefits that come at the expense of those who are excluded (DiAngelo, 2011).

IMH workers can support White families in challenging White supremacy and White privilege and in establishing foundations of family and cultural pride that are built not on the fault lines of disidentification, disavowal, and obfuscation but on the solid ground of human interconnectedness.

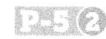

Tenet # 3: Work to Acknowledge Privilege and Combat Discrimination

In working with most families, the IMH worker can usefully support the identification and celebration of family and other cultures and can aid parents in recognizing the importance of this concept to their children. Each of the other PCRCs may be strengthened when PCRC 16 is firing.

Vignette 16.1

Richard, the father of 4-year-old Orion, calls the IMH worker to initiate treatment at the urging of the director of Orion's preschool. He explains that he and Orion's mother, Anne, have recently divorced and that Orion is "falling apart" when transitioning between households, and he is getting into trouble in his preschool classroom. Richard feels that the teachers and the preschool director are not sufficiently understanding the impact of the recent divorce on Orion. "I think it's partly a culture thing," Richard explains. "A lot of the kids in the class don't come from two-parent homes, so I think the teachers just don't understand how tough divorce can be on a kid."

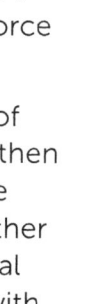

The IMH worker conducts an assessment that consists of first meeting with each parent individually in her office, then observing Orion in his classroom, then meeting with the preschool director, and finally meeting with Orion together with each of his parents in their respective homes several times. She then holds feedback meetings in her office with each parent individually.

The IMH worker, who is herself White, comes to agree with Richard that culture plays a part in the difficulties that Orion is having in the classroom, although her analysis of the situation differs from Richard's. In the course of the assessment, she learns that both parents have histories of anxiety and that there was a high degree of conflict in the marital relationship, with frequent arguments. She also learns that the family is White and that Orion had previously attended a preschool serving primarily White families. As a result of the financial strains associated with the divorce, Orion switched preschools to one that is much more racially diverse with respect to both staff and the families. Both parents associate primarily with White people, and both disclose some discomfort and anxiety around the families of color at the school, especially the African American families. Each parent independently expresses to the IMH worker a worry that the African American teachers may be more familiar with African American children and may be "hard" on Orion because he is White. Both parents see the change of schools as an unfortunate necessity resulting from the divorce, and both express guilt about Orion's attending.

During the classroom observation, the IMH worker observes Orion alternating between actively avoiding interactions with African American children and acting out aggressively with two children (in one instance pushing away a child who approached wishing to join in play and later running up to an easel and painting over a child's work). In both instances, the teacher sets limits with Orion in a clear but compassionate manner and attempts to engage him in conversation about his feelings and the antecedents of his actions. Orion appears fearful and withdraws from the teacher. Orion does not attend when the teacher is reading a story out loud, instead appearing absorbed in pulling a loose thread from his sweater.

All the adults who were consulted (the preschool director and both parents) reported that Orion tends to be irritable and contrary, and the IMH worker observes instances of this behavior in both homes. Whereas Richard states that these behaviors are new since the divorce, Anne contends that they predate the divorce, linking them to the high degree of conflict in the household that had mounted over the past 2 years.

The IMH worker discusses her impressions with each parent separately, including her sense that the parents' discomfort with the African American families at the school and lack of confidence in the African American staff may be exacerbating and providing a target for Orion's anxiety, which has its roots in the atmosphere of conflict and discord that predated the divorce and which has been exacerbated by the separations and disruptions in routine necessitated by the divorce. The worker suggests that focusing on culture may provide a helpful fulcrum for addressing Orion's anxiety. Both parents are receptive to this approach.

DC:0–5 diagnosis: Other Anxiety Disorder of Infancy/Early Childhood

DSM–5 diagnosis: Other Specified Anxiety Disorder

ICD–10–CM code: F41.8: Other Specified Anxiety Disorder

Relational Clinical Formulation

The identified client is a 4-year-old White boy who meets criteria for a diagnosis of Other Anxiety Disorder of Infancy/Early Childhood, as evidenced by intermittent inattention, frequent irritability and contrariness, and alternating between avoidance of and hostility in interactions with peers and teachers. The client's anxiety-based aggressive and avoidant behaviors are directed primarily toward African American peers and teachers, whereas his irritability is not relationship specific. He alternates between two households and demonstrates separation distress around transitions. The client's difficulties at school are exacerbated by his parents' discomfort with the school, which is partly based in their lack of confidence in or respect for the African American teachers. This attitude is conveyed to the client. These difficulties are best addressed in the context of the parent–child relationships so that both households may implement changes toward reducing the client's anxiety. The client will benefit from IMH treatment with each parent participating as a collateral partner on an alternating weekly basis.

Goal: Resolve symptoms of anxiety by strengthening PCRC 16.

Sample collaboratively generated objectives include the following:

1. At present, the client's parents report that there is no consistency between the client's mother's and father's households, resulting in unnecessary anxiety-producing disruption for the client. The client's parents will identify elements of family culture (e.g., routines or activities) that can be positively implemented in both households on a daily basis for the next 3 months.

2. The client, at present, has no language for talking about race, which exacerbates his anxiety in interracial exchanges. During weekly dyadic IMH sessions, the client's parents will engage the client in conversation about race-related topics (e.g., discussing the skin color of dolls in the treatment room, family, friends, acquaintances, as well as children and teachers at school).

3. Although they do not meet with her, the client's parents have little confidence in the client's teacher, which exacerbates the client's anxiety at school. The client's parents will each meet with the client's teacher on a monthly basis and will report experiencing a collaborative rapport with her by [date].

4. The client's daily aggressive acting out with peers will cease within 1 month.

5. The client's parents both report never having reflected on the connections between anxiety and race in their respective families or lives, which hampers their ability to support the client in resolving his difficulties. Each is

willing to work to understand these patterns. Each parent will identify during a monthly collateral meeting with the IMH worker at least one connection between anxiety and race in their own lives.

6. The client will be able to verbally identify three things he is proud of about his family within 3 months (current baseline: zero).

Vignette 16.2

Eric, a gay White man in his 40s, calls the IMH worker because he is worried about the impact on his son of "things going on at the child care center." During an office-based assessment period that includes individual meetings with Eric and dyadic meetings with Eric and his son, Randy, together, the IMH worker learns that Eric began caring for Randy 1 year ago and that the adoption was recently finalized. Randy is 2½ years old. He spent his first year of life with a different foster family, and then he was placed with Eric when his birth mother's parental rights were terminated. Eric reports that Randy has been attending the same child care center since coming to live with him and that he was recently switched into a new classroom composed of 2- and 3-year-olds. Eric is not comfortable with the teacher, fearing that she may be homophobic. "It's always 'Mommy and Daddy this' and 'Mommy and Daddy that' with her," he states. He describes that Randy has been clingy, whiney, and irritable since the transition, and he fears that the teacher is behaving with Randy in ways that are discriminatory. "But then I've been irritable too, so it's a chicken-and-egg thing, I guess."

In response to the IMH worker's inquiry, Eric explains that he has had extremely distant relationships with his family of origin since he came out in his 20s because of their bigoted and rejecting response. Eric also discloses that several months ago he broke up with a man he had been dating for the preceding 5 years. "He just wasn't up for parenting, and to me it was the most important thing in the world," Eric explains tearfully. Eric has also lost contact with many friends because the break-up strained relations with their mutual friends. "Plus," Eric added with derision, "when you're under the social worker's microscope, you don't want a bunch of old faggots hanging around."

The IMH worker suggests that Eric is suffering from depression connected with the break-up, the multiple adjustments demanded by parenthood, and the fresh experiences of homophobia he is contending with now that he is a parent. She affirms that encountering homophobia and heteronormativity in children's worlds is a painful part of gay parenting. She also shares that internalized homophobia often presents itself in new ways when gay people parent for the first time. Furthermore, she suggests that although it is not unusual for a child Randy's age to have a hard time with a transition to a new classroom, Randy has good reasons to be extra sensitive to change and to negative messages about his family. Together, Eric and the IMH worker develop a plan that involves continuing a pattern of parallel individual and dyadic meetings.

DSM−5 diagnosis: Adjustment Disorder with Depressed Mood

ICD−10−CM code: F43.21

Relational Clinical Formulation

The identified client is a 43-year-old gay White man who has recently adopted a 2½-year-old son. The client meets criteria for a diagnosis of Adjustment Disorder with Depressed Mood secondary to a recent break-up combined with the stresses related to the adoption process. Symptoms include low mood, tearfulness, and irritability. The client's condition is exacerbated by homophobia and heteronormativity encountered in the world (in the child welfare system and his son's preschool) as well as internalized homophobia (including the idea that gay people are damaging to children) but ameliorated by his love for and pleasure in his relationship with his son. These circumstances contribute to the client's social isolation, which compounds his depression. The client will likely benefit from IMH services aimed at strengthening PCRC 16. A combination of individual and dyadic sessions are recommended so that the client can freely explore grown-up matters that may be negatively affecting his sense of self as a parent and also practice engaging with his son in ways that consolidate their positive identification as a family.

Goal: Reduce symptoms of depression by strengthening PCRC 16.

Sample collaboratively generated objectives include the following:

1. The client is concerned that school personnel may not be providing a welcoming environment for gay families, but he reports not having been able to muster the confidence to speak with them about these concerns. The client will schedule a meeting with the child care director by [date].

2. The client's internalized homophobia undermines his confidence in himself as a parent, exacerbating his experience of depression. During weekly individual IMH meetings, the client will verbally identify historical roots of internalized homophobia, resulting in a decrease of the frequency of homophobic thoughts from X per day to Y per week by [date].

3. Since breaking up with his partner several months ago, the client has had zero contact with friends. The client will report following through with at least one social contact per week over the course of the next 3 months.

4. At present, the client and his son participate in no activities with other gay families, compounding the client's isolation and constraining his son's opportunities

to build affirmative identifications with LGBTQ (lesbian, gay, bisexual, transgender, and queer) culture. The client will report participating in one family activity sponsored by the LGBTQ center each month in the course of the next 6 months.

CHAPTER 18

PCRC 17—Trauma: The Rent World and the Restoration of Hope

She remembered what Mother had said back to him. "Fear has made this country do something she will one day regret, Mr. Kurihara, but we cannot let this terrible mistake poison our hearts. If we do, then we will be the ones to destroy ourselves and our children as well."

—Yoshiko Uchida (1971, p. 90)

PCRC 17: Parent is able to act to restore a sense of safety, hope, trust, and well-being for self and child following a distressing, disturbing, or **traumatic event** AND child is able to respond to parent's actions and to calm, restore, and heal.

Parent–Child Relationship Competency (PCRC) 17 describes how the protective function core to parent–child relationships under ordinary circumstances makes those relationships into an apparatus for healing when circumstances are injurious. This PCRC is closely linked to PCRC 3, which describes the operation of the protective function under ordinary circumstances.

As attachment research has conclusively demonstrated, infants and young children are born ready to seek safety and security from their primary caregivers, and caregivers tend to be intrinsically motivated to provide this refuge. PCRC 3 describes these complementary motivational systems. Daily life provides myriad opportunities for parent–child dyads to trace and retrace this territory together in ever-widening developmental spirals as infants, toddlers, and young children navigate exploration of the world, consistently safeguarded and refueled by interactions with the protective caregiver. Life generously provides silly mishaps, major frustrations, minor injuries, bitter disappointments, scary near-misses, and painful humiliations to most of us. When PCRC 3 is functioning well, the parent–child relationship absorbs and absolves all these encounters, ensuring ongoing safety and a good enough balance between growth-promoting exploration and protective "safe haven" (Powell et al., 2014) experiences. When PCRC 3 is functioning well, both parents and children are able to draw satisfaction from both components of this dialectic—exploration and connection.

All families contend with PCRC 3–level challenges on a regular basis. PCRC 17, by contrast, comes into play when families are confronted with negative experiences of more grave proportions. When parent–child dyads do experience distressing, disturbing, or traumatic events, they draw on their reservoir of successfully weathering PCRC 3–grade challenges to manage the more dysregulating challenge or crisis. A dyad that has built up an abundant supply of successful PCRC 3 circuits will benefit when PCRC 17 is activated by circumstance.

The epigraph at the beginning of this chapter illustrates PCRC 17 functioning well. In *Journey to Topaz*, Uchida (1971) has recounted in the voice of a child, Yuki Sakane, the historical trauma of the U.S. internment of Japanese Americans during World War II. Throughout the story, Yuki is repeatedly shielded by her mother's love from the devastating effects of the xenophobic criminalization, incarceration, dispossession, and dehumanization to which her family and community are subjected. Mrs. Sakane builds on her family's well-established PCRC 3–level capacities for the interpersonal maintenance of safety, protection, and comfort to preserve their sense of safety, hope, trust, and well-being in the face of traumatic events.

In an article examining trauma in the context of immigration, Foster (2001) noted the powerful moderating function of parental emotional states in determining children's experiences in crisis situations. Foster wrote,

these phenomena are probably embedded in basic aspects of the parent–child interaction, wherein parents, despite the context of crisis, are able to maintain a semblance of both the physical and emotional holding environment that is nodal to the child's psychic stability. (p. 158)

This powerful influence cuts both ways, however. When a dyad has struggled with PCRC 3, they will be exponentially more vulnerable in the face of malignant challenge because they will not have a deep reserve of successful experiences navigating the benign realm of challenge. Also, in some instances, the nature of the dyad's difficulty with PCRC 3 may actually predispose them to being in harm's way, increasing the likelihood that they will suffer traumatic experiences. Examples of this phenomenon would include a parent who experiences herself as helpless and does not act protectively with her child, resulting in the child being harmed by someone, or a child who does not seek safety through proximity but instead bolts into traffic and is hit by a car.

Regardless of a family's baseline capacities to navigate safety issues, trauma by definition overwhelms these. Trauma affects infants and young children in developmentally specific ways, and there is a role for infant mental health (IMH) workers in helping parents and others in a child's world to respond in ways that will promote healing. P-5 2 Alicia Lieberman and her colleagues at the University of California, San Francisco, Child Trauma Research Program developed trauma-focused child–parent psychotherapy, an adaptation of infant–parent psychotherapy specially tailored to treat children exposed to trauma (Lieberman et al., 2015; Lieberman & Van Horn, 2008). They emphasized the importance of working directly with the parent and child together to support the parent in restoring protective functioning following a trauma. Trauma-focused child–parent psychotherapy specifically guides IMH workers in addressing the psychological and relational complexities of family violence. Lieberman and Van Horn (2008) wrote, "When the parent becomes the agent of the trauma, as in child abuse or domestic violence, the child faces an intractable emotional dilemma because the perpetrator and the protector are one and the same" (p. 23). IMH workers can help parents to understand the nature of this dilemma faced by their child and to replace endangering interactions with protective patterns.

In the context of interlocking systems of oppression, many families are exposed to chronic stress of traumatic proportions. It is important for IMH workers to consider the impact of historical and contemporary trauma and complex stress on families, even when this is not at first glance part of the presenting issue (Andermahr, 2016; Visser, 2015). Ken V. Hardy (2013) wrote, for example, that "racial oppression is a traumatic form of interpersonal violence which can lacerate the spirit, scar the soul, and puncture the psyche" (p. 25). Hardy continued,

> *Rarely is unmasking and treating the hidden wounds of racial trauma a focal point of intervention. Instead, conventional approaches attend to family problems, individual psychological issues, behavioral problems, affect disorders, and substance misuse. These are salient factors but skirt issues of race which are powerful dynamics in the lives of youth of color.* (p. 25)

Hardy has advocated for intervention that explicitly addresses the effects of racial oppression and has offered a framework for doing so.

In a similar vein, the Center for Excellence in Children's Mental Health (2010) issued an e-review addressing contemporary manifestations of historical trauma for American Indian and Alaskan Native children. In it, the center cited Brave Heart's (1999) definition of *historical trauma* as "a constellation of characteristics associated with massive cumulative group trauma across generations" (p. 1). The review also summarized the contributions of

Evans-Campbell and Walters (2006), who delineated specific decolonizing practices that can be deployed by practitioners serving American Indian and Alaskan Native families toward healing from historical trauma.

Tenet # 8:
Allocate Resources to Systems Change

The language of PCRC 17 implies a discreet traumatic event and a baseline of well-being. Brave Heart's (1999) phrase cited earlier—"massive cumulative group trauma across generations"—makes it clear that for many peoples who have suffered historical trauma the scope of the damage is nearly unfathomable, and the idea of a baseline of well-being may seem like a lost dream. Nevertheless, there can be a role for the IMH worker in supporting parents in identifying the specific effects of historical and contemporary collective trauma on themselves and their families, and doing so can open pathways toward self-determination and healing.

Tenet # 3:
Work to Acknowledge Privilege and Combat Discrimination

Vignette 17.1

Deandre, a 3-year-old African American boy, and his mother, Chrystal, are referred to the IMH clinic by a child welfare worker. The child welfare worker explains that Deandre had come to the attention of the system a couple of months ago when his father was arrested and jailed. Deandre had been in the car with his father and had not been in a car seat. He spent 24 hours in emergency foster care shelter before being placed at home with Chrystal as an in-home dependent. The worker describes Chrystal as "hostile and help-rejecting." She states, "Frankly, my concerns have increased over time, because Deandre is really acting out, and Chrystal interacts with him in ways that escalate him." The child welfare worker is hoping that the clinic can teach Chrystal parenting skills.

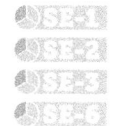

The IMH worker, who is also African American, conducts a clinical assessment that consists of several meetings with Chrystal alone and several home visits with Chrystal and Deandre together. Chrystal is enraged at the events that have befallen her family. She explains that Deandre's father, Melvin, had been previously incarcerated and was on probation at the time of the arrest. He had been pulled over by two White police officers for a tail light failure, but when the officers saw that Deandre was not in a car seat they stated that they would need to detain the child. Melvin had responded by verbally insisting that he would not be separated from his son. The police officers interpreted his statement and stance as aggressive and forcefully handcuffed him in front of Deandre. Deandre was taken into emergency foster care in one car, and Melvin was taken to jail in another.

Chrystal says that Deandre has been altered since the incident. She worries that he was abused during the 24 hours he spent in emergency foster care, and she is irate that her concerns about this possibility have been dismissed by child welfare. She describes behaviors in Deandre such as "acting hyper," "being violent," "being clingy," and "waking up screaming" that were not present before the incident. The IMH worker observes Deandre becoming extremely dysregulated on several occasions when his mother attempts to set minor limits with him. She observes a quickly escalating pattern in which Chrystal becomes alarmed and emphatic, demanding, "What is the matter with you?" and Deandre becomes increasingly dysregulated. Chrystal says to the IMH worker, "They did this to him. Something is not right with him. He was a happy baby. They messed him up."

The IMH worker meets with Chrystal alone for a feedback session. She tells her that she does not know what did or did not happen during the 24 hours in the shelter, but she believes that Deandre was traumatized by seeing his father arrested in front of him and being forcedly separated. She states that she thinks the family is contending with several systems at the same time that target African American people and hurt their families, with forced separation and the threat of forced separation being some of the mechanisms of injury. She thinks Deandre misses his father and is worried that he is being hurt. She also believes that one of the ways this whole thing is affecting the family is that it has driven a wedge between Chrystal and Deandre. The worker describes the vicious cycle she has observed. When Deandre demonstrates behaviors that are trauma symptoms, he is in those moments unrecognizable to Chrystal. Chrystal conveys her alarm and horror to Deandre, who, in turn, becomes frightened by his mother's response to him, likely feeling her emotional distance and estrangement, and he then acts in ways that are even more foreign and alarming to Chrystal. Chrystal recognizes this pattern when the IMH worker describes it and agrees to meet with the IMH worker together with Deandre to work to change this behavior.

The IMH worker suggests that she and Chrystal talk with Deandre together about the fact that he was very frightened when the White police officers hurt his daddy and took him to jail, that he was scared when he went to the strange place and did not see his mama or daddy all night, and that he is very worried about his daddy now. She proposes that they tell him that because he was so scared and is so worried he sometimes has scary dreams and sometimes becomes very angry and upset. Mama gets angry and upset too, and then everybody is even more scared and angry and upset. She suggests that they explain that she, the IMH worker, is going to visit once a week and help Deandre and his mama talk and play about the scary things that have happened to their family so that they can feel safe together again. She suggests also that they make plans to maximize contact with Melvin and help Deandre understand as much as he can about what is happening with his father day by day. She shares resources with Chrystal, including the Bill of Rights for Children With Incarcerated Parents (https://www.sfcipp.org/), to develop a family plan for navigating Melvin's incarceration.

DC:0–5 diagnosis: Posttraumatic Stress Disorder

DSM–5 diagnosis: Posttraumatic Stress Disorder for Children 6 Years and Younger

ICD–10–CM code: F43.10: Posttraumatic Stress Disorder

Relational Clinical Formulation

The identified client is a 3-year-old African American boy who meets criteria for a diagnosis of Posttraumatic Stress Disorder after witnessing his father being arrested, being forcedly separated from his father, and being held for 24 hours by child protective services in a shelter with strangers before being placed at home with his mother. Since this incident, the client has experienced nightmares and has displayed clinginess, angry acting out, proneness to states of dysregulation, and a general reduction of expression of positive emotions. These changes in the client's behavior suggest significant emotional distress and also cause significant distress to his mother, who finds his new behaviors alarming and alienating. The family is contending with racial oppression, as manifest in the pattern of targeting African American families for forced separation by the criminal justice and child welfare systems. These difficulties are best addressed in the context of the parent–child relationship to mitigate adverse relational and developmental sequelae of trauma. The client will benefit from services that include his parents as collateral partners and that focus on strengthening PCRC 17. Advocacy on the family's behalf with collateral providers and systems is also indicated.

Goal: Reduce symptoms of Posttraumatic Stress Disorder by strengthening PCRC 17.

Sample collaboratively generated objectives include the following:

1. At present, the client's mother reports never speaking with the client about his feeling afraid when he engages in acting-out behaviors (instead, she admonishes him to stop). During each weekly home-based IMH meeting over the next 3 months, the client's mother will practice holding the client and talking with the client about his underlying experiences of fear when he engages in trauma-based behaviors such as acting out.

2. At present, the client and his mother engage in cycles of escalating mutual dysregulation multiple times each day. The client's mother will report elimination of interactions that escalate the client's dysregulation by [date].

3. The client's mother reports frequently talking about race and racism in the client's presence but not talking with him directly about these topics, which may contribute to the client's generalized fear and worry. The client's mother will make use of IMH meetings over the next 3 months to create and share directly with the client developmentally informed narratives about racial oppression and family strength.

4. At present, the client has no contact with his father, which likely exacerbates his fear for his father's well-being. Over the course of the next 3 months, the client's mother will facilitate daily opportunities for the client to experience contact with his father via telephone or in-person visits and by creating video greetings on the phone to be shared with his father when possible.

5. The client's nightmares will cease by [date] (current baseline: one per night).

Vignette 17.2

Missy is a 25-year-old White woman with a 2-year-old daughter named Sissy. The dyad is referred for treatment by the case manager at the transitional housing facility where they reside. They moved into this facility from a domestic violence shelter to which Missy fled when she left Sissy's father, who had been physically violent with her beginning when she was pregnant with Sissy. The referral is prompted by the fact that although Missy has made good progress on many fronts during her 6 months of residency in the transitional program, it recently came to light that she had become involved with a man she met in her employment training program who has a history of interpersonal violence with romantic partners and allegations of physical abuse of

a 7-year-old daughter with whom he now has no contact. The case manager is worried about Missy's judgment. She reports that Missy is a very dedicated mother but has struggled around putting Sissy in child care, expressing fears that she might be molested in the care of strangers. Missy has refused individual therapy, stating, "I don't want to talk about what they'd want me to talk about," but she is open to the referral for treatment together with her daughter. In the early IMH sessions, Missy discloses the details of the violence she suffered without regard for the impact of this discussion on Sissy. At the same time, Missy is observed to be quite controlling of Sissy's behaviors and limiting of her explorations. Sissy alternates between precocious compliance and disobedience that the IMH worker sees as having a provocative, "I-dare-you-to-stop-me" quality.

DSM–5 diagnosis: Posttraumatic Stress Disorder

ICD–10–CM code: F43.10

Relational Clinical Formulation

The identified client, a 25-year-old White woman, has suffered interpersonal violence resulting in injury, dislocation, assaults on her sense of identity, economic hardship, and relationship rupture. The client meets criteria for a diagnosis of Posttraumatic Stress Disorder, as evidenced by her persistent difficulty relaxing, including frequent nightmares and night wakings, avoidance of talking about her abuse history alternating with unfiltered disclosure of the details of her abuse, and her global distrust of "strangers." The client's capacity to distinguish between safety and danger has been disabled by traumatic experiences such that she is overprotective of her toddler (e.g., limiting exploration) and at the same time puts them both in harm's way (getting involved with romantic partners who have histories of interpersonal violence). The client's sense of fearfulness is ameliorated by her love for her daughter and her determination to provide a safe and secure home for them, which has motivated her to pursue and succeed at job training. Her progress is threatened by her vulnerability to becoming involved with partners who may themselves be vulnerable to violent acting out. The client's daughter also demonstrates confusion about safety and danger, alternating between "good behavior" that is inconsistent with developmentally expectable emotional needs and "acting-out" behavior that leaves her at risk for negative and punitive interactions with adults. These difficulties are best addressed in the context of the parent–child relationship (with individual parent meetings meant to discuss material that might be disturbing for the client's child to hear). The dyad will likely benefit from treatment aimed at strengthening PCRC 17.

Goal: The client will effectively protect herself and her child from exposure to interpersonal violence, as evidenced in the strengthening of PCRC 17.

Sample collaboratively generated objectives include the following:

1. At present, the client communicates to her daughter that things are dangerous when in fact they are not multiple times per the weekly IMH session. Over the course of the next 2 months, the client will identify together with the IMH worker during each weekly session exploratory activity on the part of the toddler that is growth promoting, not dangerous.

2. At present, the client avoids talking directly with her daughter about family violence, instead frightening and overstimulating the child by talking about it to others when the client is within earshot. The client will, with the support of the IMH worker, develop a narrative about the interpersonal violence she experienced and the subsequent separation from the child's father that is developmentally appropriate by [date].

3. The client's child will cease provocative disobedience by [date], as observed by the IMH worker (current baseline: one to two incidents per weekly IMH session).

4. The client's child will accept help from the client rather than executing tasks such as cleaning up toys on her own during each IMH session over the next 2 months (current baseline: zero).

CHAPTER 19

PCRC 18—From Melancholia to Mourning, Together

Sarah loved her boots. They were as shiny as a wet slicker and as yellow as a bathtub duck. When Sarah jumped into puddles her boots went SQUISH and the water went KERSPLAT! One day, Sarah tried to put on her boots....She scrunched her toes into tight little balls. She pushed her heels with all her might. But Sarah's boots did not fit Sarah's feet....Sarah was very sad.

—Paulette Bourgeois (1987), pp. 1–16

PCRC 18: Parent is able to mourn losses and support child in **mourning** losses AND child is able to make use of parent's support to mourn losses in keeping with developmental level.

Mourning is not reserved for death; it is part of life. To the degree that we cherish something or someone, we are likely to experience grief when we lose it. For parents, this concept means that child rearing is often marked by an undercurrent of heartache, as each developmental phase passes, giving way to the next. Picture, for example, the parade of shoes, beginning with a tiny pair of booties and getting bigger month by month, that marks the rapid and irreversible passage of developmental time. For children, too, each developmental phase entails loss as well as reward. Both parents and children suffer losses stemming not only from developmental transitions but also from external factors.

The capacity to mourn is part of psychological health, and it is not to be taken for granted. To experience relationships and life endeavors as rewarding, we must be psychologically capable of investing them with value, but this investment means that we are by the same token exposed to loss. Complex processes are constantly underway, largely outside of conscious awareness, whereby we connect with and invest internal resources such as hope, love, and energy into people and experiences and also manage the myriad losses that we sustain as moments pass, people go away, landscapes change, and circumstances shift. When we are able to accept and express the painful feelings associated with loss, our internal resources are freed up again to be invested anew.

When an adult loses a job they have valued, they will be able to bring their vital energies to a new job to the degree they have been able to mourn the loss of the old job. If the process of mourning the old job is incomplete, they may find themselves doing their work in a half-hearted way, being irritated with their new coworkers for not being their previous coworkers, or otherwise being unable to embrace their new situation—or to seek employment that is truly fitting and rewarding for them. In many family structures, when a child is faced with the birth of a younger sibling and must give up the "baby" position in the family, they will be emotionally open to forming a relationship with the sibling and to experiencing the satisfactions of being a "big kid" in the family to the degree that they are able to experience and express their feelings of loss and to feel understood. (Note that this construal of the psychological meaning of having a younger sibling represents a particular, culturally inflected value system that may be common but is not universal. In some family systems, the birth of a younger sibling would not represent a loss; instead, a different life event would be tied to the human susceptibility to experiencing loss.)

Experiencing loss is painful. People have many creative ways of protecting ourselves from reckoning with and accepting loss, and each strategy has a price. Some are inclined to keep very busy or buoyant out of fear of being dragged down by sorrow. Others tend toward anger and may remain embroiled in embattled states. Some suffer from anxiety that may be diffuse or apparently linked to one worrisome prospect or another, whereas its roots in the warded-off loss remain veiled. Moreover, some people are prone to depression, which is not mourning but precisely the inability to mourn (Freud, 1917/1955). Often, interpersonal harm is caused as a result of a person's psychological difficulty experiencing loss, as others in their sphere must contend with the consequences.

This process plays out in problematic ways in parent–child relationships, because children organize themselves partly in response to their parents' patterns of managing the prospect of loss. Young children tend to believe that they are to blame when a parent displays distress for any reason. A child whose parent tends toward depression may attribute this state to an imagined deficiency of their own and may attempt to enliven their parent or, conversely, may join the parent in an experience of hopelessness, feeling they have meager internal resources and grim prospects. A child whose parent is haunted by anxiety may believe that it is something about themselves—the child—that is causing the parent anxiety and may also take on the conviction that menace lurks at every bend, confusing internal and external sources of worry, dread, and fear. A child whose parent is chronically resentful or embattled will likely believe that they are to blame for this anger and may seek to appease the parent, to "walk on eggshells," or, ironically, incite the parent's rage as a way of becoming active rather than passive in this relational battlefield.

By contrast, when a parent is able to experience and mourn losses, the child is freed from the burden of playing a part in the parent's project of defending against the loss. Also, the relational stage is set for the child to be able to experience and mourn losses in keeping with their developmental capacities. A neonate is not expected to experience loss in the same way that an older child or adult should be able to, but if the adults caring for that newborn can imagine (consciously or implicitly) that there may be experiences akin to loss (as well as, potentially, joy) even in the birth process, it is likely that this practice will inform caregiving interactions in ways that lay the foundation for the infant to experience and express loss down the line. An infant is aided in coming to terms with the infinite succession of losses that maturation entails—and in benefiting from the new experiences ushered in by each passing developmental phase—when his parent is able to recognize these emotional experiences.

Infants and toddlers are helped to experience and move through losses, bringing their full vitality to new experiences, when parents can resonate with and respect the psychological significance of such "minor" ordinary occurrences as ending a pleasurable activity, surrendering a toy that belongs to another child, saying goodbye when a parent leaves for work, or no longer fitting into their beloved rain boots—let alone monumental developmental milestones such as weaning, walking, talking, and potty training. It is not necessary for parents to consciously address or explicitly aid children with such losses. Indeed, overly solicitous caregiving interactions around ordinary losses can lead to difficulties, giving children the message that there is something wrong with their being exposed to loss and that they are somehow set apart from the rest of humanity and should be shielded from loss. Instead, parents can resonate with and recognize the psychological significance of minor losses in ways that simply convey that loss is part of life.

When a family is contending with bereavement, it is critical that the child's experience be considered (Lieberman, Compton, Van Horn, & Ippen, 2003). Often, this practice is challenging because adults in the family are likely consumed by their own grief and sorrow. In his groundbreaking study on the subject of loss, John Bowlby (1980) wrote,

> *Whereas most adults have learned that they can survive without the more or less continuous presence of an attachment figure, children have no such experience. For this reason, it is clearly more devastating still for a child than it is for an adult should he find himself alone in a strange world....[Also,] a child is entirely dependent*

for information [about the death] on the decision of his surviving relatives, [and] whereas an adult can, if he wishes, seek further for understanding and comfort should his first exchanges prove unhelpful, a child is rarely in a position to do so, [and] is at an even greater disadvantage…should his relatives or other companions prove unsympathetic to his yearning, his sorrow, and his anxiety. (pp. 290–291)

There is often a role for the infant mental health (IMH) worker in helping a family maintain a focus on the child's experience in the context of family loss.

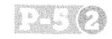

Intersecting systems of oppression frequently conspire both to cause grief and to impede mourning. People suffer losses of all kinds as a result of systems of oppression: loss of life and limb, loss of one another as a result of forced separation, loss of land possessed by conquering nations, loss of cultural continuity as a result of deracination and colonization, and loss of dignity as a result of dehumanization. Losses of such catastrophic proportions are commonplace. People lose material things—land, natural resources, possessions, homes, money, mobility, and economic opportunity—as a result of access disparities and discriminatory policies. Furthermore, people sustain devastating blows to their hopes, identities, ideals, prospects, aspirations, relationships, and sense of self as a result of systemic oppression (Andermahr, 2016; Visser, 2015).

Tenet # 10:
Advance Policy That Supports All Families

Tenet # 2:
Champion Children's Rights Globally

Sometimes, these losses are mourned. In the opening page of his famous essay distinguishing between healthy mourning and "melancholia" (depression), Sigmund Freud (1917/1955) wrote, "Mourning is regularly the reaction to the loss of a loved person, or to the loss of…one's country, liberty, an ideal, and so on" (p. 243). Frequently, however, mourning is impeded. Freud continued, "In some people the same influences produce melancholia instead of mourning" (p. 243).

Widespread cultural disregard for and disavowal of the losses sustained by particular social groups can block mourning processes. When a shopping mall is erected over a Native American burial ground, for example, pathways to mourning are literally eviscerated. Widespread devaluation of girls and women can lead to melancholia, as individuals forfeit their existential claim on physical safety, equal pay, authority, esteem, and so forth (Silverman, 1988, pp. 155–159). Homophobia and heteronormativity produce an environment in which homosexual ties are simultaneously condemned and invisibilized, proliferating losses that cannot be grieved (Butler, 1995). Moreover, colonialism, racism, and xenophobia, all of which are reproduced in part by purporting not to exist, impede mourning processes for people of color even as they incite them. Eng and Han (2000) wrote, "In the United States…assimilation into mainstream culture for people of color still means adopting a set of dominant norms and ideals—whiteness, heterosexuality, middle class family values—often foreclosed to them" (p. 670). Eng and Han continued, "The loss of these norms—the reiterated loss of whiteness as an ideal, for example—establishes… assimilation and racialization processes in the United States as a series of failed and unresolved integrations" (p. 670). Whereas mourning leads to healing and renewal, the state of irresolution described here can be chronically debilitating.

Infants and young children suffer the consequences when their families' losses remain unmourned. This process is captured in Selma Fraiberg's (1980) famous phrase "ghosts in the nursery." It is core to the role of the IMH worker to assess what losses may remain unmourned in a family; to facilitate a process of recognizing and honoring all that has been subjected to devaluation, debasement, or dispossession; and to support the family in establishing pathways out of melancholia.

P-5-4

Vignette 18.1

Linda, a 38-year-old White woman, calls the IMH worker because she is worried about her 2-year-old daughter, Mona. In this initial phone call, she explains that Mona has been having an extremely difficult time adjusting to a new child care provider. Linda says, "She used to be really a delight to care for, but now she is just so hard to please. We have gone through three nannies in 3 months! We just don't understand it." The IMH worker conducts an assessment with Mona, Linda, and Linda's husband, Brad, and learns the following.

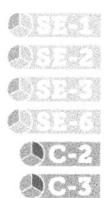

Linda and Brad both work in demanding professional jobs requiring long work hours and frequent travel. Since her birth, Mona had been cared for by Graciela, a Mexican woman who did housekeeping and child care in the family home and who stayed there overnight to care for Mona on occasions when both of her parents were traveling at the same time. Graciela left suddenly 3 months ago to return to Mexico when the cousin with whom she lived was deported. Since then, Linda and Brad have hired two replacement child care providers. The first quit after several weeks, and the second has recently raised with Linda and Brad the question of whether she is a good fit for the child.

The parents describe that Mona is irritable, easily frustrated, cries frequently, and has "gone backward" with sleep and toileting routines. Whereas she used to sleep through the night, rarely awakening before Graciela arrived at 7:30 in the morning, she now resists bedtime and wakes often at 3 or 4 a.m., having a hard time going back to sleep. She has been extremely resistant to both new child care providers, crying intensely when left with them and stating, "I want Ella [Graciela]!" She refuses to play games that she formerly enjoyed with Graciela with anyone else. She frequently refuses food and becomes distraught when any adult does something in the home that is inconsistent with the way Graciela would have done it. She has stated on several occasions when upset that she wants to "go Me-co [go to Mexico]."

When the IMH worker suggests to Brad and Linda that Mona is experiencing difficulties in grieving the loss of Graciela as would be expected, they are at first shocked, because it had seemed to them that her grief was excessive. However, on further reflection, they come to recognize that their own need to minimize Graciela's importance to Mona has left her alone. They had expected Mona to accept a replacement caregiver in a way they would never have expected if she had lost one of her parents. As they consider this possibility with the IMH worker, they realize that they have avoided the subject for two reasons: (a) guilt over not being able to protect Mona from loss and (b) shame regarding the disparity between their family's economic privilege and Graciela's economic vulnerability. In discussing possible goals and objectives for treatment, Jack and Linda realize that their own minimization of Graciela's importance to Mona has left her alone with her sorrow. They request the IMH worker's help in supporting Mona through a mourning process.

DC:0–5 diagnosis: Complicated Grief Disorder of Infancy/Early Childhood

DSM–5 diagnosis: Other Specified Trauma- and Stressor-Related Disorder

ICD–10–CM code: F43.8: Other Reactions to Severe Stress

Relational Clinical Formulation

The identified client, a 2-year-old White girl, has recently lost an important attachment figure—the provider who had cared for her since birth—and meets criteria for a diagnosis of Complicated Grief Disorder of Infancy/Early Childhood. The client is frequently distraught; seeks her lost caregiver; refuses the ministrations of other caregivers; and demonstrates regression regarding previously established sleep, eating, and toileting routines. These symptoms and behaviors worry her parents a great deal and have presented barriers to establishing a new care context, because prospective child care providers find these behaviors challenging to manage. The family faces financial and logistical stresses as a result of the upheaval to the household routine, leading to employment strain for the parents. The client will likely benefit from participating in weekly IMH sessions together with her parents as collateral partners. The purpose of the sessions will be to resolve the client's grief and restore her to her former level of developmental functioning by strengthening Parent–Child Relationship Competency (PCRC) 18.

Goal: Resolve grief by strengthening PCRC 18.

Sample collaboratively generated objectives include the following:

1. The client's parents report feeling baffled by the client's current developmental and behavioral difficulties. During each weekly triadic IMH session over the course of the next 3 months, the client's parents will verbally identify at least one plausible meaning (based on their emerging understanding of social–emotional development) for the client's behavior in the moment.

2. The client's parents have imagined that talking about the absent caregiver would increase the client's distress, and so they have entirely avoided mentioning her in the client's presence, likely exacerbating the client's frightening sense that the caregiver has completely disappeared. The client's parents will report engaging in at least one activity per day with the client over the course of the next 2 months to acknowledge, remember, and honor the caregiver (e.g., look at pictures of her, write letters to her, talk about things they love about her) and to reassure the client that the caregiver is okay.

3. The client's parents report that they have not acknowledged the magnitude of the client's loss, instead conveying to her that she is overreacting, which likely compounds her sense of isolation. In the course of the

next 2 months, the parents will report acknowledging the reasons for the client's grief (e.g., "You love Graciela, and you miss her so much.") at least three times per day when the client cries or seeks the absent caregiver.

4. The client will accept emotional comfort from her parents either in play themes (e.g., bringing baby dolls to them for tending) or physically (e.g., cuddling when feeling sad) at least one time per each weekly IMH session, as observed by the clinician over the course of the next 3 months.

5. The client's help-rejecting behaviors with her new caregiver will reduce from 10 times per day to two times per day by [date] per the parents' report.

6. Incidents of the client refusing sleep (presently occurring 7 days per week) will cease within 6 months per the parents' report.

Vignette 18.2

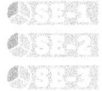 A social worker associated with an obstetrics practice contacts the IMH clinic with a referral. She explains that a tragedy has befallen a 27-year-old pregnant woman in their care: Her partner was shot and killed 1 month ago. "Needless to say, she is devastated," the social worker reports. "I am really worried because she used to be very engaged in her prenatal care, but she has stopped coming in for her check-ups." She explains that during a recent outreach phone call to the patient following a missed appointment, she declined to reschedule but did give permission to be contacted by the IMH worker, who schedules a home visit.

Salina is at the beginning of her third trimester of pregnancy. Her partner was a victim of community violence—he was shot and killed apparently randomly. Since his death, Salina describes that she has had a hard time getting out of bed or feeling motivated to do anything. Whereas she had been excited about the coming baby, she now feels "un-pregnant." She knows she should eat "for its sake," but she has no appetite. She denies suicidal ideation but says in response to the IMH worker's inquiry, "I'm not going to kill myself, but I wish they had killed me along with him." She has barely left her apartment since the funeral.

DSM−5 diagnosis: Major Depressive Disorder, single episode, severe, with peripartum onset

ICD−10−CM code: F32.2

Relational Clinical Formulation

The client is a 27-year-old pregnant woman who has recently suffered the traumatic loss of her partner, the father of the expected baby. She meets criteria for a diagnosis of Major Depressive Disorder, as evidenced by low mood, loss of appetite, anhedonia, fatigue, psychomotor retardation, hypersomnia, and a pervasive sense of hopelessness. Her capacity to feel excited about the birth of the expected baby is impaired, and she has been avoiding prenatal care. Despite these challenges, she exhibits protective impulses toward the expected baby. For example, she states wishing to be able to eat for the sake of the expected baby and avoiding medication for fear that it would be harmful to the baby. Twice-weekly home-based IMH services are recommended to strengthen PCRC 18 in support of the client's preparation for parenthood.

Goal: Decrease symptoms of depression by strengthening PCRC 18.

Sample collaboratively generated objectives include the following:

1. The client avoids prenatal care appointments, likely because focusing on the expected baby is a traumatic reminder of her lost partner. The client will identify in twice-weekly meetings with the IMH worker over the next 2 weeks things that might make it tolerable for

her to attend a prenatal care appointment (e.g., being accompanied by a friend, alerting obstetrics staff to avoid asking her certain questions).

2. The client states that she has not consulted a psychiatrist about her symptoms of depression because she assumed that psychotropic medication would be counterindicated during pregnancy. The client will consult with a psychiatrist to discuss possible risks and benefits of medication by [date].

3. The client is, at present, very isolated, which is likely exacerbating her depression. During twice weekly meetings with the IMH worker over the next month, the client will identify people she might want to make contact with who could support her when her baby is born.

4. Because of the depression-related feeling that "nothing matters," the client has avoided making a birth plan, which exposes her to the risk of being further disempowered during labor and delivery. The client will collaborate with her obstetrics social worker to develop a birth plan by [date].

5. The client's depression-related hypersomnia is reflected in her sleeping an average of 16 hours per day at present. This symptom will decrease such that the client sleeps an average of 8 hours per day by [date].

CHAPTER 20

PCRC 19—Efficacy: The Importance of Being Someone Who Can Make a Meaningful Contribution

Along with a few other young black men, Jude had gone down to the shack where they were hiring. Three old colored men had already been hired, but not for the road work, just to do the picking up, food bringing and other small errands....it was a shame to see those white men laughing with the grandfathers but shying away from the young black men who could tear that road up....Jude himself longed to be taken. Not just for the good money, more for the work itself. He wanted to swing the pick or kneel down with the string or shovel the gravel....More than anything he wanted the camaraderie of the road men: the lunch buckets, the hollering, the body movement that in the end produced something real, something he could point to. "I built that road," he could say.

—Toni Morrison (1973, pp. 81–82)

PCRC 19: Parent has the ability to work or otherwise contribute to society/the world AND child shows developmentally expectable signs of a sense of **efficacy**, confidence, and competence.

Parent–Child Relationship Competency (PCRC) 19 posits a link between the parent's ability to engage meaningfully with the wider world and the development of that same sense of efficacy in the child. The fundamental contention is that people suffer when internal or external barriers prevent them from contributing positively to relationships, society, and the world, and this experience affects the children.

P-5 2

The forms that individual contributions may take are literally infinite. Volunteering as a crossing guard before and after school hours in one's neighborhood may be the activity that satisfies this need in one person, whereas the next person's psychological need to contribute is met by pursuing particular activities such voting, recycling, or singing in a group.

Community activities or religious or social service organizations often provide opportunities for meaningful engagement. The majority of people may find more individual ways of making contributions. For some people, the form is altruism; for others, artistic expression; for others, activities that provide a sense of being one among a number with others; and for some, it is a solitary activity. This need does not have to be productive in any dramatic or obvious way. Simply building a sand castle that will be washed away with the tide may serve this need. Some people are psychologically organized such that much of their self-esteem is bound up only with being recognized as making a contribution. For others, recognition may be incidental or perhaps even uncomfortable. What matters is the sense that meaningful engagement occurs, whatever the form or scale.

One's employment may or may not satisfy the urge to contribute to society and the world. People often feel that the work they do is meaningless or injurious, perhaps even pitted against the greater good in some way. Employment is unavoidably political, and patterns of social injustice perpetuate barriers to access, opportunity, and mobility along absolutely predictable lines. It is important to be aware of this injustice as a frame for appreciating the status and stresses of those with whom we work. In a report titled *Systemic Inequality: How America's Structural Racism Helped Create the Black/White Wealth Gap*, Hanks, Solomon, and Weller (2018) documented the history of the wealth gap between Black and White Americans and noted that

Tenet # 3:
Work to Acknowledge Privilege and Combat Discrimination

persistent labor market discrimination and segregation...force blacks into fewer and less advantageous employment opportunities than their white counterparts. Thus, African Americans have less access to stable jobs, good wages, and retirement benefits at work—all key drivers by which American families gain access to savings. (p. 1)

Hanks et al. (2018) further noted that "Hispanic families have only slightly more wealth than black families" (p. 2). Social injustice is organized along all axes of difference such that people endure employment discrimination and economic inequity on the basis of gender, sexual orientation, immigration status, ability status, age, and other identity markers. It is important to consider these powerful impediments in dealing with every family and to take what actions one can toward social justice.

Tenet # 10:
Advance Policy
That Supports
All Families

Having the capacity to provide for one's child is, after all, a core concern for most parents. However, for many working people, jobs come along not with benefits but instead with hidden costs. This concept is captured by the powerful lyrics to the song "More Than a Paycheck" by Ysaye M. Barnwell of the group Sweet Honey in the Rock (1983, track 5): "We bring more than a paycheck to our loved ones and family. We bring asbestosis, silicosis, brown lung, black lung disease. And radiation hits the children before they've even been conceived." The chilling specter of work-related hazards harming children prenatally is captured in Juana Alicia's 1983 mural *Las Lechugueras*, which depicts a pregnant migrant worker laboring in a field that is being sprayed with pesticides by a prop plane (Jacoby, 2009, pp. 36–37).

Work-related injury and illness are issues parents in many circumstances must face and endure. Children are affected materially and psychologically by their parents' sense of what work offers them. Young toddlers often delight in handling dustpans and brooms, buckets, and rakes as much as any toy. They imitate the necessary task-oriented behaviors they see their parents doing. Furthermore, they note the particular spirit in which a parent leaves for work (i.e., whether it is with a sense of dread, burden, or pleasant anticipation) and how a parent feels when returning home.

D. W. Winnicott (1963/1965a) theorized that very young infants have a psychological need to "contribute-in" within their relationships with primary caregivers. He suggested that when all goes well enough and caregivers are able to convey that what the baby "offers" to them is received and valued, the baby develops confidence in her ability to contribute-in. In Winnicott's words, the baby's "growing confidence that there will be opportunity for contributing-in, for giving...

provides one of the fundamental constructive elements of play and work" (p. 77).

What infants can offer—the particular way in which they contribute-in—is not quantifiable or necessarily even observable, but it is felt and understood between the infant and the parent that something valuable has been offered and accepted. Perhaps an infant's appreciative gurgle while nursing leads her mother to say, "I'm glad you like it!" Or perhaps a toddler adds her shoe to the line of shoes sitting by the front door or calls out "ding dong!" when the doorbell rings, and the family enjoys this demonstration of his game participation in family life. In a different mode, toddlers distribute their blocks or raisins to people who are gathered in the room. Often, if another baby is crying, a mobile infant will crawl over and try to do something about it.

Although the act of contributing-in may be a helpful or game action such as the previous examples, it may also be a subtler form of communication and participation in the ongoing relational flow of the family. The critical ingredients are a spontaneous expression on the part of the child that is seen and responded to by the parent such that the child feels her impact. Such exchanges produce in the child a sense of efficacy, confidence, and competence. The baby develops a sense that they have an effect on other people that is valued and that they can do this volitionally and well: "What I do matters. I am felt and seen."

Winnicott (1957/1965b) postulated that the infant's later capacities to derive satisfaction from play and to work are based in part on building up sufficient experiences of being a person with something to offer that is valued. He imagined a set of concentric circles with the infant at the center and the wide world at the periphery. Winnicott wrote,

> The existence of a family and the maintenance of a family atmosphere result from the relationship between the parents in the social setting in which they live. What the parents can "contribute-in" to the family that they are building up depends a great deal on their general relationship to the wider circle around them, their immediate social setting. One can think of ever-widening circles, each social group depending for what it is like inside on its relation to another outside social group. (p. 41)

This image of concentric circles makes clear the degree to which threat from the outer circles directed at parents—for example, racial targeting for criminalization or xenophobic policies leading to threats of deportation—can undermine parents' capacities to work or contribute to society and the world, which is likely to reverberate in the inner circle of the family and can thwart a developing infant's sense of efficacy, confidence, and competence. When PCRC 19 is functioning well, even parents contending with extreme stress or oppression feel that avenues are open to them for meaningful engagement, and they are able to register and benefit from their children's offerings, promoting in their children a sense of confidence in their power to have a positive effect on their parents despite adversity.

When this PCRC is not functioning well, there is a role for the infant mental health (IMH) worker in helping families mitigate adverse effects of these "concentric circle" difficulties. P-5 6 The child is likely to feel helpless in the helplessness of his parents. The baby is infected by what ails the parents. This condition is part of why we are not working with either separately—the unit needs care. Intervention at the level of any of the concentric circles may be warranted—for example, advocacy around employment discrimination that is threatening a family's financial stability, treating parental depression secondary to being blocked from opportunities to contribute to society and the world, or working to amplify a baby's attempts to contribute-in and addressing impediments to parents' capacities to receive and value the baby's gifts.

Vignette 19.1

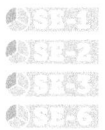

The mental health consultant at Nuevo Dia child care center refers 3-year-old Marisol and her mother, Anna, to an IMH clinic because they are at risk of losing their subsidized spot at the center because of low attendance. "I've really advocated on their behalf with the director because I know the family needs child care, but the center can only stretch so far. The bottom line is 'use it or lose it.' I have tried to explain this to Anna, and she says she understands, but then she calls saying Marisol is sick, or they just don't show up. And sometimes when they do come, Marisol gets so upset at drop-off that Anna ends up not leaving her at the center." When the bilingual–bicultural Cuban American IMH worker meets with Anna, she learns that the family is contending with chronic fear because they are undocumented immigrants from Guatemala and Marisol's father, Fernando's, current job requires that he drive his employer's truck on a regular basis. Anna is afraid that Fernando will be pulled over by the police and deported. She wants him to seek employment with the janitorial service she works for, which does not require driving. Fernando feels that it is his responsibility to provide for his family, and he earns more at his present job than he would working for the janitorial service. He feels he must tolerate the risk. Anna and Fernando argue about this topic frequently.

Anna reports that Marisol has difficulty falling asleep unless one of her parents lies down with her, and she frequently becomes distraught on waking if her father is not home.

She often complains of stomachaches in the morning and expresses reluctance or fear about going to school, which mounts to highly distressed crying on a regular basis when Anna attempts to leave her at Nuevo Dia.

DC:0–5 diagnosis: Separation Anxiety Disorder

DSM–5 diagnosis: Separation Anxiety Disorder

ICD–10–CM code: F93.0

Relational Clinical Formulation

The identified client is a 3-year-old Latina girl who meets criteria for a diagnosis of Separation Anxiety Disorder, as evidenced by becoming highly distressed at the prospect of separating from her parents, fighting sleep, school refusal, and somatic symptoms (stomachaches when facing separation). These difficulties strain family relationships, restrict school attendance (thus limiting opportunities for learning and engaging in growth-promoting experiences), and involve a high degree of stress and emotional pain for the client and her family. The client's school placement is at risk as a result of low attendance, and dismissal would undermine the client's mother's capacity to work. Contributing to the client's worry about separation is the real threat of deportation with which the family contends. The parents are in a catch-22: They must work to provide for the family, but working exposes them to the risk of deportation and forced separation. The client's anxiety is rooted in her awareness of these dangers, and it is amplified by her sense of powerlessness and unpredictability. These difficulties are best addressed in the context of the parent–child relationships so that the parents can develop strategies for increasing the client's sense of security despite the real dangers faced by the family. Treatment aimed at strengthening PCRC 19 is recommended, as an increase in client's sense of efficacy will likely lead to reduced anxiety. Collateral parent sessions not involving the client may be helpful to grapple with risk issues. Collateral meetings involving the parents and the mental health consultant as well as other child care staff members may be warranted to support school attendance.

Goal: Decrease the client's anxiety via strengthening PCRC 19.

Sample collaboratively generated objectives include the following:

1. The client's parents will report zero incidents per week of arguing within earshot of the client about the danger of family separation (current baseline: two to four incidents per week).

2. Within [specify time frame], the client's parents will develop an emergency family safety plan in keeping with National Traumatic Stress Network recommendations so that they know what steps to take in the event that a parent is detained.

3. At present, client's anxiety is exacerbated by feeling little capacity to have a positive effect. During each weekly IMH session in the course of the next [specify number] weeks, the client's parents will verbally identify actions that she takes that have a positive effect.

4. The parents and IMH worker will meet with the mental health consultant and client's teachers by [date] to develop intervention strategies teachers can use on a daily basis to increase client's sense of efficacy.

5. Client's worries that her father may disappear are heightened by her lack of knowledge regarding his comings and goings. The parents will report informing the client on a daily basis at bedtime about the father's schedule for leaving for work and returning home the next day.

6. Incidents of the client crying on waking will decrease to one to two per month within [specify number] months (current baseline: three to four per week) per the parents' report.

7. The client's school attendance will increase from 2 to 3 days per week to 5 days per week by [date] per the child care consultant's report.

Vignette 19.2

Gerome, who is 26 years old, and his 18-month-old son, Billy, are referred to an IMH clinic by the case manager at the transitional housing facility where they reside. Gerome is in recovery and has recently assumed custody of Billy following a period of child welfare involvement. Billy's mother, Mary, resides in a different state. She is addicted to heroin and has lost reunification services. The case manager reports, "I'm worried about Gerome. Since Billy has been living with him, he has stopped going to 12-Step meetings as consistently, even though we provide child care for that. He doesn't want to let the kid out of his sight, but pretty much all they do, as far as I can tell, is watch TV in their room. We try to get him to bring Billy to activities, but he just isolates with the kid." When the IMH worker meets with Gerome, he learns that Gerome is very worried about being judged negatively in relation to his parenting of Billy. He is afraid he could lose custody of his son again, but he is also overwhelmed by the responsibility of parenting. He describes a couple of occasions in which Billy became dysregulated in public, and Gerome had a hard time comforting him and was afraid child protective services would be notified. "Seems best we stay in here," Gerome stated with a worried expression. Billy was meanwhile engaged in slipping plastic forks and spoons under the door of their room into the hallway. When Gerome becomes more comfortable with the IMH worker, he confides that he despairs of being able to stay sober and protect and provide for his son, and he dreads his time at the transitional housing facility running out. Together, they identify some objectives that Gerome believes would help him feel less daunted by the uncharted territory he faces.

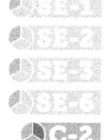

DSM–5 diagnosis: Adjustment Disorder with Anxiety

ICD–10–CM code: F43.22

Relational Clinical Formulation

The identified client is a 26-year-old White man in early recovery from polysubstance abuse who has recently assumed custody of his 18-month-old son. He is having difficulty adjusting to parenting and meets criteria for a diagnosis of Adjustment Disorder with Anxiety. He worries constantly about being judged negatively by others and ultimately losing custody of his son. These concerns lead him to avoid going out in public with his son. He is also very worried about being separated from his son, needing to reassure himself through constant proximity to the child. The dyad is primarily confined to their shared room in a transitional housing facility. This pattern is threatening the client's recovery, because he is not able to attend 12-Step meetings or other recovery-oriented activities. His anxiety-based withdrawal also prevents him from pursuing employment. His child is also missing out on opportunities for growth-promoting engagement with other people and environments. The client expresses worry that he will not succeed in maintaining his recovery, finding a way to earn a living, and raising his child. The client will benefit from services aimed at reducing anxiety by strengthening PCRC 19. It will be important to include the client's son in the treatment so that the client can increase comfort with parenting skills and the dyad can develop confidence together in their capacity to explore and contribute to the broader environment. Collateral involvement with transitional housing staff, child care staff, and recovery support people may be warranted to coordinate services around family adjustment.

Goal: Increase confidence in parenting and decrease anxiety via strengthening PCRC 19.

Sample collaboratively generated objectives include the following:

1. During each weekly IMH session in the course of the next [specify time frame], the client and his son will practice emerging from their room to explore the facility or the neighborhood together with the IMH worker.

2. When on his own in public with his son, the client will report remaining calm when his son is distressed, as evidenced by not fleeing to their room [specify number of times] by [specify date] (current baseline: zero).

3. The client will report attending [specify number] 12-Step meetings (and leaving son in child care) per week by [date] (current baseline: zero).

4. The client will report meeting with the case manager to review vocational programs by [date].

CHAPTER 21

PCRC 20—Reflective Functioning and the Capacity for Concern

Dear Daughter,

This letter has taken an extraordinary time getting itself together. I have all along known that I wanted to tell you directly some of the lessons I have learned and under what conditions I have learned them. My life has been long, and believing that life loves the liver of it, I have dared to try many things, sometimes trembling, but daring, still. I have only included here events and lessons that I have found useful. I have not told how I have used the solutions, knowing that you are intelligent and creative and resourceful and you will use them as you see fit.

—Maya Angelou (2008, p. xi)

PCRC 20: Parent is able to **reflect** upon/think about his or her own experience, including how his or her past experiences may be impacting his or her experiences as a parent and can recognize the child's experience as that of a separate person AND child shows developmentally expectable signs of experiencing him- or herself as a unique person with interest in and concern for others as separate people.

Parent–Child Relationship Competency (PCRC) 20 describes the parent's and child's developmentally grounded capacities to appreciate each other's separateness. As with all PCRCs, the ways in which this manifests are highly socioculturally variable. Some societies expect and foster a sense of individual subjectivity that is interdependent with and indivisible from connectedness with others, whereas other societ-ies prize and socialize for autonomy and independence (Bernstein, Harris, Long, lida, & Hans, 2005). Within this spectrum, PCRC 20 focuses on the degree to which a parent is able, in socioculturally meaningful ways, to recognize the child as a unique person, and the child is able, as develop-ment unfolds, to likewise see the parent as a unique person.

Attachment theorists have identified *reflective functioning* as an important ingredient in parents' capacities to interact with infants and young children in ways that promote secure attachment, which, in turn, is associated with many felicitous developmental outcomes (Fonagy, Steele, Steele, Moran, & Higgitt, 1991).

Reflective functioning is defined as "the essential human capacity to understand behavior in light of underlying men-tal states and intentions" (Slade, 2005, p. 269). Dan Siegel (2001) described *mindsight*, which is a similar capacity, as "the capacity of the mind to create a representation of the mind of others, and of the self" (p. 78). These conceptu-alizations describe intersubjective processes that are both ordinary and subtle. A parent's reflective functioning or mindsight supports their capacity to experience empathy for their child and carves out space for the child to grad-ually grow into themselves out of the neonatal state of complete dependence.

Winnicott (1952/1958) described this process from the baby's side. Winnicott famously asserted that "there is no such thing as a baby" (p. 99), meaning that a baby cannot be conceptualized separate from the caregiver who supports her existence and also that a baby does not initially experience herself as a separate person. Winnicott (1966/1987) wrote, "The important thing is that *I am* means nothing unless *I* at the beginning *am along with another human being* who has yet to be differentiated off" (p. 11). This process of the parent's becoming "differentiated off" as a separate person in the perception of the infant happens gradually in situations of health, according to Winnicott.

When all goes well enough, the baby develops what Winnicott (1963/1965a) called the *capacity for concern*, which is a state of recognition of the separateness of the parent that would have been too frightening for the child at an earlier stage of dependence and is—according to this theory—blessedly beyond the scope of imagination of the neonate.

Although these processes are ordinary, they do represent important psychological and interpersonal achievements, and they are not to be taken for granted. For example, Abram (1996) described a situation in which difficulties arise in the area of a parent's capacity to appreciate her infant's separateness, and the resulting confusion for the developing child. Abram wrote,

> *It is not the infant's responsibility if the mother is persecuted by his crying. However, if the mother is continually persecuted by her infant's needs because of her own difficulties, the infant is likely to grow up convinced that he is responsible for his mother's feelings.* (p. 100)

A parent feeling "persecuted" in this way by a dependent infant would be an example of a deficit of reflective functioning, because if the parent had recourse to reflective functioning, they would recognize the infant's needs as a developmental phenomenon rather than a personal attack or indictment. In Winnicott's (1963/1965a) own words, "I am trying to describe what happens between mothers and their babies and between parents and their children when there is no separation" (p. 77).

Everyone has moments when our reflective capacities abandon us and also some themes or realms of experience are more opaque to reflection than others. In such moments and instances, it is challenging for us to fully appreciate the "otherness" of other people; we tend to feel that they are to blame for our struggles or that their struggles define our existence. For most people, such collapsed moments pass, and interpersonal relating between two separate subjects is restored.

When parents have chronic and global difficulties with reflective functioning, this issue is often part and parcel of a problematic pattern of personal and interpersonal challenge. Sometimes, people habitually feel themselves to be at the mercy of others' realities or that other people are extensions of themselves, and they deal in action rather than reflection. These types of patterns create trying circumstances for those in their sphere. Infants and developing children are especially vulnerable to bearing the burden of parents' deficits in reflective functioning, because they are primed by virtue of their dependence to organize themselves around their attachment figures. Therefore, the infant described earlier whose mother feels persecuted by his needs is likely to experience himself, as he develops, as injurious and to build that idea of himself into his sense of who he is as a person.

These types of interpersonal patterns can create difficulties for children, because they tend (a) to apply to new relation-ships the "rules" or templates for interacting that they have learned with parents and (b) to present themselves to others as they have come to experience themselves to be with their parents. Infant mental health (IMH) workers can interrupt these types of problematic patterns, supporting parents to de-personalize some of the most trying aspects of caregiv-ing, to open up routes to empathy, to expand their capacities for reflection, to deepen their understanding of develop-ment, and to sharpen their perceptiveness regarding their child's unique and separate subjectivity.

P-5 2

Efforts toward these ends will also open pathways for the child to experience himself independently—for example, to understand that it is not dangerous or harmful to have a perspective that is different from their parent's or that a parent's ill humor does not need to dampen their own high spirits. Sometimes, an IMH worker can help a parent to construct a narrative about their own challenges that will be developmentally meaningful to the child. A parent who struggles with bouts of depression, for example, might say to a child, "Sometimes, I do not feel well, and you notice that I am different, and I don't play with you so much. I love you all the time, even when I don't feel well. When I don't feel well, Grandma takes care of me so that I can get better and play with you again." A reflective narrative such as this one can support the child toward ultimately understanding that their subjectivity is interconnected with but differentiated from that of the parent. This awareness enables the development of the capacity for concern, which is the foundation for the child's caring relationship with the world.

> **Tenet # 6:**
> Understand That Language Can Hurt or Heal

Vignette 20.1

The mental health consultant at Parkside Preschool refers Pedro, a 26-month-old boy of Mexican descent, to the IMH clinic because of developmental and behavioral concerns. She reports that teachers in the 2-year-olds' classroom are having a hard time managing Pedro's behaviors, and she is concerned that his parents, Jorge and Maryella, may be interacting with him in ways that are not helpful. The IMH worker, who is of Mexican descent and who is bilingual–bicultural herself, meets with Jorge and Maryella, who grant her permission to observe Pedro in the classroom and to meet with his teachers and the mental health consultant. Following this assessment, the worker meets with Maryella and Pedro at home several times.

The IMH worker hears and sees that Pedro is a very active, highly physical toddler and that his impulsive and chaotic behaviors are leading to difficulties at home and at school. She observes Pedro throw crackers across the table at snack time and then run around the room screeching when his teacher invites him to join her in picking them up; attempt to climb the bookshelf in the book corner as though it were a ladder; and grab a toy car that another little boy is playing with and then say "no, no!" reflexively when teachers attempt to engage him in conversation. At home, Pedro displays similar disruptive and avoidant behaviors. In both settings, the IMH worker has the sense that Pedro is anxious about his own behaviors and the negative feedback he gets from caregivers, but he appears unable to slow himself down. In fact, his anxiety about caregivers' disapproval and anger seems to escalate his frenzied activity level and send him running away from them.

Maryella reports that she and Jorge argue frequently about Pedro and that she feels blamed by Jorge, who thinks she is spoiling Pedro and that he needs to learn to behave or he will "end up in jail." She explains that several of Jorge's male relatives are incarcerated. Although the family attends church on a regular basis, they avoid participating in church-related activities because they feel embarrassed about Pedro's behavior in comparison with other children his age. Maryella worries that perhaps Pedro is "confused" because he is being raised bilingually, and the "American teachers" at the school do not know how to teach children to be "respectful."

The IMH worker tells Maryella that she believes Pedro wishes very much to be able to comply with the adults' expectations of him and to play with the other children but that he has a condition some children suffer from that makes calming down and cooperating very challenging. She states that she does not think that bilingualism is a problem for Pedro—on the contrary, it is a source of richness in his life—but that sometimes there are cultural differences among grown-ups that can indeed be confusing for children. She also states that Latino boys and men are sometimes misperceived by those outside their culture as being aggressive, so it is very important to help others understand that Pedro is struggling to control his impulses and needs help; he is not trying to hurt others. She proposes weekly home-based IMH sessions with regular meetings with school personnel so that everyone can arrive at a common understanding about Pedro's challenges and can help Pedro learn to accept help from others in calming down, waiting, and taking turns.

Maryella discusses this with Jorge, and the parents agree to this proposal.

DC:0–5 diagnosis: Overactivity Disorder of Toddlerhood

DSM–5 diagnosis: Attention Deficit Hyperactivity Disorder, predominantly hyperactive–impulsive presentation

ICD–10–CM code: F90.1: Disturbance of Activity and Attention

Relational Clinical Formulation

The identified client is a 26-month-old boy of Mexican descent who meets criteria for a diagnosis of Overactivity Disorder of Toddlerhood, as evidenced by his extremely high level of agitation, impulsivity, and physical activity. These behaviors strain his relationships with peers and teachers at school as well as with his parents, and the family's social life is restricted as a result. Client appears not to be able to reflect before taking action, and he seems baffled by and anxious about the ways others respond to him, apparently lacking an understanding of his impact on others. The client is at risk of developing a negative self-image and is avoidant of interpersonal engagement as a result of the frequent interpersonal discord and punitive responses that he encounters. He is also at risk of being misperceived as aggressive rather than impulsive in the context of racism toward Latino males. The client will likely benefit from home-based IMH services (together with his parents as collateral partners) aimed at expanding his capacity to reflect rather than act and to rely on others for help rather than fleeing interactions with caregivers. Collateral meetings with the mental health consultant and other school personnel will also likely be important in order to develop helpful strategies that may be implemented at school.

Goal: Reduce impulsivity and increase self-calming capacities by strengthening PCRC 20.

Sample collaboratively generated objectives include the following:

1. The client attempts to move physically away from adults when they call his name 100% of the time. The client will allow his mother to get physically close to him without resistance four out of five times by [date] per the mother's report.

2. The client's mother reports almost always feeling blindsided by the client's impulsive behaviors. During each weekly IMH meeting over the next 3 months, the client's mother will identify early signs that the client may be about to act impulsively at least one time.

3. At present, the mother reports never engaging in connected calming-down strategies together with the client, instead threatening separation by attempting to put him on time-outs when he engages in disruptive behavior. The client's mother will report practicing calming-down strategies with the client, such as blowing a pinwheel at the first sign that the client is "revving up" five times per day over the course of the next 3 months.

4. At present, the mother reports having no strategies to engage with the client proactively around his impulsivity, instead intervening after he acts out. During each weekly home-based IMH meeting, the client's mother will practice mutually pleasurable proactive inhibition response activities with the client (e.g., "Simon Says").

5. At present, the client engages in disruptive behaviors in the classroom 10 times per school day. Incidents of disruptive behavior will reduce to one to two per school day per the teacher's report by [date].

Vignette 20.2

Shirley, a 28-year-old White woman, calls the IMH clinic requesting "support." She has three young children: Bo, 9 months old; Angie, 2 years old; and Manny, 3½ years old.

In response to the IMH worker's inquiries about presenting problems, Shirley is not able to be more specific than having her "hands full" with three young children. During a home-based assessment period that also involves several trips into the community, the IMH worker learns that each of the children has a different father, but none of these men are directly involved in the children's lives, although Manny's father pays child support, and Shirley is involved in court proceedings attempting to secure child support from the other two men. Shirley informs the IMH worker that she is currently dating a man in her building, but this relationship is secret because he is married to another woman and has a child with her. Shirley's financial resources are meager, but she is quite familiar with the community and social service resources available to her, organizing the family's days around accessing soup kitchens and other free services and activities. She takes pride in her ability to make use of these resources, and the family is well known to many providers. She states coyly, "We are stars!"

Although Shirley has a hard time articulating specific areas of concern, the IMH worker observes patterns of interaction with the children that seem problematic. Shirley is clearly happiest when the whole family is in physical contact—for example, on the sofa watching cartoons or squeezed into a single seat on the bus, almost like an amoeba. She tends to thwart the children's impulses for independent activity—for example, becoming subtly punishing or expressing mock injury—when Manny moves to play on his own. She is breastfeeding Bo and tends to initiate breastfeeding in response to a range of expressions from Bo, some of which might be more fruitfully responded to with verbal interactions or play. She has rigid ideas about gender differences, referring to Angie as "Mommy's little helper" and imploring her frequently to share in caregiving tasks, even though she is younger than Manny. She has many somatic complaints, and she often puts the children in a psychological bind by encouraging physical contact and then complaining of aches and pains. When the IMH worker inquires about the possibility of accessing group care for some or all of the children, Shirley says, "I've looked into that, but you hear such bad things about what happens to kids in child care. I'd rather keep them safe with me."

At the same time, Shirley expresses a sense of being overrun by her children, and when in public, she will often seek sympathy from and enlist the aid of strangers—for example, asking for "a hand" lifting the stroller. She seems in such moments to be broadcasting her wish for male partnership. She is quite preoccupied with her single status, talking with the IMH worker in the children's presence about longing to be in a relationship and feeling betrayed and mistreated by all the children's fathers. The IMH worker notices that Manny tends to become dysregulated and aggressive toward Angie when the conversation goes in this direction.

The IMH worker arranges a feedback session with Shirley alone and describes some of the patterns she has observed. She suggests that Shirley has learned some ways of be-ing that undoubtedly developed for good reasons but that may not be serving her and her children well. She states that she has heard the theme of loneliness in what Shirley has shared with her, and she thinks that Shirley may use her children as a buffer against loneliness, which may be ham-pering the children's development by encouraging them to remain more dependent on her than is best for them. She explains that this pattern can easily take hold for parents who have experienced challenges and disappointments in relationships such as Shirley has described in her own per-sonal history. She proposes that they meet together with the children to examine these patterns and work to foster each child's individual developmental path in the best pos-sible way, with one-on-one sessions scheduled as needed to discuss grown-up topics such as dating. Shirley agrees to this, and together they develop treatment objectives reflecting the overarching goals of enhancing reflective functioning and celebrating each family member's auton-omy and uniqueness.

DSM–5 diagnosis: Dependent Personality Disorder

ICD–10–CM code: F60.7

Relational Clinical Formulation

The identified client, a 28-year-old White woman, meets criteria for a diagnosis of Dependent Personality Disorder, as evidenced by her extreme avoidance of being alone; her pervasive sense that others are to blame for her circumstances; her pattern of going to great lengths to receive care, sustenance, and approval from others; and her preoccupation with perceived abandonment. These patterns play out with her children in ways that hamper their development, deprive them of potentially growth-promoting experiences, and put them at risk of likewise developing problematic patterns of relating. The client's capacity to reflect on and alter such patterns would likely be enhanced by IMH services that include her children as collateral partners so that developmentally appropriate independence can be fostered for all family members. Weekly home- and community-based IMH services aimed at strengthening PCRC 20 are recommended.

Goal: Increase tolerance for reflection, separation, and independence by strengthening PCRC 20.

Sample collaboratively generated objectives include the following:

1. The client redirects her children toward interaction with her when they initiate independent exploration several times per each weekly IMH session. The client will verbally acknowledge to the IMH worker one such incident during each weekly IMH session over the course of the next 3 months.

2. Within 6 months, the client will be able to support each child in one developmentally appropriate independent activity during each weekly IMH session.

3. At present, the client reports not being able to tolerate being alone "even long enough to go to the bathroom by myself" and instead keeps her children with her at all times. The client will report being able to enjoy being alone for an interval of 1 hour while her children are safely in the care of someone else by [date].

4. At present, the client's extreme avoidance of separation prevents her from considering potentially growth-promoting early care and education settings available to her children. The client will visit three child care sites or preschools and discuss their potential merits with the IMH worker by [date].

AFTERWORD

Reflective Supervision, Transference–Countertransference, and the Unique Singularity of Each Practitioner in the Relational Matrix

The Parent–Child Relationship Competencies (PCRCs) are bidirectional, unfolding between parents and children, but they take shape in a multidirectional, relational context. For example, James McHale (e.g., McHale, 2007; McHale & Fivaz-Depeursinge, 2010) has emphasized the degree to which an individual's parenting style and capacities are affected by their co-parenting relationships. Furthermore, many researchers have noted how influential the provider relationship is on parents and families and—also, in a parallel fashion—how supervisor–supervisee relationships influence the therapist–client or provider–family relationship (Frawley-O'Dea & Sarnat, 2001; Heffron & Murch, 2010, 2012). Infant mental health (IMH) work tends to stir powerful transference–countertransference dynamics (Wright, 1992), and reflective supervision can be a critical ingredient for ensuring ethical and appropriate practice and preventing secondary traumatization and other hazards. A growing body of research attests to the powerful beneficial effects of embedding reflective supervision and consultation in IMH services and systems (Eggbeer, Shahmoon-Shanok, & Clark, 2010). Appendix I—Questions to Guide Reflection—offers a series of reflective prompts that might aid supervisors and consultants in integrating the PCRCs with supervisees.

P-5 3

Tenet # 8:
Allocate Resources to Systems Change

One thing that is often stressed in discussions of reflective supervision in the context of IMH work is the concept of *parallel process.* It is suggested that the supervisor should interact with the IMH worker in ways one hopes the IMH worker will interact with the parent, in the hopes that the parent, in turn, will then interact in these ways with the child. This model, which we might call the "nesting doll" model of supervision, holds great merit. There is probably no better method of learning new ways of interacting than to experience them directly in the context of a relationship.

However, this model also has some limitations, because it suggests a hierarchical, unidirectional flow of influence, with the supervisor at the top and the child at the bottom. Of course, it is important to acknowledge that supervision, intervention, and family life all exist within power structures and to recognize who holds what power where. However, it is also important to be aware that there are many forms of power and influence. Children teach parents a great deal, parents teach IMH workers, and supervisors learn from IMH workers. Much of what supervisors offer may have value, surely, but IMH workers and families likely bring important life experiences and knowledge bases to which the supervisor does not have access. Hernández and McDowell (2010) wrote,

> Supervision informed by a critical postcolonial perspective disputes theories and practices that reproduce the status quo of inequities generated and maintained by the cultural and social capital of dominant groups. The cultural knowledge and life experiences of clients and supervisees is centered alongside developing field knowledge, supporting cultural democracy within the microsystems of therapy and supervision. (p. 29)

Also, it must be acknowledged that not only good things flow from supervisors to cascade through the tiers of influence. Problematic things—for example, prejudices, biases, blind spots, unresolved conflicts, ungrieved losses, harmful patterns of identification and disidentification—can also issue from the supervisor, complicating or imperiling the IMH work. It is critical that these processes be acknowledged and subjected to analysis and challenge just as much as other forces that may put a worker or a family at risk or negatively affect the work (Noroña et al., 2012). Supervisors must not be left out when plans are made for embedding a matrix for reflection in a program or system of care. Supervisors also require and deserve opportunities for consultation: thinking and talking with another person in the service of deepening personal awareness so as to expand professional competence.

Ken Hardy has described the process of personal and professional development that led him to develop the *Multicultural Relational Perspective*—"a worldview that provides an in-depth and comprehensive framework for clinical supervision" (Hardy & Bobes, 2017, p. 4). He stated that clinical necessity led him to act in ways that were

> *counter to how I'd been trained and how I was supposed to conduct therapy at the clinic....I was finding a voice that had been dormant during my formal training, with its narrow focus on diagnostic thinking and psychological functioning.* (Hardy & Bobes, 2017, p. 27)

This voice was embodied and socially located, the voice of an African American man, whose clinical skill led him beyond the strictures of therapist non-self-disclosure into which he had been indoctrinated. Instead, he recognized the clinical and ethical imperative of addressing the African American father with whom he was speaking in a way that explicitly acknowledged some of their shared experiences—as well as some points of difference—as African American men and family members in a racist society. As a result of this process, Hardy and Bobes (2017) arrived at the following core principles of supervision from the Multicultural Relational Perspective:

- The centrality of relationships and the notion that human suffering is located within relationships;
- Cultural factors are salient contextual variables in our lives and must be attended to with humility, sensitivity, and competence;

- Our understanding of sociocultural trauma and the hidden wounds associated with it are essential to clinical effectiveness;

- An acute exploration of the self of the therapist and the self of the supervisor are critical issues to the provision of effective therapy and supervision; and

- Clinicians explore and understand the role that their biases (conscious and otherwise) may have on therapy and supervision (pp. 4–5).

The concept of the "acute exploration of the self of the therapist and the self of the supervisor" supports the vision of "cultural democracy in the microcosms of therapy and supervision" articulated by Hernández and McDowell (2010) earlier. Clearly, supervisors have power and responsibilities by virtue of their role that necessitates caution. The supervisory context is not an even playing field, and its primary purpose is to support the supervisee in the service of their clinical work. However, whereas this method has historically meant that the supervisor remains disembodied and cloaked behind a veneer of professional distance, these insights garnered from critical race theory and postcolonial theory demand a disciplined examination and use of the supervisor's singular embodiment and social location. Twenty years ago, we wrote a book titled *How You Are Is as Important as What You Do...in Making a Positive Difference for Infants, Toddlers, and Their Families* (Pawl & St. John, 1998). We continue to believe this assertion to be true and easily lost sight of. In addition, we have come to understand that *who* you are is also of vital importance—that the IMH worker's and the supervisor's embodied and socially located experiences must be recognized, reflected on, and factored in.

These principles are very much in keeping with the *Diversity-Informed Tenets for Work With Infants, Children, and Families* (© Irving Harris Foundation; hereafter, "the Tenets"; see www.diversityinformedtenets.org). In closing, it is important to return to the Tenets and to consider once again Tenet #8:

"*Allocate Resources to Systems Change: Diversity and inclusion must be proactively considered when doing any work with or on behalf of infants, children, and families. Resource allocation includes time, money, additional/alternative practices, and other supports and accommodations, otherwise systems of oppression may be inadvertently reproduced. Individuals, organizations, and systems of care need ongoing opportunities for reflection in order to identify implicit bias, remove barriers, and work to dismantle the root causes of disparity and inequity.*"

This book is very much about resources. The PCRCs are natural resources belonging to children and parents that support health, development, and well-being. The preceding chapters have sought to illustrate how IMH workers can direct their efforts at strengthening the PCRCs as needed. As such, it is hoped that this book will be a useful tool in the hands of those undertaking this important and challenging work. In addition, a primary focus of this volume is to equip workers and programs to be able to document their efforts in ways that readily facilitate being paid, and so it is intended as a resource for the workforce and the field.

Tenet #8 emphasizes the responsibility that everyone in the field has in making sure that resources are allocated in ways that further social justice. Because interlocking systems of oppression are continually reproduced in systems, institutions, discourses, and practices, even individuals, programs, and systems of care with the most altruistic intentions will find themselves complicit with reproducing injurious dynamics unless we incorporate the discipline of diversity- and inclusion-focused reflection into our daily work lives. Embedding diversity-informed reflective supervision and consultation into programs and systems can serve this function.

If this book helps to promote clarity and efficiency, liberate time for creative clinical efforts, and secure remuneration for IMH work—as it is hoped that it will—then let us direct these resources toward building in reflective structures and practices dedicated to advancing social justice.

Maria Seymour St. John and Jeree H. Pawl

APPENDIX A

The Parent–Child Relationship Competencies (PCRCs)

PCRC 1: Parent is able to register and respond effectively to child's **needs** AND child is able to signal needs clearly in keeping with age level.

PCRC 2: Parent is able to maintain his or her own **health and well-being**, promote child's health, and access pediatric (or other culturally meaningful) care as needed AND child is able to grow in keeping with developmental expectations and maintain physical health.

PCRC 3: Parent has the capacity to provide **safety, protection, and comfort** for child AND child seeks out and accepts comfort and protection from parent and has a developmentally expectable ability to register security, anxiety, and fear.

PCRC 4: Parent is able to be **emotionally attuned** to/empathize with child AND child is able to experience and express a developmentally expectable range of human emotion.

PCRC 5: Parent has the capacity to self-regulate and to engage in **mutual regulation** with child AND child is able to participate in mutual regulation with the parent and is developing the capacity to self-regulate.

PCRC 6: Parent has the capacity to identify, act on, and also control **impulses** sufficiently to have rewarding relationships and life experiences and can foster these abilities in child AND child demonstrates an age-expectable capacity to identify, act on, and also control impulses.

PCRC 7: Parent is able to pay attention and focus as needed and to engage child in attending and focusing AND child demonstrates a developmentally expectable capacity for

shared focus/mutual attention and is on a path toward being able to focus and attend on his or her own.

PCRC 8: Parent possesses and conveys to child reasonable confidence that many things can be figured out/worked out successfully AND child demonstrates age expectable **problem-solving** capacities.

PCRC 9: Parent talks to child and otherwise facilitates child's entry into **language and literacy** (including multilingualism as appropriate) and confidence in communication AND child is developing at age level the capacity for two-way gestural and/or verbal communication.

PCRC 10: Parent is able to take satisfaction from **symbolic activities** and may use conversation, narration, play, and/or other practices to promote these capacities in child AND child is able to use symbols in developmentally expectable ways to play, process, and partake in meaning-making.

PCRC 11: Parent is able to **access resources** on behalf of child and family AND child is able to make use of resources accessed by parent and is on a path toward accessing resources as developmentally expectable.

PCRC 12: Parent is able to maintain and enjoy a **network of family and/or friends**, that may include a co-parent, and to support child's relationships with this circle AND child is able to enjoy developing relationships with this network of people.

PCRC 13: Parent is able to manage frustration and channel **aggression** in appropriate directions, and to promote these capacities in child AND child is developing these capacities at age level.

PCRC 14: Parent is able to set limits with child in ways that promote development AND child is able to make good use of **limit-setting** interactions in working toward internalizing the ability to avoid danger, consider others, follow rules, defer gratification, etc.

PCRC 15: Parent has the capacity to plan for and support the child around **separations** in ways that promote development and well-being AND child displays an age-expectable capacity to manage and benefit from developmentally reasonable separations from parent.

PCRC 16: Parent takes pride and pleasure in his or her (or family) **culture(s)**, respects other cultures, and has the capacity to promote a sense of cultural identity and respect for other cultures in child AND child is able to take pleasure and pride in family culture(s) and demonstrates respect for other cultures.

PCRC 17: Parent is able to act to restore a sense of safety, hope, trust, and well-being for self and child following a distressing, disturbing, or **traumatic event** AND child is able to respond to parent's actions and to calm, restore, and heal.

PCRC 18: Parent is able to mourn losses and support child in **mourning** losses AND child is able to make use of parent's support to mourn losses in keeping with developmental level.

PCRC 19: Parent has the ability to work or otherwise contribute to society/the world AND child shows developmentally expectable signs of a sense of **efficacy**, confidence, and competence.

PCRC 20: Parent is able to **reflect** upon/think about his or her own experience, including how his or her past experiences may be impacting his or her experiences as a parent and can recognize the child's experience as that of a separate person AND child shows developmentally expectable signs of experiencing him- or herself as a unique person with interest in and concern for others as separate people.

APPENDIX B

Parent–Child Relationship Competencies (PCRCs) Scoring Sheet

Parent–Child Relationship Competencies Scoring Sheet: A Tool for Reflection

Include no identifying or protected health information (PHI) on this form.* Not to be included as part of chart/ medical record.

Case Code:				
Assessment Date:				
What Assessment Is This? (Circle)	Initial	6-Month	1-Year	Other (specify)
Child's Age at Present Assessment	Years:		Months:	
Child – Salient Social Location Markers				
Parent's Age at Present Assessment				
Parent – Salient Social Location Markers				
Family Language(s)				
Case Open on Child or Adult? (Circle)	Child		Adult	
Diagnosis:				

This form records the infant mental health (IMH) worker's impressions and level of concern. It is to be used for clinical reflection as part of an assessment or reassessment process and may inform collaborative treatment planning with parents. It should not be considered an empirically established rating of functioning.

---

* Find a printable copy of this form on www.zerotothree.org/PCRCresources

Complete a separate form for each parent or caregiver if more than one is involved in treatment. Complete on the basis of observation, parent report, and (with parent's permission) input gathered from others. Score as follows:

0—Bidirectional competency is present and functioning well to facilitate child development, relationship satisfaction, and family well-being. All elements of the competency description must be present and functioning well for this rating to be appropriate.

1—Bidirectional competency is present but strained such that support may be needed in this area. Some elements of the competency description may be functioning better than others.

2—Bidirectional competency functions unevenly or inconsistently or needs strengthening or refining. It may be that one element of the competency description is present and functioning, but another is inconsistent or underdeveloped.

3—Bidirectional competency is absent or seriously impaired. This rating is appropriate if one or more elements of the competency description are absent or seriously impaired, even if another element is present and functioning.

N—No (or not enough) information.

No.	Parent–Child Relationship Competency (PCRC)	0	1	2	3	N
1	Parent is able to register and respond effectively to child's **needs** AND child is able to signal needs clearly in keeping with age level.					
2	Parent is able to maintain his or her own **health and well-being**, promote child's health, and access pediatric (or other culturally meaningful) care as needed AND child is able to grow in keeping with developmental expectations and maintain physical health.					

No.	Parent–Child Relationship Competency (PCRC)	0	1	2	3	N
3	Parent has the capacity to provide **safety, protection, and comfort** for child AND child seeks out and accepts comfort and protection from parent and has a developmentally expectable ability to register security, anxiety, and fear.					
4	Parent is able to be **emotionally attuned** to/ empathize with child AND child is able to experience and express a developmentally expectable range of human emotion.					
5	Parent has the capacity to self-regulate and to engage in **mutual regulation** with child AND child is able to participate in mutual regulation with the parent and is developing the capacity to self-regulate.					
6	Parent has the capacity to identify, act on, and also control **impulses** sufficiently to have rewarding relationships and life experiences and can foster these abilities in child AND child demonstrates an age-expectable capacity to identify, act on, and also control impulses.					
7	Parent is able to pay attention and focus as needed and to engage child in attending and focusing AND child demonstrates a developmentally expectable capacity for **shared focus/mutual attention** and is on a path toward being able to focus and attend on his or her own.					
8	Parent possesses and conveys to child reasonable confidence that many things can be figured out/ worked out successfully AND child demonstrates age expectable **problem-solving** capacities.					
9	Parent talks to child and otherwise facilitates child's entry into **language and literacy** (including multilingualism as appropriate) and confidence in communication AND child is developing at age level the capacity for two-way gestural and/or verbal communication.					

No.	Parent–Child Relationship Competency (PCRC)	0	1	2	3	N
10	Parent is able to take satisfaction from **symbolic activities** and may use conversation, narration, play, and/or other practices to promote these capacities in child AND child is able to use symbols in developmentally expectable ways to play, process, and partake in meaning-making.					
11	Parent is able to **access resources** on behalf of child and family AND child is able to make use of resources accessed by parent and is on a path toward accessing resources as developmentally expectable.					
12	Parent is able to maintain and enjoy a **network of family and/or friends**, that may include a co-parent, and to support child's relationships with this circle AND child is able to enjoy developing relationships with this network of people.					
13	Parent is able to manage frustration and channel **aggression** in appropriate directions, and to promote these capacities in child AND child is developing these capacities at age level.					
14	Parent is able to set limits with child in ways that promote development AND child is able to make good use of **limit-setting** interactions in working toward internalizing the ability to avoid danger, consider others, follow rules, defer gratification, etc.					
15	Parent has the capacity to plan for and support the child around **separations** in ways that promote development and well-being AND child displays an age-expectable capacity to manage and benefit from developmentally reasonable separations from parent.					
16	Parent takes pride and pleasure in his or her (or family) **culture(s)**, respects other cultures, and has the capacity to promote a sense of cultural identity and respect for other cultures in child AND child is able to take pleasure and pride in family culture(s) and demonstrates respect for other cultures.					

No.	Parent–Child Relationship Competency (PCRC)	0	1	2	3	N
17	Parent is able to act to restore a sense of safety, hope, trust, and well-being for self and child following a distressing, disturbing, or **traumatic event** AND child is able to respond to parent's actions and to calm, restore, and heal.					
18	Parent is able to mourn losses and support child in **mourning** losses AND child is able to make use of parent's support to mourn losses in keeping with developmental level.					
19	Parent has the ability to work or otherwise contribute to society/the world AND child shows developmentally expectable signs of a sense of **efficacy**, confidence, and competence.					
20	Parent is able to **reflect** upon/think about his or her own experience, including how his or her past experiences may be impacting his or her experiences as a parent and can recognize the child's experience as that of a separate person AND child shows developmentally expectable signs of experiencing him- or herself as a unique person with interest in and concern for others as separate people.					

APPENDIX C

Elements of Clinical Formulation Justifying Parent–Child Relationship Competencies (PCRCs)-Focused Intervention

In most systems of care, a clinical formulation is required to make the case for why treatment is indicated and how it may help. It is a pivotal statement in pinpointing what has been learned during the assessment that the parent agrees treatment may help address. Common necessary elements include the following:

1. a description or statement of the presenting problem or issue;

2. a diagnosis;

3. a list of the symptoms of distress or impairment that meet criteria for assigning the diagnosis;

4. a description of impairments in significant areas of life functioning;

5. a description of any exacerbating or ameliorating factors, including strengths; and

6. a statement of recommended intervention in light of items 1–5.

When recommending dyadic (or triadic) intervention, it is important to also include

7. A statement regarding the relational implications of the difficulty.

An individual's functioning (Item 4) may be assessed using various frameworks. Infant mental health (IMH) workers should think together with reflective supervisors or consultants and with those responsible for quality assurance and utilization review within their program or system of care to determine relevant domains within their practice setting and scope of practice. Brief descriptions of several common frameworks for establishing a client's level of functioning follow.

The *Diagnostic and Statistical Manual of Mental Disorders* (5th ed.; DSM–5; American Psychiatric Association, 2013) adopts the World Health Organization Disability Assessment Schedule 2.0 (WHODAS 2.0; World Health Organization, 1992) for determining level of functioning, which identifies the following domains (Gold, 2014):

1. Understanding and communicating,

2. Getting around (mobility),

3. Self-care,

4. Getting along with people (social and interpersonal functioning),

5. Life activities (home, academic, and occupational functioning), and

6. Participation in society (participation in family, social, and community activities).

The Social Security Administration (www.ssa.gov) lists the following domains of functioning to determine children's eligibility for disability services:

1. Acquiring and using information,

2. Attending and completing tasks,

3. Interacting and relating with others,

4. Moving about and manipulating objects,

5. Caring for yourself, and

6. Health and physical well-being.

The *DC:0–5™: Diagnostic Classification of Mental Health and Developmental Disorders of Infancy and Early Childhood* (DC:0–5; ZERO TO THREE, 2016) provides frameworks for assessing the relational context (Axis II) and also the child's developmental competence (Axis V)—both critical areas of functioning to consider and support.

Many *10th Revision of the International Classification of Diseases* (ICD–10; World Health Organization, 1992) codes describe challenges related to areas of functioning relevant to IMH work, including the following:

- Failure to thrive;
- Child abuse problems;
- Child neglect and abandonment problems;
- Child in welfare custody;
- Parent–child problems;
- Parent–biological child conflict;
- Parent–foster child conflict;
- Parent–adopted child conflict;
- Parent–child estrangement;
- Parental overprotection;
- Inappropriate (excessive) parental pressure;
- Encounter for mental health services for parental child abuse;
- Encounter for mental health services for victim of parental child abuse;
- Encounter for mental health services for victim of nonparental child abuse;
- Encounter for mental health services for perpetrator of parental child abuse;
- Problems in relationship with spouse or partner;
- Problems in relationship with in-laws;
- Problems related to negative events in childhood;
- Problems related to upbringing;
- Problems related to unwanted pregnancy;
- Upbringing away from parents;
- Other absence of family member;
- Maternal care for fetal problem;

- Supervision of high-risk pregnancy due to social problems;
- Other stressful life events affecting family and household;
- Problem related to primary support group, unspecified;
- Phase of life problem;
- Problems of adjustment to life-cycle transitions;
- Other problems related to primary support group, including family circumstances; and
- Other problems related to social environment.

In creating a clinical formulation that sets the stage for IMH treatment, it is important also to include a clear justification for including the other family member(s) as collateral partners in the treatment. When the child is the identified client, inclusion of the parent as collateral partner in the treatment is often justified on the basis of (a) the importance of making changes in the caregiving environment to further treatment goals and objectives and (b) the potential for the parent to implement interventions in the naturalistic environment on a daily basis. When the parent is the identified client, inclusion of the child as collateral partner in the treatment is often justified on the basis of (a) the importance of having in vivo opportunities to implement changes in role functioning as a parent and (b) mitigating the risk of adverse developmental outcomes following from the parent's mental health difficulty. In both instances— when the child is the identified client and when the parent is the identified client—dyadic intervention is justified by (c) the idea of strengthening the Parent–Child Relationship Competencies (PCRCs) to promote family well-being.

Adaptation is another important factor to consider in arriving at dyadic (or triadic) clinical formulations. In all relationships, there is a degree of adaptation such that one partner makes adaptations to accommodate the other's needs or behaviors. When one partner struggles with a diagnosable condition, often the symptoms or impairments lead the other relationship partner to make adaptations or accommodations. This occurrence can be helpful but can also be problematic if it causes distress or puts healthy development at risk. For example, a parent may make lifestyle adaptations when a child with autism is averse to being in social situations, but these adaptations can lead to parental distress (e.g., isolation) and place the child at developmental risk (e.g., missing out on opportunities to learn relating and communicating skills). When a parent suffers from depression, a child may make adaptations such as suppressing needs or attempting to care for or enliven the parent, which lead to distress and developmental risk (e.g., restricted range of affect, missed opportunities to learn to experience and express emotion, role reversal).

Here are important elements of a relational clinical formulation:

Identified client is [add demographic descriptors] who meets criteria for a **diagnosis** of [insert qualifying diagnosis], as evidenced by [behavioral **symptoms** in keeping with DC:0–5 or DSM–5]. These impairments/symptoms negatively affect [insert **domain of life functioning**; e.g., functioning as a parent/developmental functioning/ family functioning] in the following way: [briefly describe, setting the stage for which PCRCs need strengthening]. These problems are **exacerbated/ameliorated** by [insert compounding factors and/or strengths, which could include well-functioning PCRCs]. These difficulties are best addressed in the context of the parent–child relationship because/so that [briefly state **rationale** for recommending dyadic intervention; e.g., to support daily implementation of intervention strategies]. Weekly home-based dyadic IMH services [or substitute **recommended modality and frequency**] including [parent/child] as **collateral partner** are recommended to [reduce symptoms/improve functioning] by **strengthening PCRC** [insert appropriate number].

APPENDIX D

Library of Sample Parent–Child Relationship-Based Manifestations of Child Symptoms and Functional Impairments

This library of sample relationship-based manifestations of child symptoms and functional impairments[D1] is organized according to the Parent–Child Relationship Competency (PCRC) most obviously affected. Note, however, that many of the relational/behavioral difficulties listed here would negatively affect several PCRCs. Also, this library is suggestive, not exhaustive; any symptom or functional impairment that a child struggles with might strain any PCRC.

Remember that in PCRC-focused treatment planning and documentation of clinical work, it is important to make clear on an ongoing basis (a) how the diagnosis or condition that meets service/medical necessity requirements is linked to difficulties in the parent–child relationship and (b) how the intervention will help or is helping. This library offers examples of child behaviors that may be a target of intervention. Because, according to Winnicott (1958), there is no such thing as a baby separate from the caregiving context, some child behaviors are irreducibly dyadic.

Documentation would incorporate these types of behaviors by linking the diagnosis with the symptom/functional impairment and spelling out the problematic consequences for the child/relationship/family.

For example, the first item in this library is "Difficulty signaling needs."

[D1] Inspiration for some items in this library was drawn from Axis II of the *DC:0–5™: Diagnostic Classification of Mental Health and Developmental Disorders of Infancy and Early Childhood* (DC:0–5; ZERO TO THREE, 2016) and the Functional Emotional Assessment Scale (S. I. Greenspan & DeGangi, as cited in DeGangi, 2000, pp. 341–360).

Here are a few ways this item might be linked to a diagnosis and included in documentation:

1. Undereating Disorder involves the client's tendency to fall asleep quickly when given a bottle, apparent lack of interest in eating, and *lack of signaling the need for food*, which leaves the parent confused about when to offer the bottle, exacerbating lack of developmentally expectable weight gain.

2. The client's trauma-based tendency to miscue leads to consistent *failure to signal need for emotional closeness*, instead behaving in ways that leave the parent feeling rejected and kept at bay, perpetuating a cycle of thwarted social–emotional development.

3. The client's autism-based aversion to social interaction *prevents him from signaling his need* for relational help connecting with others, compounding his and his family's isolation.

The following phrases may be useful in describing the symptom/functional impairment:

- Absence of
- Aversion to
- Avoidance of
- Challenged to
- Contends with
- Demonstrates
- Difficulty
- Engages in
- Exhibits
- Failure to
- Inability to
- Incapacity to
- Inflexibility regarding
- Intolerance of
- Lack of

- Overreliance on
- Pattern of
- Paucity of
- Persists in
- Preoccupation with
- Proneness to
- Refusal of/to
- Reliance on
- Tendency to
- Unable to
- Vulnerability to

The following phrases may be useful in describing the problematic/negative relational impact of the symptoms/impairments:

Child's behavior or parent's accommodation to child's behavior...

- Makes it challenging for parent to facilitate social–emotional development
- Makes it challenging for parent to support health/growth
- Makes it challenging for parent to ensure physical safety
- Results in stress for parent
- Requires intensive supervision by parent
- Requires intensive remediating intervention by parent
- Undermines parental confidence
- Taxes parent/family resources
- Leads to family discord
- Exacerbates discord between co-parents
- Contributes to family isolation
- Impinges on siblings' developmental needs
- Puts family at risk of child welfare involvement/forced separation

- Complicates/impedes family reunification
- Results in excessive focus on limit setting
- Results in missed opportunities for learning
- Limits opportunities for growth-promoting interaction
- Strains peer relationships
- Leads to risk of exclusion from child care

PCRC 1: Parent is able to register and respond effectively to child's **needs** AND child is able to signal needs clearly in keeping with age level.

Child behavioral symptoms and functional impairments that might negatively affect PCRC 1 include the following:

- Difficulty signaling needs because of, for example,
  - Sensory underresponsivity
  - Failure to thrive
  - Withdrawal
  - Anxiety
  - Inhibition
  - Limited communicative repertoire
  - Lack of social reciprocity
  - Depressive muting of emotion
- Fear that needs will not be met, leading to help-rejecting behaviors
- Difficulties with expressive language lead to frustration communicating needs
- Tendency to miscue, signaling the opposite of actual emotional needs
- Suppression of needs because of, for example,
  - Parentification
  - Role-reversal
  - Fear of overwhelming parent

- Somaticizes or gets in accidents to attract care when emotional needs go unmet

PCRC 2: Parent is able to maintain his or her own **health and well-being**, promote child's health, and access pediatric (or other culturally meaningful) care as needed AND child is able to grow in keeping with developmental expectations and maintain physical health.

Child behavioral symptoms and functional impairments that might negatively affect PCRC 2 include the following:

- Congenital medical condition leads to family grief and stress
- Medical condition leads to intensification of need for care that taxes family system
- Birth complications lead to family stress
- Neonatal abstinence syndrome exacerbates parental guilt and shame
- Constitutional vulnerability leads to complex needs for care
- Failure to thrive leads to parental anxiety
- Feeding/eating difficulties lead to parental stress
- Overeats—uses bottle or food rather than interaction with parent for comfort/stimulation/regulation
- Picky eater—challenging to feed
- Medical trauma-based phobia leads to resistance around pediatric care
- Enuresis/encopresis leads to discord
- Bedwetting leads to discord
- Power struggles around diapering or potty training
- Resists parent's attempts to administer breathing treatments
- Refuses parent's attempts to administer medication/physical therapy exercises/other intervention

- Avoidance of grooming ministrations (clipping nails, doing hair, and so forth)
- Oppositional behavior leads to lack of cooperation around hygiene routines
- Phobias complicate hygiene routines (e.g., water phobia complicating bathing)
- Avoids physical activity—challenging to engage in physical activity
- Sleep disturbance (sleep resistance, night wakings, and so forth) lead to sleep deficit
- Resists interventions geared to address developmental delay
- Sensory processing irregularities lead to frequent struggles around engaging with physical environment (e.g., dressing, bathing, being buckled into car seat)

PCRC 3: Parent has the capacity to provide **safety, protection, and comfort** for child AND child seeks out and accepts comfort and protection from parent and has a developmentally expectable ability to register security, anxiety, and fear.

Child behavioral symptoms and functional impairments that might negatively affect PCRC 3 include the following:

- Incapacity to register danger
- Disinclination to seek protection from parent
- Difficulty trusting parent to protect
- Engages in trauma-/anxiety-based reckless behaviors, for example,
  - Bolting
  - Being accident prone
  - Moving toward rather than away from risk/danger
  - Ignores danger signals
- Engages in depression- or anxiety-based self-harming behaviors, for example,

- Flailing
- Head banging
- Lurching from parents arms
- Putting fist down throat
- Holding breath
- Engages in behaviors that endanger others (e.g., biting, hitting, throwing things)
- Exhibits disinhibited social engagement
- Does not seek comfort from parent
- Difficulty accepting comfort from parent
- Exhibits lack of appropriate wariness with unfamiliar adults
- Fails to use appropriate social referencing/track parent when in public

PCRC 4: Parent is able to be **emotionally attuned** to/empathize with child AND child is able to experience and express a developmentally expectable range of human emotion.

Child behavioral symptoms and functional impairments that might negatively affect PCRC 4 include the following:

- Escalates to states of being extremely upset quickly
- Resists parent's attempts to provide comfort
- Signals emotional states weakly or in confusing ways (miscues)
- Collapses emotionally when frustrated or disappointed
- Subject to intense moods, straining household atmosphere
- Difficulty accepting parent's help in shifting mood
- Prone to panic, as evidenced by freezing
- Demonstrates emotional numbing
- Emotionally constricted
- Rarely evidences pleasure

- Delayed, convoluted, or incoherent expression of emotional upset
- Engages in reversal of affect
- Withdraws from parent
- Demonstrates clinginess
- Whines, pouts, and is difficult to cajole
- Difficult to soothe
- Challenged to read emotional cues of others
- Stifles emotion for fear of burdening parent

PCRC 5: Parent has the capacity to self-regulate and to engage in **mutual regulation** with child AND child is able to participate in mutual regulation with the parent and is developing the capacity to self-regulate.

Child behavioral symptoms and functional impairments that might negatively affect PCRC 5 include the following:

- Relies on self-stimulating behaviors, limiting opportunities for growth-promoting interactions with parent
- Relies on self-soothing behaviors, missing opportunities for soothing interactions with parent
- Difficulty relaxing
- Arches/does not mold
- Averts gaze/avoids eye contact
- Locks gaze—cannot break eye contact
- Low tolerance for being put down—prefers to be held constantly
- Resists/avoids touch
- Exaggerated startle response
- Difficult to calm/soothe
- Difficult to rouse/engage
- Easily overstimulated
- Tendency to be overwhelmed/"go limp"

- Challenged to join others with socially appropriate energy level
- Sleep-related difficulties strain parent/family, for example,
  - Frequent wakings
  - Resists bedtime
  - Prone to nightmares
- Toileting-related difficulties strain parent/family, for example,
  - Refuses diaper
  - Resists toilet training
  - Touches/smears feces
  - Enuresis
  - Encopresis
- Finds transitions challenging—requires intensive preparation and support
- State transitions are not fluid, requiring intensive facilitation

PCRC 6: Parent has the capacity to identify, act on, and also control **impulses** sufficiently to have rewarding relationships and life experiences and can foster these abilities in child AND child demonstrates an age-expectable capacity to identify, act on, and also control impulses.

Child behavioral symptoms and functional impairments that might negatively affect PCRC 6 include the following:

- Difficulty inhibiting impulses, constantly getting into things, requiring close supervision
- Difficulty acting on impulses—withdrawn, inhibited, fearful—requires intensive encouragement/scaffolding
- Prone to angry outbursts
- Intrusive with others, requiring close supervision

- Demonstrates lack of developmentally expectable negative capabilities (e.g., capacity to wait, hold one's tongue, defer gratification), requiring intensive parental management
- Anxiety around impulses imagined to be "bad" leads to:
  - Somatic complaints
  - Counterphobic or compulsive acting out
  - Avoidance
  - Phobias
  - Compensatory "good" behavior
  - Need for reassurance
- Difficulty remembering/cooperating with a plan, requiring intensive parental management
- Incapacity to make use of parent as auxiliary impulse control mechanism
- Incapacity to take turns

PCRC 7: Parent is able to pay attention and focus as needed and to engage child in attending and focusing AND child demonstrates a developmentally expectable capacity for **shared focus/mutual attention** and is on a path toward being able to focus and attend on his or her own.

Child behavioral symptoms and functional impairments that might negatively affect PCRC 7 include the following:

- Difficulty attending, requiring intensive parental scaffolding
- Withdrawn, difficult to engage
- Easily upset/difficulty remaining calm, requiring intensive help maintaining equilibrium
- Easily overstimulated, making it challenging to focus
- Easily distracted, requiring frequent redirection/refocusing

- Cautious to explore, requiring intensive encouragement
- Limited ability to sustain shared focus with others, requiring constant re-engagement
- Need to be in control; difficulty sharing/being with
- Challenged to balance internal and external focus
- Challenged to sustain interest in others
- Restricted range of interests
- Preoccupation with limited repertoire of objects/activities
- Incapacity to be flexible—becomes fixated
- Requires precise routines/things to be "just so"
- Sensory sensitivities/sensory processing irregularities lead to retreat from learning opportunities without intensive parental mediation of environment
- Reliance on self-stimulating behaviors blocks opportunities for focusing and attending
- Reliance on self-soothing behaviors blocks opportunities for focusing and attending

PCRC 8: Parent possesses and conveys to child reasonable confidence that many things can be figured out/worked out successfully AND child demonstrates age expectable **problem-solving** capacities.

Child behavioral symptoms and functional impairments that might negatively affect PCRC 8 include the following:

- Low frustration tolerance, requiring intensive scaffolding
- Easily feels defeated/gives up, requiring intensive affirmation/coaxing
- Cognitive delay, requiring remediation
- Demonstrates depression-based hopelessness
- Lack of flexibility, requiring intensive reassurance/cajoling

- Passive, lacking a sense of agency
- Preoccupied with worries
- Frozen/constricted by fear
- Difficulty rousing/engaging/rising to challenge, requiring intensive encouragement
- Demonstrates anxiety-based perfectionism
- Hypervigilance prevents exploration/learning

PCRC 9: Parent talks to child and otherwise facilitates child's entry into **language and literacy** (including multilingualism as appropriate) and confidence in communication AND child is developing at age level the capacity for two-way gestural and/or verbal communication.

Child behavioral symptoms and functional impairments that might negatively affect PCRC 9 include the following:

- Evidences language delay, requiring intensive remediating intervention by parent
- Restricted sounds/utterances
- Selectively mute
- Avoids one language in bilingual household
- Hearing impairment necessitates intervention
- Challenged to participate in back-and-forth gestural or verbal communication
- Resists being read to/interacting with books
- Unable to respond to parent in contingent manner
- Problems with accurately reading social cues leads to interpersonal conflict/social isolation
- Withdraws/avoids communicative interaction
- Talks incessantly, unable to engage in back-and-forth flow
- Overreliance on "screens" restricts opportunities for social exchange

- Unable to take pleasure/solace in language-based interactions

PCRC 10: Parent is able to take satisfaction from **symbolic activities** and may use conversation, narration, play, and/or other practices to promote these capacities in child AND child is able to use symbols in developmentally expectable ways to play, process, and partake in meaning-making.

Child behavioral symptoms and functional impairments that might negatively affect PCRC 10 include the following:

- Restricted repertoire of play themes/interests
- Engages in traumatic play (repetitious, violent or alarming, distressing rather than pleasurable, transformative or growth promoting)
- Unable to take pleasure/solace in symbolic activity
- Unable to appreciate/enjoy elaboration and nuance
- Unable to make use of narrative to process experience
- Appears not to expect to be considered or consulted
- Missed opportunities for engagement in symbolic activities because of, for example,
  - Withdrawal
  - Agitation
  - Hyperactivity
  - Distractability
  - Somberness
  - Fear/timidity/anxiety
- Demonstrates developmentally inappropriate concrete thinking
- Troubled unduly by frightening fantasies/imaginary experiences
- Relies on fantasy to the exclusion of engaging with others/benefiting from shared symbolic activities

- Suffers from delusions
- Suffers from hallucinations
- Appears to believe that one must override or be overridden; incapacity to trust in shared meaning-making endeavors

PCRC 11: Parent is able to **access resources** on behalf of child and family AND child is able to make use of resources accessed by parent and is on a path toward accessing resources as developmentally expectable.

Child behavioral symptoms and functional impairments that might negatively affect PCRC 11 include the following:

- Resists engaging in learning opportunities/intervention services provided by parent
- Avoids novel, potentially growth-promoting experiences
- Paucity of internal resources
- Incapacity to marshal internal resources
- Demonstrates behaviors that lead to risk of exclusion from group care
- Engages in behaviors that lead to family restriction of social engagement
- Vulnerable to states of being extremely upset such that participation in recreational activities is limited
- Engages in behaviors that lead to family isolation
- Resists participation in intervention
- Refuses to accept help from trustworthy others
- Demonstrates disregard for offerings (e.g., toys, activities, materials) provided by parent
- Picky eater, making it difficult for parent to provide nutrition
- Demonstrates low curiosity, requiring intensive facilitation to benefit from learning opportunities

PCRC 12: Parent is able to maintain and enjoy a **network of family and/or friends**, that may include a co-parent, and to support child's relationships with this circle AND child is able to enjoy developing relationships with this network of people.

Child behavioral symptoms and functional impairments that might negatively affect PCRC 12 include the following:

- Clingy with parent
- Separation avoidant
- Demonstrates lack of flexibility
- Engages in sibling conflict
- Antagonistic with stepparent
- Attention-dependent; incapacity to enjoy being "one in the number"
- Evidences socially indiscriminate behavior
- Vulnerable to displaying loyalty to parent by cutting ties with/disavowing attachment to others from whom parent is estranged
- Requires intensive wooing/facilitation of relationships because of being, for example,
  - Withdrawn
  - Somber
  - Aggressive
  - Fearful
  - Demanding
  - Excessively shy
  - Highly reactive
  - Socially avoidant
  - Disruptive
  - Uncooperative
  - Difficult to manage
- Challenged to engage in pro-social behaviors

- Tends to misread social cues, resulting in discord with or alienation from peers
- Sensory sensitive such that unfamiliar environments are aversive

PCRC 13: Parent is able to manage frustration and channel **aggression** in appropriate directions, and to promote these capacities in child AND child is developing these capacities at age level.

Child behavioral symptoms and functional impairments that might negatively affect PCRC 13 include the following:

- Vulnerable to being misperceived as aggressive by others (e.g., through a racist lens)
- Challenged to discharge aggressive impulses along pathways that bring reward
- Inability to inhibit aggressive impulses toward others, requiring intensive supervision around, for example,
  - Biting
  - Grabbing
  - Kicking
  - Hitting
  - Throwing objects
- Inability to channel aggressive impulses in appropriate directions, requiring intensive monitoring/facilitation/ intervention
- Tendency to direct aggressive impulses toward self, for example,
  - Flailing
  - Head banging
  - Biting self
  - Breaking valued toys/objects
  - Behaving in ways geared to incite parental disapproval/recrimination

- Shame or anxiety regarding aggressive impulses leading to, for example,
  - Inhibition/withdrawal
  - Somatic symptoms (e.g., enuresis)
  - Reaction formation—aggressive acting out
- Vulnerable to angry outbursts
- Tendency to behave in ways that incite anger/ aggression in others

PCRC 14: Parent is able to set limits with child in ways that promote development AND child is able to make good use of **limit-setting** interactions in working toward internalizing the ability to avoid danger, consider others, follow rules, defer gratification, etc.

Child behavioral symptoms and functional impairments that might negatively affect PCRC 14 include the following:

- Difficulty complying with limits
- Tendency to heed limits out of compliance rather than cooperation
- Difficulty trusting that parent will be consistent about slimits
- Tendency to engage in power struggles with parent
- Vulnerable to emotional collapse around limit setting
- Prone to experiencing shame in response to limit setting
- Tendency to plead with parent/pursue negotiation
- Impaired capacity to register satiation/fatigue/ oversaturation necessitates parental imposition of limits
- Challenges in understanding risk/danger necessitate extensive focus on limits
- Displays frequent challenging behavior, resulting in inordinate focus on limits

- Impulsivity or sensory sensitivity leads to inordinate focus on limit setting from caregivers
- Engages in behaviors that tend to trigger limit-setting response from parent, when something else is truly needed (e.g., comfort, affection, nurture)

PCRC 15: Parent has the capacity to plan for and support the child around **separations** in ways that promote development and well-being AND child displays an age-expectable capacity to manage and benefit from developmentally reasonable separations from parent.

Child behavioral symptoms and functional impairments that might negatively affect PCRC 15 include the following:

- Social–emotional development/well-being threatened because of forced separation/parental deprivation (e.g., because of incarceration, deportation, child welfare involvement)
- Despondent because of forced separation/parental deprivation
- Emotional strain due to extended separation from parent (e.g., parent traveling)
- Social–emotional development taxed by co-parent separation/dissolution/divorce
- Difficulty tolerating growth-promoting separations from parent
- Reliance on constant contact with parent to maintain equilibrium
- Developmentally problematic reliance on parent for coregulation
- Challenged to move between solo, dyadic, and triadic or group interactions
- Emotional numbing leads to apparent indifference to separation
- Traumatic separation has led to emotional detachment
- Becomes dysregulated around "good-byes"

- Hypervigilant around separations
- Avoids physical proximity and emotional closeness
- Displays undue separation anxiety
- Resists sleep, which taxes parent/family system
- Clingy

PCRC 16: Parent takes pride and pleasure in his or her (or family) **culture(s)**, respects other cultures, and has the capacity to promote a sense of cultural identity and respect for other cultures in child AND child is able to take pleasure and pride in family culture(s) and demonstrates respect for other cultures.

Child behavioral symptoms and functional impairments that might negatively affect PCRC 16 include the following:

- Demonstrates learned fear of/negative attitudes toward particular cultural groups
- Demonstrates entitlement
- Shows signs of negative identifications/self-representations related to culture
- Evidences shame-based avoidance of family cultural practices/activities/experiences
- Blames self/parent for problems attributable to forces of oppression
- Narrow repertoire of idioms of respect
- Paucity of racial literacy
- Evidences wounds of racial or historical trauma
- Immigration challenges strain development or well-being
- Acculturation challenges strain development or well-being
- Evidences confusion/anxiety secondary to being placed in binds related to differing cultures (e.g., cultural differences between co-parents or

between generations, expectations at child care are different from home)

- Impaired capacity to take pleasure/pride in family cultural traditions/experiences
- Exhibits behaviors that lead parent to restrict engagement with potentially enriching social/cultural experiences

PCRC 17: Parent is able to act to restore a sense of safety, hope, trust, and well-being for self and child following a distressing, disturbing, or **traumatic event** AND child is able to respond to parent's actions and to calm, restore, and heal.

Child behavioral symptoms and functional impairments that might negatively affect PCRC 17 include the following:

- Disrupted regulatory capacities complicate caregiving demands
- Disabled capacity to discern safety and danger leads to risky/reckless behavior
- Vulnerability to flooding leads to, for example,
  - Hyperactivity
  - Hyperarousal
  - Emotional inaccessibility
  - Traumatic play (repetitious, violent or alarming, distressing rather than growth promoting)
- Tendency to experience parent as a trauma trigger
- Collapse of faith in parent's protective functioning
- Incapacity to experience joy
- Evidences hopelessness
- Demonstrates developmentally problematic self-reliance
- Altered presentation frightens/alienates parent
- Hypervigilance/inability to relax impedes capacity to, for example,

- Play
- Rest
- Trust
- Be silly
- Experience joy
- Phobic avoidance limits opportunities for learning and exploration
- Emotional numbing leads to failure to signal need for comfort

PCRC 18: Parent is able to mourn losses and support child in **mourning** losses AND child is able to make use of parent's support to mourn losses in keeping with developmental level.

Child behavioral symptoms and functional impairments that might negatively affect PCRC 18 include the following:

- Disturbed regulatory capacities (e.g., sleep, appetite) complicate caregiving demands
- Avoids experiences that trigger reminders of loss
- Depressive anhedonia impedes capacity to enjoy experiences/relationships
- Manic defense against loss leads to hyperactivity/ emotional inaccessibility
- Self-recrimination erodes confidence
- Hopelessness dampens capacity for motivation, excitement, joy, and so forth
- Irritability taxes parent's patience and empathy
- Developmentally based inconsistent remembering that object is lost leads to repeated re-experiencing of loss, which can tax parent's patience and empathy
- Fear of loss/abandonment impedes capacity to trust/ rely on parent
- Experiences parent as reminder of lost other

- Impeded capacity to accept comfort from parent due to experiencing parent as altered following loss
- Anger at parent (based in irrational belief that parent could have prevented loss) perplexes and hurts parent
- Evidences developmental setback/regression, which can frustrate/dishearten/anger parent

PCRC 19: Parent has the ability to work or otherwise contribute to society/the world AND child shows developmentally expectable signs of a sense of **efficacy**, confidence, and competence.

Child behavioral symptoms and functional impairments that might negatively affect PCRC 19 include the following:

- Little confidence in capacities, as evidenced by inhibition in the face of novelty
- Lack of relational confidence reflected in rarely making bids for interaction
- Lacks persistence—quickly despairs of being able to succeed at something
- Appears not to expect to be noticed or considered, for example, seeming startled/confused when addressed
- Rough or reckless management of body and objects reflecting sense that success is hit-or-miss leads to frequent conflict/discord
- Frenzied, fervent quality to play or enjoyable interactions, suggesting fear that they may end precipitously at any moment
- Listlessness
- Lack of vocalization
- Helplessness out of keeping with what would be developmentally expectable
- Vagueness/blankness to facial expression suggesting little experience with/low expectations for face-to-face interaction

- Rarely takes initiative
- Underdeveloped sense of curiosity as reflected in inhibited exploratory behaviors
- Restricted sense of agency or entitlement as reflected in not making bids for participation
- Passive, expecting to be manipulated and managed physically rather than participating actively in care, for example, around being diapered, dressed, and bathed

PCRC 20: Parent is able to **reflect** upon/think about his or her own experience, including how his or her past experiences may be impacting his or her experiences as a parent and can recognize the child's experience as that of a separate person AND child shows developmentally expectable signs of experiencing him- or herself as a unique person with interest in and concern for others as separate people.

Child behavioral symptoms and functional impairments that might negatively affect PCRC 20 include the following:

- Prone to entering "freeze/fight/flight" mode
- Prone to impulsive acting out
- Challenged to inhibit impulses
- Lacks a sense of humor
- Lacks curiosity
- Hesitates to differentiate self from parent (e.g., express opinions or preferences that may differ from parent's)
- Displays developmentally inappropriate concrete thinking
- Limited capacity to identify what others may be thinking or feeling
- Paucity of imagination
- Restricted symbolic capacities (e.g., play themes less elaborate or varied than would be developmentally expectable)

- Insensitive to the impact of own actions on others
- Cannot settle: keeps things "topsy-turvy" in the environment and interpersonal sphere
- Organized around parent's moods, for example,
  - Attempts to enliven depressed parent
  - "Walks on eggshells" with irritable parent
  - "Nurses" fragile/easily injured parent

APPENDIX E

Library of Sample Parent–Child Relationship-Based Manifestations of Parent Symptoms and Functional Impairments

This library of sample relationship-based manifestations of parental symptoms and functional impairments[E1] is organized according to the Parent–Child Relationship Competency (PCRC) most obviously affected. Note, however, that many of the relational/behavioral difficulties listed here would negatively affect several PCRCs. Also, this library is suggestive, not exhaustive; any symptom or functional impairment that a parent struggles with might strain any PCRC.

Remember that in PCRC-focused treatment planning and documentation of clinical work, it is important to make it clear on an ongoing basis (a) how the diagnosis or condition that meets service/medical necessity requirements is linked to difficulties in the parent–child relationship and (b) how the intervention will help or is helping. This library offers examples of parent behaviors that may be a target of intervention.

Documentation would incorporate these types of behaviors by linking the diagnosis with the symptom/functional impairment and spelling out the problematic consequences for the child/relationship/family.

For example, the first item in this library is "Challenged to provide for child's concrete needs." Here are a few ways this item might be linked to a diagnosis and included in documentation:

[E1] Inspiration for some items in this library was drawn from Axis II of the *DC:0–5™: Diagnostic Classification of Mental Health and Developmental Disorders of Infancy and Early Childhood* (DC:0–5; ZERO TO THREE, 2016) and the Functional Emotional Assessment Scale (S. I. Greenspan & DeGangi, as cited in DeGangi, 2000, pp. 341–360).

1. Depression-based low energy (hypersomnia and psychomotor retardation) leave the client *challenged to provide for the child's concrete needs* because he cannot marshal the energy to complete daily activities, such as going to the grocery store, placing the child's health and well-being at risk.

2. When experiencing Bipolar II–based manic states, the client becomes very internally preoccupied and is *unable to register or provide for the child's concrete needs*, such as eating at regular intervals, placing the family at risk of child welfare involvement/forced separation.

3. Substance abuse disorder leads the client to alternate between "tunnel vision" focus on procuring substance of choice and "tuned out" states when under the influence, leaving the client *unable to register or provide for the child's concrete needs* (e.g., diapering, feeding) and thus endangering the child.

The following phrases may be useful in describing the symptom/functional impairment:

- Absence of
- Aversion to
- Avoidance of
- Challenged to
- Contends with
- Demonstrates
- Difficulty with
- Engages in
- Exhibits
- Failure to
- Inability to
- Incapacity to
- Inflexibility regarding
- Intolerance of
- Lack of

- Overreliance on
- Pattern of
- Paucity of
- Persists in
- Preoccupation with
- Proneness to
- Refusal of/to
- Reliance on
- Tendency to
- Unable to
- Vulnerability to

The following phrases may be useful in describing the problematic/negative relational impact of the symptoms/impairments:

Parent's behavior or child's accommodation to parent's behavior...

- Negatively affects child's social–emotional development
- Negatively affects child's health/physical development
- Places child at risk of illness
- Places child at risk of injury
- Places child's safety at risk
- Leads to family isolation
- Strains/impedes child's relationship with co-parent
- Deprives child of opportunities to participate in growth-promoting exploration
- Restricts learning opportunities for child
- Impedes child's capacity to develop internal resources
- Negatively affects child's capacity to trust others
- Thwarts child's curiosity
- Limits child's participation in growth-promoting social interactions

- Places family at risk of child welfare involvement/forced separation
- Complicates family reunification
- Negatively shapes child's self-concept
- Thwarts child's developmental expectable strivings for exploration/autonomy

PCRC 1: Parent is able to register and respond effectively to child's **needs** AND child is able to signal needs clearly in keeping with age level.

Parental behavioral symptoms and functional impairments that might negatively affect PCRC 1 include the following:

- Symptoms of mental health disorder impede capacity to meet child's needs
- Grave disability extends to incapacity to meet child's basic needs
- Displays disorganization/executive functioning difficulties such that they are challenged to provide for child's concrete needs
- Trauma-based fear of dependency leads to incapacity to tolerate child's dependence
- Limited emotional resources lead to limited capacity to meet child's emotional needs
- Vulnerable to feeling antagonistic or competitive with child
- Difficulty reading or responding to child's needs, for example,
  - Tendency to feel overwhelmed
  - Tendency to feel persecuted
  - Tendency to feel ineffectual
  - Tendency to minimize
  - Tendency to exaggerate
  - Tendency to react punitively
  - Tendency to ignore/tune out

- Prone to misreading child's cues
- Incapacity to conceptualize child's behavior as signaling emotional need

PCRC 2: Parent is able to maintain his or her own **health and well-being**, promote child's health, and access pediatric (or other culturally meaningful) care as needed AND child is able to grow in keeping with developmental expectations and maintain physical health.

Parental behavioral symptoms and functional impairments that might negatively affect PCRC 2 include the following:

- Repeats with child problematic historical patterns of interacting around health-related matters
- Grave disability extends to incapacity to ensure child's health and well-being
- Challenged to maintain child/family health, for example,
  - Challenged to maintain recovery
  - Challenged to engage in self-care
  - Challenged to secure/provide nutrition for child/ family
  - Challenged to provide opportunities for recreation/ physical exercise for child/family
- Avoids pediatric (or other culturally appropriate) care on child's behalf
- Interacts around grooming ministrations or hygiene routines in ways that incite discord and struggle
- Incapacity to support child in maintaining and participating in hygiene routines
- Disorganization impedes capacity to follow through with child's medical needs or implement needed supports such as:
  - Asthma treatments
  - Wearing glasses

- Completing exercises as recommended by early intervention specialist
- Getting enough sleep
- Presents child for unnecessary medical care as a way of engaging helping professionals
- Depressive guilt prevents parent from grappling forthrightly with child's disability
- Trauma-based avoidance prevents parent from speaking openly with child about medical condition
- Depression-based lethargy prevents family engagement in health-promoting activities
- Lack of confidence prevents parent from advocating for family health
- Devaluation of inherited cultural healing practices deprives family of potential wellness resources
- Prioritizes other things (e.g., productivity, romantic relationships) over health and well-being of child
- Incorporates child in disordered eating patterns
- Avoids open spaces, depriving child of opportunities to be outdoors

PCRC 3: Parent has the capacity to provide **safety, protection, and comfort** for child AND child seeks out and accepts comfort and protection from parent and has a developmentally expectable ability to register security, anxiety, and fear.

Parental behavioral symptoms and functional impairments that might negatively affect PCRC 3 include the following:

- Repeats with child patterns from past involving interpersonal failures of safety, comfort, or protection
- Experiences child as dangerous
- Acts in ways (e.g., impulsive, poor judgment, risk taking) that place family in harm's way

- Emotional numbing leads to inability to register or respond effectively when child is afraid
- Engages in abusive interactions with child (physical, sexual, or emotional)
- Engages in neglectful interactions regarding child
- Incapacity to effectively address hazards in home environment
- Exhibits lack of protective impulses toward child
- Inhibition of protective impulses toward child
- Incapacity to act on protective impulses toward child
- Believes self to be endangered by child
- Acts in ways that are overly protective/limiting of child's exploration
- Abandons child (physically, financially, or emotionally)
- Frightens child
- Endangers child; for example,
  - Unable to maintain a safe environment
  - Driving while intoxicated
  - Engaging in verbal or physical altercations in child's presence
  - Failing to protect from others who harm child
  - Reliance on untrustworthy others to care for child
- Exploits child; for example,
  - Requiring developmentally inappropriate or emotionally harmful labor
  - Using child as a lure
  - Using child to meet emotional needs
  - Engaging in role reversal/promoting parentification

PCRC 4: Parent is able to be **emotionally attuned** to/empathize with child AND child is able to experience and express a developmentally expectable range of human emotion.

Parental behavioral symptoms and functional impairments that might negatively affect PCRC 4 include the following:

- Repeats with child patterns of failed attunement parent experienced in relation to caregivers growing up
- Unresponsive to signs of distress in child (e.g., does not seem to hear infant's cries)
- Tends to be preoccupied with/lost in child's emotional experience
- Difficulty emotionally attuning to child
- Difficulty experiencing empathy for child
- Difficulty taking child's point of view
- Difficulty tolerating ambivalent feelings in parent–child relationship
- Difficulty tolerating a range of emotional expressiveness in child/family
- Limited affection for child
- Limited psychological investment in child
- Limited capacity to take pleasure in child
- Reliance on child to meet emotional needs
- Misreads child's emotions
- Flat affect/restricted range of affect prevents emotional joining/mirroring
- Is easily emotionally injured, conveying to child that they are injurious
- Engages in rivalry with child
- Prone to negative attributions toward child
- Is emotionally brittle, depriving child of opportunities to experience "repair"

- Tends to be emotionally withholding/constricted/withdrawn
- Tends to be histrionic, for example responding in exaggerated or self-serving ways to child's imagined distress
- Mood is like "weather" in household, overshadowing child/family experiences
- Overly affected by child's emotions, abdicating parental authority/judgment

PCRC 5: Parent has the capacity to self-regulate and to engage in **mutual regulation** with child AND child is able to participate in mutual regulation with the parent and is developing the capacity to self-regulate.

Parental behavioral symptoms and functional impairments that might negatively affect PCRC 5 include the following:

- Repeats with child problematic patterns around coregulation that parent experienced with caregivers growing up
- Challenged to engage in mutual regulation with child
- Difficulty calming/relaxing
- Difficulty rousing/activating
- Tendency to overstimulate child
- Tendency to understimulate child
- Erratic pacing (e.g., going from "zero to 60") undermines child's capacity to regulate
- Tendency to be overwhelmed/"go limp" in the face of child's energy
- Energetic mismatch with child
- Affective mismatch with child
- Difficulty matching pacing with child
- Difficulty registering subtle cues from child (responds only at "boiling point")
- Challenged to notice when child is tired

- Inability to capitalize on windows of alertness in child
- Challenged to accurately perceive state transitions in child
- Difficulty establishing/maintaining routines
- Difficulty establishing predictability for child
- Incapacity to support child through transitions
- Unable to read bodily and behavioral signs of child's physiological, arousal, and/or emotional states
- Challenged to comprehend and adjust to child's sensory integration needs
- Relies on child for coregulation

PCRC 6: Parent has the capacity to identify, act on, and also control **impulses** sufficiently to have rewarding relationships and life experiences and can foster these abilities in child AND child demonstrates an age-expectable capacity to identify, act on, and also control impulses.

Parental behavioral symptoms and functional impairments that might negatively affect PCRC 6 include the following:

- Repeats with child problematic patterns of interacting from past involving impulse control
- Difficulty inhibiting impulses for the sake of child's well-being
- Difficulty acting on impulses for the sake of child's well-being
- Incapacity to inhibit impulses to use substances negatively affecting child/family
- Prone to angry outbursts
- Tends to intrude on child's play
- Handles child's body in ways that startle/disorient child/undermine child's sense of agency
- Responds punitively to child's developmentally expectable impulses (e.g., sexual, aggressive)

- Responds with alarm or an expression of being overwhelmed in response to child's impulses
- Challenged to help child learn to identify, check, act on, or redirect impulses
- Encourages impulsive behavior in child
- Experiences child's impulsivity as being the source of parent's challenges
- Unable to make/follow through on plans for/with child
- Disrupts child's play/learning activities
- Unable to support child in anticipating and managing transitions
- Lack of planning and follow-through places child/family in dangerous/taxing/compromised situations
- Demonstrates lack of negative capabilities (e.g., capacity to wait, stand by, hold one's tongue, defer gratification) leading to discord/mishap/lost opportunity for child/family

PCRC 7: Parent is able to pay attention and focus as needed and to engage child in attending and focusing AND child demonstrates a developmentally expectable capacity for **shared focus/mutual attention** and is on a path toward being able to focus and attend on his or her own.

Parental behavioral symptoms and functional impairments that might negatively affect PCRC 7 include the following:

- Repeats with child problematic patterns around shared focus and mutual attention from parent's past
- Difficulty attending to things that are important to/growth promoting for child
- Incapacity to turn off cell phone, television, etc., to make space for connection and interaction with child
- Incapacity to support child in engaging in activities other than television or other "screens"

- Challenged to manage transitions between solo, two-person, and three-person (or more) interactions
- Difficulty settling into focused exchanges with child
- Limited ability to enjoy shared focus with child
- Incapacity to follow child's lead
- Lack of patience with child's appetite for repetition
- Incapacity to suspend/alter grown-up agenda
- Difficulty imagining or appreciating what captures child's interest
- Limited tolerance for input along one or more sensory modalities (e.g., sound, sight, touch) leads to restricted sensory environment for child
- Conveys to child conviction that the world holds no attraction/reward
- Overstimulates/overwhelms/overpowers/overrides child
- Provides understimulating environment for child
- Provides overstimulating environment for child
- Underresponsive to child's bids for attention/interaction
- Difficulty attending and focusing leads to problems in role functioning such as:
  - Incapacity to hold a job
  - Incapacity to follow through with reunification requirements
  - Incapacity to cooperate with co-parent
- Difficulty pursuing, retaining, or implementing information pertinent to care of child

PCRC 8: Parent possesses and conveys to child reasonable confidence that many things can be figured out/worked out successfully AND child demonstrates age expectable **problem-solving** capacities.

Parental behavioral symptoms and functional impairments that might negatively affect PCRC 8 include the following:

- Repeats with child problematic patterns around problem solving from parent's past
- Difficulty problem solving on behalf of child/family, for example,
  - Tendency to be incapacitated by worry
  - Difficulty organizing thinking
  - Difficulty mustering/channeling energy to tackle problems
  - Tendency to externalize/blame others
  - Prone to catastrophic thinking
  - Prone to globalization
  - Difficulty planning for child/family activities
- Personalization/internalization prevent recognition of external contributions to family difficulty (e.g., how systems of oppression harm family)
- Shame/stigma prevent parent from seeking help
- Tendency to mask rather than secure needed assistance in relation to deficits
- Tendency to become lost in the problems of others (e.g., co-parent)
- Tendency to feel overwhelmed in relation to child's difficulties leads to incapacity to act (e.g., engage in medical or educational advocacy on child's behalf)
- Little patience for promoting child's problem-solving efforts
- Challenged to provide adequate stimulation/learning experiences for child
- Conveys fear/helplessness/hopelessness to child

PCRC 9: Parent talks to child and otherwise facilitates child's entry into **language and literacy** (including multilingualism as appropriate) and confidence in communication AND child is developing at age level the capacity for two-way gestural and/or verbal communication.

Parental behavioral symptoms and functional impairments that might negatively affect PCRC 9 include the following:

- Repeats with child problematic patterns related to language and literacy from parent's past
- Avoidance of talking to child
- Challenged to listen to child
- Does not engage in vocal exchanges with infant
- Demonstrates a lack of awareness that infant/child is listening when adults talk or argue
- Incapacity to recognize/value family literacies
- Devaluation of bilingualism
- Prone to shame in relation to reading and/or speaking
- Inability to promote racial literacy in child resulting from proneness to:
  - Internalized racism
  - Disavowed racism
  - Unacknowledged privilege
- Paucity of opportunities for literacy development
- Traumatic avoidance of reading-related activities
- Shame-based avoidance of reading-related activities
- Problems with accurately reading social cues leads to interpersonal conflict/social isolation
- Impeded capacity to construct family narratives regarding important/difficult family experiences
- Refusal to talk about subjects child needs help processing
- Talks incessantly, unable to engage child in back-and-forth flow

- Overreliance on "screens" to occupy child restricts child's opportunities for social exchange
- Engages in noncontingent interactions with child
- Ignores/misses opportunities to respond to child's bids for communicative exchange

PCRC 10: Parent is able to take satisfaction from **symbolic activities** and may use conversation, narration, play, and/or other practices to promote these capacities in child AND child is able to use symbols in developmentally expectable ways to play, process, and partake in meaning-making.

Parental behavioral symptoms and functional impairments that might negatively affect PCRC 10 include the following:

- Repeats with child problematic patterns from past related to symbolic activity and meaning-making
- Avoidance of playing with child/engaging in culturally appropriate symbolic activity
- Unable to take pleasure/solace in symbolic activity
- Gravely disorganized thinking endangers child/leads to environmental deprivation
- Traumatic re-experiencing collapses symbolic matrix, exposing child to impoverished and frightening worldview
- Concrete thinking prevents facilitation of symbolic capacities in child
- Subject to delusions that may lead to child endangerment
- Subject to hallucinations that may lead to child endangerment
- Subject to depression-related flattening of perception (e.g., color appears dulled), impeding ability to facilitate symbolic capacities in child

- Withdrawal/isolation/fear/depression results in maintaining a symbolically impoverished environment for child/family
- Conviction that life is meaningless prevents engaging child in meaning-making exchanges/activities
- Lack of understanding of interpersonal influence prevents co-construction of meaning
- Lack of capacity for contingent interaction prevents child from developing a sense that meaning can be made in relationships

PCRC 11: Parent is able to **access resources** on behalf of child and family AND child is able to make use of resources accessed by parent and is on a path toward accessing resources as developmentally expectable.

Parental behavioral symptoms and functional impairments that might negatively affect PCRC 11 include the following:

- Repeats with child problematic patterns from parent's past regarding accessing resources
- Limited recognition of external/systemic barriers to family well-being
- Devaluation of family/cultural resources
- Repeats undermining patterns regarding management of family resources
- Challenged to seek and/or apply knowledge regarding child's condition
- Challenged to secure resources on behalf of child/family
- Tendency to waste resources that might benefit child/family
- Holds pathological belief that some people succeed without help from others
- Believes that reliance on others is a trap

- Pervasive sense of helplessness/emptiness impedes agency
- Avoidance of self-care measures that would make accessing resources easier
- Shame- or stigma-based avoidance of securing needed resources
- Tendency to alienate resource gatekeepers
- Incapacity to imagine that the world holds promise
- Focused on external resources to the exclusion of internal or interpersonal experiences
- Incapacity to marshal internal resources
- Difficulty nurturing child's capacity to build internal resources

PCRC 12: Parent is able to maintain and enjoy a **network of family and/or friends**, that may include a co-parent, and to support child's relationships with this circle AND child is able to enjoy developing relationships with this network of people.

Parental behavioral symptoms and functional impairments that might negatively affect PCRC 12 include the following:

- Repeats with child problematic patterns from parental past regarding family and friends
- Difficulty establishing/maintaining relationships
- Prioritizes other things (work, substance use, recreation) over nurturing family's social network
- Disregard for ties that are important to child (e.g., with peers, neighbors, relatives)
- Problematic patterns of relating from family of origin repeated in contemporary family
- Devaluation of family/community/culture
- High degree of conflict with co-parent
- Incapacity to cooperate or communicate effectively with co-parent

- Tendency to engage in gatekeeping or parental alienation regarding co-parent
- Challenged to establish effective role definition in blended/extended family
- Engages in conflict rather than co-operation with other caregivers
- Tendency to "burn bridges"/engage in emotional cutoff
- Tendency to withdraw/isolate

PCRC 13: Parent is able to manage frustration and channel **aggression** in appropriate directions, and to promote these capacities in child AND child is developing these capacities at age level.

Parental behavioral symptoms and functional impairments that might negatively affect PCRC 13 include the following:

- Repeats with child problematic patterns from parent's past regarding aggression
- Discomfort with aggressive impulses leads to disavowal and problematic modes of expression of aggression
- Tendency to feel threatened/endangered/controlled by child
- Vulnerable to angry/aggressive outbursts with child
- Exposes child to frightening interpersonal antagonism or violence
- Exposes child to frightening/overwhelming representations of aggression or violence
- Challenged to tolerate or celebrate child's aggressive impulses
- Holds the belief that some people (e.g., girls/women) ought not to experience or express aggression
- Incapacity to advocate for child when child is mis-perceived as aggressive (e.g., through a racist lens)

- Inhibited from action due to fear of being perceived as aggressive through a racist lens (e.g., stereotype of angry Black woman or violent Black man)
- Incapacity to provide growth-promoting outlets for child's aggressive impulses
- Inability to help child recognize and symbolize/be fueled by aggressive impulses
- Mocks/shames/humiliates/teases/frustrates child
- Aggrandizes self by belittling child
- Incites aggression in child
- Incites "bad" behavior in child to be able to discharge aggression through punishment
- Tendency to compete with child

PCRC 14: Parent is able to set limits with child in ways that promote development AND child is able to make good use of **limit-setting** interactions in working toward internalizing the ability to avoid danger, consider others, follow rules, defer gratification, etc.

Parental behavioral symptoms and functional impairments that might negatively affect PCRC 14 include the following:

- Repeats with child problematic patterns from parent's past regarding limit setting
- Incapacity to exercise moderation, leading to chaos in household
- Difficulty heeding limits (e.g., speed limits, spending, alcohol consumption) endangers child/family
- Difficulties around limit setting with co-parent/ extended family
- Disagreements with co-parent around limit setting leads to incoherent messages for child
- Difficulty setting growth-promoting limits with child
- Challenged to implement developmentally meaningful limits with different-aged siblings

- Relies on separation (e.g., "time out") to set limits, which is eroding relational solutions
- Tendency to engage in power struggles with child
- Tendency to plead with child
- Tendency to threaten child
- Tendency to escalate rather than remain calm and firm around limit setting
- Confuses limit setting with punishment
- Alternates between being overly permissive and then punitive

PCRC 15: Parent has the capacity to plan for and support the child around **separations** in ways that promote development and well-being AND child displays an age-expectable capacity to manage and benefit from developmentally reasonable separations from parent.

Parental behavioral symptoms and functional impairments that might negatively affect PCRC 15 include the following:

- Repeats with child problematic patterns from parent's past around separation
- Challenged to maintain connection with child despite forced separation (incarceration, deportation, child welfare involvement)
- Challenged to support child's connection with absent family member in situation of forced separation (incarceration, deportation, child welfare involvement)
- Challenged to make decisions with child's best interests in mind in the context of separation/dissolution/divorce
- Lack of empathy around child's separation-related struggles
- Tendency to feel overwhelmed/stifled by child's dependence leads to developmentally problematic emotional or physical separations

- Subject to separation rage, leading to problematic interpersonal patterns that undermine family stability
- Confuses separation with abandonment, undermining capacity to support growth-promoting separations for child
- Difficulty tolerating growth-promoting separations from child
- Difficulty tolerating child's difference/being a separate person
- Reliance on constant affirmation from child undermines child's differentiation
- Reliance on child for coregulation prevents differentiation
- Fear/worry leads to restrictive supervision/impedes child's growth-promoting exploration
- Uses separation (e.g., "time out" or emotional cutoff) as punishment
- Difficulty trusting others prevents development of social milieu for child
- Emotional numbing leads to developmentally harmful separations

PCRC 16: Parent takes pride and pleasure in his or her (or family) **culture(s)**, respects other cultures, and has the capacity to promote a sense of cultural identity and respect for other cultures in child AND child is able to take pleasure and pride in family culture(s) and demonstrates respect for other cultures.

Parental behavioral symptoms and functional impairments that might negatively affect PCRC 16 include the following:

- Repeats with child problematic patterns from parental past regarding culture
- Internalized stigma/shame prevents promotion of positive cultural identifications

- Devalues family's sociocultural resources, traditions, etc.
- Challenged to advocate on child's behalf to ensure culturally responsive care from pediatric, early intervention, early care and education providers and the like
- Difficulties in co-parenting relationship regarding cultural differences
- Difficulties in blended/extended family relationships regarding cultural differences
- Promotes in child fear of/negative attitudes toward particular cultural groups
- Blames self/child for problems attributable to forces of oppression
- Narrow repertoire of idioms of respect prevents socialization of child toward respect
- Paucity of racial literacy impedes capacity to promote racial literacy in child
- Evidences wounds of racial or historical trauma negatively impacting parenting
- Acculturation challenges undermine parental role functioning
- Immigration challenges undermine parental role functioning
- Challenged to support child's developing bicultural identity
- Misattributes problematic parenting practices to cultural tradition (e.g., harmful patterns of interacting that may derive from internalized systems of oppression)
- Complies with dominant cultural conventions harmful to self/child/family
- Socializes child in keeping with harmful cultural mores
- Fails to cultivate in child respect for others perceived as different

- Promotes in child the pathological belief that privilege is based in merit
- Isolates child/family from potentially enriching cultural connections
- Imposes culturally inappropriate expectations on child

PCRC 17: Parent is able to act to restore a sense of safety, hope, trust, and well-being for self and child following a distressing, disturbing, or **traumatic event** AND child is able to respond to parent's actions and to calm, restore, and heal.

Parental behavioral symptoms and functional impairments that might negatively affect PCRC 17 include the following:

- Repeats with child problematic trauma-related patterns from parent's past
- Inability to recognize wounds of racial trauma in self or child impedes empathic functioning
- Inability to recognize wounds of historical trauma for family impedes empathic functioning
- Inability to recognize wounds of immigration trauma for family impedes empathic functioning
- Inability to tolerate the fact that child has been harmed leads to emotional abandonment of child
- Limited understanding of the relational impact of trauma
- Lack of understanding of developmental impact of trauma
- Disabled capacity to discern safety and danger leads to child endangerment
- Vulnerability to flooding prevents empathic attunement
- Tendency to experience child as a trauma trigger
- Collapse of protective functioning
- Altered presentation following trauma frightens child

- Hypervigilance leads to overly restrictive supervision
- Ruptured protective functioning leads to inadequate supervision
- Sense of foreshortened future prevents planning on behalf of child and family
- Phobic avoidance restricts child's opportunities for learning and exploration
- Emotional numbing prevents empathic attunement/emotional responsiveness

PCRC 18: Parent is able to mourn losses and support child in **mourning** losses AND child is able to make use of parent's support to mourn losses in keeping with developmental level.

Parental behavioral symptoms and functional impairments that might negatively affect PCRC 18 include the following:

- Repeats with child problematic patterns from parental past related to loss and mourning
- Internalizes rather that recognizing systems of oppression that have led to injury, loss, and trauma for self/child/family
- Capacity to engage in rituals and processes that would facilitate family mourning is impeded
- Depressive anhedonia impedes capacity to enjoy child
- Believes that infants and children cannot be depressed
- Challenged to register or respond to child's depressive symptoms
- Unable to identify sources of sorrow in past, instead perceiving present life with child as grim/empty/bereft
- Debilitated by tendency to turn aggressive impulses toward self, leaving little energy for engaging with child
- Manic defense against loss leads to failure to attune to child

- Maintains belief that sadness or negative affect will harm fetus
- Maintains belief that sadness or negative affect will harm infant
- Maintains belief that sadness or negative affect will render milk harmful
- Self-recrimination erodes confidence in parenting capacities
- Hopelessness dampens capacity to facilitate growth opportunities
- Nurturing capacities sapped
- Depressive lethargy leads to abdication of parenting responsibilities
- Withdraws from child
- Depressive isolation limits child's opportunities for growth-promoting exploration and learning
- Emotionally disconnected from child

PCRC 19: Parent has the ability to work or otherwise contribute to society/the world AND child shows developmentally expectable signs of a sense of **efficacy**, confidence, and competence.

Parental behavioral symptoms and functional impairments that might negatively affect PCRC 19 include the following:

- Repeats with child problematic patterns from parental past regarding a sense of efficacy, confidence, and competence
- Symptoms of mood disorder/personality disorder/ substance abuse disorder lead to recurrent problems with employment, undermining family stability
- Internalizes rather that recognizing systems of oppression that have led to blocked opportunity for self/child/family

- Sense of shame overshadows recognition of positive capacities or potential
- Lack of sense of parental agency/authority
- Disinclination to make a positive contribution restricts sense of possibility for child
- Incapacity to recognize opportunities to make a positive contribution
- Employment-related risks and hazards endanger child and family
- Incapacity to buffer child and family from work-related stressors
- Employment-related challenges undermine child and family well-being
- Incapacity to advocate on child's behalf
- Pervasive sense of helplessness prevents parent from facilitating rewarding family engagement with community/wider world
- Thwarts child's agency
- Criticizes child inordinately
- Rejecting of child
- Tends to belittle, mock, or humiliate child
- Challenged to recognize child's desire to please/make a contribution
- Lack of motivation to provide for/take care of child/family
- Sees it as someone else's responsibility to provide for/take care of child/family
- Lack of confidence in capacity to successfully provide for/take care of child/family

PCRC 20: Parent is able to **reflect** upon/think about his or her own experience, including how his or her past experiences may be impacting his or her experiences as a parent and can recognize the child's experience as that of a separate person AND child shows developmentally expectable signs of experiencing him- or herself as a unique person with interest in and concern for others as separate people.

Parental behavioral symptoms and functional impairments that might negatively affect PCRC 20 include the following:

- Repeats with child problematic patterns from parental past regarding reflective functioning
- Prone to entering "freeze/fight/flight" mode
- Lacks a sense of humor
- Confuses child with figures from parental past, including self as a child
- Believes that child is the source of life difficulties
- Reports feeling helpless to improve parent–child relationship/family circumstances
- Imposes values/beliefs that are harmful to child
- Tendency to globalize impedes capacity to tolerate painful family experiences or tackle discrete challenges
- Tendency to engage in catastrophic thinking frightens child
- Tendency to offer contradictory accounts of the same material confuses child
- Vulnerability to black-and-white thinking undermines child's and family's capacities for integration
- Limited capacity for insight regarding child's experience
- Avoidance of potential contact with painful thoughts or feelings leads to restriction of child's emotional, relational, or physical world

- Fosters fear in child of people representing particular groups (e.g., based on gender, race)
- Interacts with child in ways that foster a sense of superiority (e.g., based on gender, race)
- Interacts with child in ways that inhibit the development of awareness of privilege
- Frequent/persistent negative attributions toward child
- Blames child for...
- Upholds developmentally inappropriate expectations of child
- Prone to action rather than reflection in response to child
- Proneness to action rather than reflection continually destabilizes family
- Demonstrates lack of insightfulness, as evidenced by...
- Substitutes child for self, for example,
  - Presents child for unnecessary medical care
  - Enlists child in bringing desired attention from others
  - Neglects self-care needs, focusing exclusively on child
- Concrete/disorganized thinking impedes capacity to facilitate development of child's symbolic and communicative capacities
- Repeats rather than working through painful past experiences

APPENDIX F

Library of Sample Observable, Measurable, Relationship-Focused Objectives

Objectives are things that clients and their collateral partners do.

Objectives are generated collaboratively with parents as part of the treatment planning process. During the clinical assessment process, the infant mental health (IMH) worker joins with the parent in reflecting on what has been learned about the difficulties that affect and that are manifest in the parent–child relationship and the family. The Parent–Child Relationship Competencies (PCRCs) may be an explicit part of this conversation or may simply inform the IMH worker's thinking in engaging in this conversation. The IMH worker supports the parent in articulating overarching goals for the child, the adult-as-parent, the parent–child relationship, and the family. Together, the IMH worker and parent identify specific changes that the parent would like to see that would constitute meaningful milestones toward achieving their overarching goals.

In most systems of care, objectives need to be formulated in observable and measurable terms to be deemed coherent indicators of progress in treatment. It is critical that IMH workers have direct access to information about how documentation is evaluated within their program or system of care. Because evaluation criteria vary from state to state, county to county, and program to program, this library should not be considered a substitute for proactive, program-specific conversations about documentation requirements.

In many systems, the necessary elements of an objective are as follows:

Who (client, collateral partner, or both together) + **What** (objective-related verb—see list below—plus content) + **When** (frequency and timeframe) + **How Measured** (as observed/reported by whom?) + **Baseline** (where we are starting from?).

Remember that in the context of behavioral health or mental health systems, the objectives must make sense in connection with the diagnosable condition or functional impairments necessitating the service. Plenty of absolutely wonderful life objectives do not require the intervention of IMH workers! There must be a clear link among the following:

1. The diagnosable condition establishing medical/service necessity,

2. The behavioral symptoms and functional impairments that manifest in a PCRC in need of strengthening,

3. The family's overarching goals, and

4. The collaboratively generated relationship-focused objectives.

When all of these elements are articulated, it should be clear why the expertise of the IMH worker is specifically useful in supporting the family to pursue their goals and meet their objectives.

Vignette 1 (PCRC 2)

Imagine an underweight 3-month-old infant with a parent who is anxious about this condition, feeling criticized and blamed by pediatric providers and helpless to improve the situation. The parent and infant are engaged in frequent unsuccessful feeding interactions because the parent is not sure when the baby might be hungry, so she attempts to feed too frequently for the baby to regularly experience and express hunger, resulting in a vicious cycle.

One straightforward objective might be: "Infant's weight will be within developmentally expectable limits by the next pediatric appointment." This objective alone does not demonstrate why IMH intervention is indicated or how a diagnosable behavioral health condition plays a role in the difficulty. Therefore, this objective would need to be included along with additional objectives that do address the relational, emotional, or behavioral issues of concern.

Here is an example of how an objective aimed at establishing a growth-promoting feeding pattern for this dyad might be written with the infant as the identified client, the parent as the identified client, or either:

1. The client will clearly signal hunger to the parent by crying or rooting 8 times per day on a daily basis as reported by the parent (current baseline: 1–2 times per day) within the next month.

2. The client will report registering and responding to the infant's signals of hunger 8 times per day on a daily basis within the next month (current baseline: 1–2 times per day).

3. The client and the collateral partner will sustain feeding interactions of 20 minutes' duration every 3 hours on a daily basis within the next month (current baseline: brief interactions multiple times per day) as reported by [parent/client].

Often, it is useful to put the baseline as well as the desired outcome in the parent's own words, for example:

4. The client reports only knowing for sure that the baby is hungry once or twice a day and attempting to feed unsuccessfully every hour or so out of concern for the baby's low weight. The client will report daily successful feeding interactions with the infant of 20 minutes' duration approximately every 3 hours within the next month.

It is often important to include within the objective some of the behavioral symptoms or functional impairments related to the diagnosable condition. For example, if the parent is the identified client in this vignette and meets criteria for an anxiety diagnosis, the objective might state the following:

5. As a result of relentless worry about getting it wrong, the client reports only knowing for sure that the baby is hungry once or twice a day and attempting to feed unsuccessfully at least every hour. The client will report daily successful feeding interactions with the infant of 20 minutes' duration no more frequently than every 3 hours within the next month.

Some systems advocate **SMART** as a mnemonic device for remembering the key elements of objectives—**S**imple or **S**traightforward, **M**easurable, **A**chievable (alternatively, this letter can stand for **A**ction-oriented or **A**ction word), **R**ealistic and **R**elevant, and **T**ime-framed or **T**ime-limited. Other systems use **RUMBA**: **R**ealistic, **U**nderstandable, **M**easurable, **B**ehavioral, and **A**ttainable. IMH workers can initiate collaborative conversations with reflective supervisors and whoever may be responsible for quality assurance in their program or county to agree on helpful guidelines along these lines.

Relationship difficulties always exist for good reasons and are usually multiply determined, so change can be slow. It is often helpful to use the Stages-of-Change framework (Copeland, 2000; Taubman, 2007) for formulating objectives collaboratively with the parents so that the objectives are reasonable, meaningful, and attainable in the context of the present reality of family life. This approach articulates the following sequence for objectives:

1. The client [or collateral partner] will acknowledge the problem.

2. The client [or collateral partner] will be able to describe the problem accurately.

3. The client [or collateral partner] will identify strengths, resources, and strategies available to resolve the problem.

4. The client [or collateral partner] will act on identified strengths, resources, and strategies to resolve the problem.

5. The client [or collateral partner] will manifest ultimate outcomes.

Vignette 2 (PCRC 3)

What follows is an example of a Stages-of-Change–based series of collaboratively generated relationship-focused treatment objectives with a child welfare–involved family. The child (a toddler) is in an out-of-home placement because of findings of both neglect and physical abuse. The parent denies having harmed the child and reports not knowing how the child was injured. The family is receiving reunification services, and the dyad has 2 days of unsupervised time together at present; weekly home-based IMH visits are to take place during one of these visits. The parent is the identified client in this example. The relationship-focused clinical formulation linked a diagnosable condition (depression, with related isolation, irritability, hopelessness, anhedonia, low sense of efficacy, and low energy) with challenges in parental role functioning leading to findings of child abuse and neglect and current family separation.

1. **Acknowledge the problem:** At present, the client is outraged that the child has been removed and states seeing no reason for child welfare involvement in her family's life. During weekly home-based IMH meetings, the client will identify three things that led others to deem there to be safety concerns related to her toddler by [date].

2. **Describe the problem accurately:** At present, the client states that she does not have any parenting challenges other than "the system being in my life." During weekly home-based IMH meetings, the client will identify three pre-existing parenting challenges that may be

exacerbated by current child welfare involvement by [date].

3. **Identify strengths, resources, and strategies available to resolve the problem:** The client states that she feels alone, blamed, and without help as a parent. During weekly home-based IMH meetings, the client will identify three potential sources of support and enjoyment for herself and toddler by [date].

4. **Act on identified strengths, resources, and strategies to resolve the problem:** At present, the client engages in no community activities with the toddler. The client will report during weekly home-based IMH meetings attending story hour at the library with toddler (or another such activity) one time per week over the course of the next 3 months.

5. **Manifest ultimate outcomes:**

    A. At present, the client gets irritated with the toddler's demands and responds with verbal reprimands several times per day, resulting in an escalation of being upset for the dyad. The client will report using self-calming techniques practiced during weekly home-based IMH visits on a daily basis over the course of the next 6 months.

    B. At present, the client's toddler is in out-of-home placement, and the client has six reunification requirements to meet. During weekly home-based IMH meetings, the client will address impediments to meeting reunification requirements such that all requirements are met and the family is reunified within 6 months.

    C. At present, the client reports experiencing symptoms of depression (e.g., fatigue, irritation, lack of pleasure) that make parenting extra challenging during most hours of each day. The client will report during weekly home-based IMH meetings engaging in daily self-care routines such that she experiences entire symptom-free days at least once a week by [date].

Sample objective-related verbs: accomplish, achieve, avoid, be able to, be free of, cease to, decrease, demonstrate, establish, eliminate, increase, identify, maintain, manifest, outline, practice, prevent, plan, procure, realize, regain, reduce, report, resolve, restore, stabilize, secure, utilize

PCRC-Focused Objectives

For each of the following relationship-focused objectives, the **Who** and **What** elements are provided. The IMH worker would specify the **When, How Measured**, and **Baseline** elements as needed in keeping with documentation requirements in their practice setting. In addition, the IMH worker would specify for each objective who is the identified client and who is the collateral partner. For example, the first item in this library is "Parent will accurately verbally identify infant's physical/emotional needs." In the plan of care for an instance in which the parent is the identified client, this item would be stated this way: "The client will accurately verbally identify the infant's physical/emotional needs," whereas in the plan of care for an instance in which the child is the identified client, this item would be stated this way: "The parent as collateral partner will accurately verbally identify the client's physical/emotional needs."

Remember that, together, the objectives must make it clear why the expertise of an IMH worker is needed to help in addressing the difficulty. What are the emotional, behavioral, or relational problems linked to a diagnosable condition that make this set of objectives important?

PCRC 1: Parent is able to register and respond effectively to child's **needs** AND child is able to signal needs clearly in keeping with age level.

Sample relationship-focused objectives addressing PCRC 1 include the following:

- Parent will develop a plan to balance self-care needs with caregiving demands throughout each day.
- Parent will verbally identify child and family needs and possible sources of support.
- Parent will reflect on their own early experiences around needs being met or unmet and how this history may impact their parenting interactions with child.
- Co-parents will establish a nighttime care schedule for taking turns responding to the needs of their newborn baby so each parent can get adequate sleep.
- Parent will describe differences between instances when their toddler evidences a need versus a preference.
- Child's capacity to signal need clearly will increase, as evidenced by reaching or calling out for parent, gesturing, or using words.
- Parent will verbally identify signs of hunger in child.
- Parent will accurately verbally identify the infant's emotional needs.
- Parent will respond with holding, rocking, and so forth when infant cries.
- Incidents of child's miscuing will cease.
- Child's help-rejecting behaviors toward parent will be reduced.
- Child will accept the bottle when offered by parent.
- Parent will reduce frequency of offering bottle and expand repertoire of responsiveness.

PCRC 2: Parent is able to maintain his or her own **health and well-being**, promote child's health, and access pediatric (or other culturally meaningful) care as needed AND child is able to grow in keeping with developmental expectations and maintain physical health.

Sample relationship-focused objectives addressing PCRC 2 include the following:

- Parent will reflect on health-related experiences throughout their life that may affect their parenting interactions with child.
- Parent will implement practices they value for promoting family health and well-being that they have learned from family members or members of their culture/community.
- Parent will identify barriers to accessing nutritious food for family that may be exacerbating emotional or relational difficulties.
- Parent will verbally identify systemic barriers to their family's accessing or benefiting from care.
- Parent will implement harm reduction strategies to protect child from adverse effects of substance use.
- Parent will identify resources and opportunities for family to engage in pleasurable physical activity together in order to decrease depression-related low energy.
- Parent will support child to gain weight, resulting in child reaching developmentally expectable weight.
- Parent will engage in self-care activities so as to have energy to care for child.
- Co-parents will go on a date to have renewed energy for parenting.
- Parent will verbally identify historical experiences with health care/medical intervention that may be negatively affecting their confidence in pediatric care.

- Incidents of parent's forgetting to take medication they find helpful in maintaining parental functioning will decrease.
- Frequency of parent's participation in 12-Step meetings they find helpful in maintaining parental functioning will increase.
- Instances of parent's substance use in presence of child will cease.
- Parent will enlist landlord's or housing advocate's support in redressing conditions that trigger child's asthma.
- Parent and child will collaborate around medication-related interactions such that incidents of child's medication refusal will cease.
- Parent will create rewarding interactions around oral hygiene such that child's avoidance of brushing teeth will cease.
- Parent will reduce incidents of engaging in power struggles with child around toileting.
- Parent and child will engage in anxiety-reducing interactions at bedtime such that incidents of child's bedwetting will be reduced.
- Parent will support improvement of child's fine motor skills, as indicated by client's ability to adequately grasp, hold, and manipulate small objects.
- Parent will support improvement of child's gross motor skills, as indicated by client's ability to roll over, sit without support, and stand/walk.
- Parent will provide engaging activities that facilitate child's crossing midline.
- Parent will support improvement of child's self-help skills, as indicated by client's ability to hold a bottle, use a spoon, and participate in dressing.
- Child will demonstrate a developmentally expectable understanding of parent's medical condition.

- Child will demonstrate a developmentally expectable understanding of parent's mental health condition.
- Parent will demonstrate an understanding of child's medical condition.
- Child will cooperate in early intervention/pediatric services accessed by parent.
- Parent will facilitate child's attendance at/participation in early intervention/pediatric services.
- Child will make use of parent's help to increase use of assistive devices or aids (e.g., glasses).
- Parent will reinforce child's increased use of assistive devices or aids (e.g., glasses).
- Parent will access adaptive baby care equipment to support parenting with a disability.

PCRC 3: Parent has the capacity to provide **safety, protection, and comfort** for child AND child seeks out and accepts comfort and protection from parent and has a developmentally expectable ability to register security, anxiety, and fear.

Sample relationship-focused objectives addressing PCRC 3 include the following:

- Child will seek comfort from parent by increasing proximity/initiating cuddling/reaching to be picked up.
- Parent will offer comfort when child appears to need it by increasing proximity/initiating cuddling/holding child.
- Child will increase referencing of parent (e.g., tracking, checking back visually) when in public.
- Parent will identify experiences in their own relationship history/life history that make it difficult to recognize signs of potential danger.
- Parent will describe problematic patterns in their own upbringing related to children's need for comfort that

may be negatively affecting the current relationship with child.

- Child will cease to bolt in public, instead staying close enough to parent to be safe.
- Parent will physically restrict client from bolting when near traffic.
- Parent will intervene to ensure child's physical safety until incidents of child's self-injurious behaviors (e.g., recklessness, head banging, holding breath) cease.
- With parent's guidance and, as needed, physical intervention, incidents of child's injurious behaviors toward others (e.g., biting, kicking) will cease. Parent will hold child rather than putting her on time out when child is dysregulated.
- Parent will identify behavioral signs that infant may be experiencing anxiety or fear.
- Parent will identify behavioral signs that infant may be feeling comforted or safe.
- With parent's reassurance, child's hypervigilance will decrease.
- When infant exhibits "freezing" behavior, parent will prioritize increasing infant's sense of safety.
- Parent and child will feel safer, as evidenced by increased incidents of shared laughter.
- Parent will confirm that there are no syringes in a room before bringing infant into it.
- Parent will check to ensure that the stove is turned off before going to bed or leaving the apartment.
- Parent will check on sleeping baby at regular intervals.
- Parent will increase supervision by proactively checking on child at intervals of [number] times per [time unit] rather than waiting for a mishap before intervening.
- Parent will enlist landlord's cooperation in installing child safety equipment in apartment.

- Parent will call domestic violence shelter to find out steps for taking shelter there with infant.
- Parent will access crisis nursery rather than leaving infant with unreliable neighbor should the need arise for emergency care.
- Child will be soothed by parent's body/voice rather than relying on bottle.

PCRC 4: Parent is able to be **emotionally attuned** to/empathize with child AND child is able to experience and express a developmentally expectable range of human emotion.

Sample relationship-focused objectives addressing PCRC 4 include the following:

- Parent will respond to infant's cries with holding and verbal soothing.
- Child will calm and cease to cry when held and verbally soothed by parent.
- Child will cease miscueing when feeling the need for comfort or reassurance.
- Parent will respond to child's imagined underlying emotional need rather than their behavioral miscues.
- Parent will be able to verbalize plausible emotional motivation for child's behavior.
- Parent will practice infant massage techniques with baby when baby appears receptive.
- Parent and child will demonstrate contingent interaction.
- Parent and child will practice reparation following incidents of rupture.
- Parent will verbally describe child's imagined point of view.
- Parent and child will expand vocabulary of emotions.

- Parent will state for child what they perceive child to be feeling.
- Parent will help child put painful feelings into words.
- Parent will adjust pacing, tone, and so forth in response to child's cues of interest, fatigue, curiosity, pleasure, overstimulation, and so forth.
- Parent and child will demonstrate comfort with an increased range of expressed emotion.
- Parent will report increased pleasure in interacting with child.
- Child will demonstrate increased pleasure (e.g., animation, vocalization) in interactions with parent.
- Parent's tolerance for negative affect will increase, as evidenced by refraining from chastising child or withdrawing when child demonstrates sadness, anger, and so forth.
- Parent will describe historical antecedents to current difficulties with child's expression of particular emotions.
- Child will ask parent for help rather than treating parent as a prosthetic devise (e.g., pulling parent toward the refrigerator when wanting food).
- Child will demonstrate reduced anxiety, as evidenced by ceasing to engage in role-reversed caregiving interactions with parent when parent is in distress.
- Child will demonstrate awareness of the feelings/ responses of others (e.g., saying "excuse me" when bumping into peers).

PCRC 5: Parent has the capacity to self-regulate and to engage in **mutual regulation** with child AND child is able to participate in mutual regulation with the parent and is developing the capacity to self-regulate.

Sample relationship-focused objectives addressing PCRC 5 include the following:

- Parent will identify experiences they have had throughout their life involving regulatory capacities and how these experiences my affect their parenting interactions with child.
- Parent will accurately describe their energetic match or mismatch with child in a given moment.
- Co-parents will collaborate so that each can practice being a coregulating partner with child.
- Parent will practice self-calming techniques such as running gaze slowly over infant's face and body, noticing tiny details when parent experiences panic.
- Parent will facilitate child's practicing self-calming techniques such as placing hand on racing heart, counting, and blowing bubbles.
- Parent will follow through with self-care routines such as taking medication, eating, or exercising such that they have enough energy to match child's energy level.
- Parent will facilitate child's activation in order to benefit from opportunities for learning and connecting.
- Parent and child will engage in coregulation interactive games such as up-regulating and down-regulating finger-play and songs (e.g., "Itsy Bitsy Spider" or "Motor Boat Motor Boat Go So Slow").
- Parent will practice mindful self-regulation techniques when baby cries.
- Parent will verbally identify signs of state regulation changes in baby.

- Parent will capitalize on baby's windows of quiet alert state to [goal].
- Child will cooperate with bedtime routine established by parent.
- Parent will verbally identify impediments to establishing a bedtime routine for child.
- When dysregulated, child will be calmed by parent's soothing interactions.
- Incidents of child becoming dysregulated when in parent's care will decrease.
- Parent will use anticipatory language to support child in managing difficult transitions.
- Instances of parent's losing their temper and yelling at child will decrease.
- Parent will complete a sensory profile inventory to pinpoint areas of sensitivity for child.

PCRC 6: Parent has the capacity to identify, act on, and also control **impulses** sufficiently to have rewarding relationships and life experiences and can foster these abilities in child AND child demonstrates an age-expectable capacity to identify, act on, and also control impulses.

Sample relationship-focused objectives addressing PCRC 6 include the following:

- Parent will safeguard family well-being by managing impulses to drink/use by [date].
- Co-parents will check impulses to fight in the presence of child.
- Parent will refrain from disciplining child impulsively.
- Parent will verbally articulate rather than acting on impulses that would be harmful or detrimental to child/family.
- Parent will cease to suppress impulses toward actions that would enhance family well-being.

- Parent will verbally articulate for child growth-promoting impulses that child seems to be inhibiting.
- Parent will encourage child to act on growth-promoting impulses.
- With parent's guidance, child will use words to express anger/displeasure rather than hitting.
- Parent will praise child for inhibiting impulses toward prosocial ends.
- Parent will praise child for attempting to inhibit impulses toward prosocial ends.
- Parent will engage child in response inhibition games such as freeze tag or "Simon Says."
- Child will demonstrate spontaneous initiation of play.
- Child will engage in vigorous physical activity.
- Child will initiate physical contact.
- Parent will provide appealing acceptable alternatives when child demonstrates an impulse to take an unacceptable action.
- Child will ask parent for help when struggling with difficult impulses.

PCRC 7: Parent is able to pay attention and focus as needed and to engage child in attending and focusing AND child demonstrates a developmentally expectable capacity for **shared focus/mutual attention** and is on a path toward being able to focus and attend on his or her own.

Sample relationship-focused objectives addressing PCRC 7 include the following:

- Parent will turn cell phone off while interacting with child for intervals of [time unit].
- Parent will verbally identify signs that infant is interested in something.

- Parent will identify and expand zone of child's interest (e.g., elaborate with increasing nuance on activities of child's favorite action figure).
- Parent will decrease child's exposure to "screens."
- Child will increase incidents of social referencing with parent.
- Child's gaze aversion with parent will decrease.
- Parent will elongate intervals of shared focus with child.
- Parent will use tone of voice and facial expression to kindle child's interest in objects and activities.
- Parent will engage infant in activities that stimulate a range of sensory modalities (sight, sound, smell, taste, touch, and proprioception).
- Parent will follow child's lead to identify areas of interest.
- Duration of interval that child can sustain engagement with novel activity with parent will increase.
- Duration of interval that child can sustain engagement with an activity on their own in the presence of parent will increase.
- Parent will provide opportunities for vigorous physical play alternating with calm, focused activities.
- Increase amount of one-on-one time between child and parent.
- Parent will reduce environmental stimuli to support child's capacity to focus.

PCRC 8: Parent possesses and conveys to child reasonable confidence that many things can be figured out/worked out successfully AND child demonstrates age expectable **problem-solving** capacities.

Sample relationship-focused objectives addressing PCRC 8 include the following:

- Parent will facilitate child's problem-solving capacity by asking questions/making suggestions/providing encouragement rather than taking over.

- Parent's sense of being overwhelmed by caregiving responsibilities will decrease, as evidenced by articulating discreet needs and challenges so these can be tackled one by one.

- Child will demonstrate increased confidence in their problem-solving capacities, as evidenced by asking for help rather than collapsing into tears.

- Parent will verbally affirm child's capacity to take effective action.

- Parent's capacity to advocate on child's behalf will increase, as evidenced by writing a list of concerns to raise with pediatrician/teacher.

- Parent will limit confounding variables in order to increase child's experiences of pleasure and success with exploratory/learning activities.

- Parent will introduce increasing complexity around child's exploratory/learning activities based on reading child's readiness cues.

- Parent will practice the principle of titrated elaboration, attending to child's growing edge and continually expanding horizons.

- Parent will tolerate and articulate the value of child using toys and objects in unconventional ways (e.g., building with puzzle pieces rather than completing the puzzle or pretending a bowl is a bicycle helmet).

- Parent will refrain from bringing desired objects to infant, instead providing opportunities for infant to crawl in order to reach objects.
- Incidents of parent losing patience with child will decrease.
- Co-parents will communicate, cooperate, and compromise in child's presence rather than fighting when encountering difficulty.
- Parent will demonstrate to child that broken items may be repaired.
- Child and parent will practice "stop and think" together when frustrated, overwhelmed, or discouraged.
- Parent will offer verbal encouragement when child appears frustrated with a task.
- Incidents of child losing patience with growth-promoting challenge will decrease.
- Parent will identify impediments to their capacity to solve problems on behalf of self and family.
- Parent will verbally identify impediments to finding a job/securing housing/entering recovery toward providing for child/family.

PCRC 9: Parent talks to child and otherwise facilitates child's entry into **language and literacy** (including multilingualism as appropriate) and confidence in communication AND child is developing at age level the capacity for two-way gestural and/or verbal communication.

Sample relationship-focused objectives addressing PCRC 9 include the following:

- Parent will talk to child.
- Child will demonstrate bilingual language acquisition as supported by parent.

- Parent will strategize with early care and education providers regarding supporting child's bilingual/bicultural development.
- Co-parents will collaborate regarding promoting child's language development, considering such questions as limiting time with "screens," promoting bilingualism, speaking about hard topics, and so forth.
- Child will engage with parent in mutually contingent face-to-face interactions for episodes lasting [time unit].
- Parent will echo sounds baby makes.
- Family will identify and celebrate culturally meaningful forms of literacy, including music, art, religion, craft, trade, food, and other microcultural forms.
- Parent will promote racial literacy in child by speaking about race and racism.
- Parent will enhance child's capacity to read the social world, including systems of oppression, by providing language for experiences of oppression and adversity.
- Baby will echo aspects of parent's speech.
- Child will initiate gestural communication.
- Parent will respond verbally to child's gestural communication.
- Parent will practice the principle of titrated verbal elaboration, attending to child's growing language edge and continually expanding linguistic horizons.
- Child and parent will sing together.
- Parent will narrate child's play.
- Parent will identify books that reflect aspects of family culture.
- Parent will establish comfortable, enjoyable spaces and routines for engaging with books.
- Parent will allow child to select a book to look at/read.
- Child will use agency in engaging with books (e.g., turning pages, establishing the pace, pointing

to details of pictures, and so forth) with parent's involvement.

- Parent will create a developmentally meaningful narrative about...
- Parent and child will construct booklets documenting aspects of family life.
- Increase incidents of child's use of words to express needs and desires.
- Expand parent's use of verbal responses to child's bids for interaction.
- Parent and child will complete loops of back-and-forth gestural or verbal communication.

PCRC 10: Parent is able to take satisfaction from **symbolic activities** and may use conversation, narration, play, and/or other practices to promote these capacities in child AND child is able to use symbols in developmentally expectable ways to play, process, and partake in meaning-making.

Sample relationship-focused objectives addressing PCRC 10 include the following:

- Parent will engage with child in co-construction of meaning rather than unilaterally imposing meaning (e.g., determining what a clay shape represents).
- Parent will identify symbolic activities family might engage in that would counter (e.g., depression, hopelessness, sense of isolation).
- Incidents of family participation in symbolic activities will increase.
- Parent will articulate possible meanings of child's behavior.
- Child's engagement in traumatic play will cease.
- Parent will articulate for child possible meanings of others' behavior.

- Parent will introduce child to systems of meaning making (e.g., artistic, social, cultural, spiritual).
- Duration of child's episodes of pleasurable engagement in play will increase.
- Parent will articulate growth-promoting value of play.
- Child and parent will construct a story or drawing together to make meaning of a challenging aspect of family life.
- Parent will articulate links between their historical experiences with play and their experiences around their child's play.
- Parent will practice waiting, watching, and wondering to see what play themes child develops.
- Parent will verbally express possible meanings of child's play.
- Parent will identify readily available household objects that may serve as play materials for child.
- Parent will add nuance to child's play themes.

PCRC 11: Parent is able to **access resources** on behalf of child and family AND child is able to make use of resources accessed by parent and is on a path toward accessing resources as developmentally expectable.

Sample relationship-focused objectives addressing PCRC 11 include the following:

- Parent will identify systemic barriers to accessing resources on behalf of child and family.
- Parent will identify family/cultural resources that may be devalued or diverted away from family by dominant culture.
- Parent will take steps to preserve family/cultural resources that may be devalued or diverted away from family by dominant culture.
- Parent will identify internal impediments to accessing resources on behalf of child and family.

- Parent will identify internal resources helpful to fulfilling parenting role that are in need of cultivation/replenishment.
- Parent will develop a plan to cultivate/replenish internal resources helpful in fulfilling parenting role.
- Child's reserve of internal resources [energy, resilience, humor, curiosity, interpersonal skills, and so forth] will be deepened, as evidenced by...
- Parent will secure early intervention/medical/educational services for child.
- Parent will implement at home strategies learned from early intervention practitioners.
- Incidents of child resisting participation in early intervention activities will decrease.
- Parent will increase availability of nutritious food for child and family.
- Incidents of child refusing nutritious food will decrease.
- Parent will increase opportunities for child to play and explore outdoors.
- Incidents of child avoiding/derailing outdoor activities will reduce.

PCRC 12: Parent is able to maintain and enjoy a **network of family and/or friends**, that may include a co-parent, and to support child's relationships with this circle AND child is able to enjoy developing relationships with this network of people.

Sample relationship-focused objectives addressing PCRC 12 include the following:

- Incidents of parent engaging in gatekeeping interactions with co-parent will reduce.
- Parent will intervene effectively to reduce sibling conflict.
- Parent will speak with child about the expected baby.

- Family isolation will be reduced, as evidenced by accessing the Family Resource Center to connect with other families.
- Parent will access mediation to reduce hostility with neighbors, thus increasing child and family comfort and safety in the neighborhood.
- Parent will arrange to go to the park with a parent and child from child's care center after pick-up to support children's friendship.
- Parent and child will join in neighborhood gathering.
- Child's separation anxiety will be reduced, as evidenced by settling readily into play with relative caregiver.
- Child will identify a game she enjoys playing with uncle.
- Despite parental conflict, parent will support child's relationship with other parent.
- Co-parents will establish a custody schedule that prioritizes child's developmental and relational needs over logistical convenience.
- Co-parents will consider sibling, stepsibling, and half-sibling relationships, as well as the need for one-on-one parent–child time when creating custody schedule.
- Stepparent will yield to parent's authority regarding disciplining child.
- Child will demonstrate increasing comfort with stepparent, as evidenced by lengthened intervals of relaxed, mutually enjoyable play.
- Parent will practice a protective narrative to use in public when strangers say offensive things or ask rude questions about child's difference.
- Child will, with parent's guidance, ask to join other children in play rather than barging in.

- Parent will strategize with early care and education providers about how to support child's relationships with peers.
- Parent will talk with child about absent family member and maintain ties via phone calls, letter writing, and so forth.
- Child will, with parent's guidance, ask children if it's OK before touching them.
- Parent will arrange child care so she is able to have adult time with friends.
- Parent and grandparent will resolve conflicts sufficiently to promote child–grandparent relationship.
- Parent and grandparent will develop a plan as to daily division of labor regarding caring for child/grandchild.

PCRC 13: Parent is able to manage frustration and channel **aggression** in appropriate directions, and to promote these capacities in child AND child is developing these capacities at age level.

Sample relationship-focused objectives addressing PCRC 13 include the following:

- Child will cease to bite peers.
- Parent will cease to act out aggressively with child.
- Parent will effectively contain sibling conflict.
- Parent will identify alternate possible emotional meanings of child's behavior when at first glance child seems to be motivated by aggression.
- Parent will reframe child's behavior in terms of child's vulnerability when teachers attribute aggression to child.
- Parent will differentiate between child's and parent's own aggressive acting out versus being assertive.
- Parent will convey to child that aggressive impulses are universal and need not be discharged in damaging ways.

- Parent will cease to use corporal punishment with child.
- Decrease incidents of co-parents arguing in child's presence.
- Parent will enact safety plan if level of marital conflict rises.
- Child and parent will direct aggressive impulses into vigorous and safe family recreational activity.
- Parent will provide language for child's imagined aggressive impulses.
- Parent will refrain from censoring or sanitizing aggressive themes in child's play.
- Incidents of parent inciting aggression in child will cease.
- Parent will counter child's inhibition by encouraging rough-and-tumble play, making messes, and so forth.
- Incidents of parent conveying fragility in the face of child's developmentally expectable aggressive impulses will reduce.

PCRC 14: Parent is able to set limits with child in ways that promote development AND child is able to make good use of **limit-setting** interactions in working toward internalizing the ability to avoid danger, consider others, follow rules, defer gratification, etc.

Sample relationship-focused objectives addressing PCRC 14 include the following:

- Parent will exercise moderation/heed limits as a harm reduction strategy in order to promote child and family safety.
- Parent will set limits/exercise boundaries with other adults in the interest of promoting child and family well-being.
- Parent will articulate the difference between effective and ineffective limit setting.

- Child will co-operate with parent around a prohibition.
- Parent will articulate the difference between necessary and unnecessary limit setting.
- Parent will articulate growth-promoting aspects of effective limit setting.
- Parent will articulate links between past experiences and current struggles with limits.
- Child will accept parent's offer of an alternative instead of resisting a limit.
- Parent will articulate the difference between limit setting and punishment.
- Parent will reduce incidents of the unnecessary and diluting use of "no."
- Parent will use a unique and startling pitch in setting critical safety-related limits with child.
- Incidents of parent exposing child to danger by failing to heed limits will reduce.
- Incidents of child defying reasonable limits set by parent will reduce.
- Incidents of child "testing"/inciting limit setting interactions will reduce.
- Incidents of child and parent engaging in power struggles will reduce.
- Incidents of parent nagging child will reduce.
- Incidents of parent threatening child will reduce.
- Incidents of parent pleading with child will reduce.

PCRC 15: Parent has the capacity to plan for and support the child around **separations** in ways that promote development and well-being AND child displays an age-expectable capacity to manage and benefit from developmentally reasonable separations from parent.

Sample relationship-focused objectives addressing PCRC 15 include the following:

- Incidents of child demonstrating clinging behavior in the face of potentially growth-promoting separations will reduce.

- Parent will signal to child that separating is safe and presents growth-promoting opportunities when this is the case.

- Parent will identify difficult separation-related experiences during their own upbringing that may impede their parental functioning around present-day separations.

- Parent will identify a sleeping arrangement that works for family (e.g., co-sleeping or sleeping separately from child) and support child in understanding and habituating to this arrangement.

- Increase incidents of child entering classroom without becoming dysregulated.

- Incidents of parent disappearing without saying goodbye will cease.

- Parent will alert child 15 minutes before supervised visit is ending so child will not be taken by surprise.

- Parent's tolerance for child's independent play and exploration will increase.

- Parent will access resources to mitigate harm to child in the event of forced separation (e.g., incarceration or deportation of a family member, child welfare involvement).

- Parent will provide developmentally meaningful information for child regarding forced separations family may be experiencing (e.g., due to incarceration, deportation, or child welfare involvement).

- Child will demonstrate confidence that the parent from whom they are separated loves them.
- Parent will help child to write a letter or draw a picture to connect with a loved one across a separation.
- Parent will create a developmentally meaningful narrative regarding anticipated separation.
- Child will participate in picking out an object likely to be comforting to them during period of separation.
- Parent and child will make a plan for telephone contact during period of separation.
- Parent will report a reduction in experience of emotional numbing when separating from child.

PCRC 16: Parent takes pride and pleasure in his or her (or family) **culture(s)**, respects other cultures, and has the capacity to promote a sense of cultural identity and respect for other cultures in child AND child is able to take pleasure and pride in family culture(s) and demonstrates respect for other cultures.

Sample relationship-focused objectives addressing PCRC 16 include the following:

- Family participation in community events will increase.
- Co-parents will reflect on the effect that cultural and other differences between them may have on their parenting styles.
- Parent will construct a family tree and talk with child about ancestors.
- Parent will select and read with child books celebrating aspects of family culture.
- Instances of parent saying disparaging things about women in child's presence will cease.
- Instances of parent condoning interpersonal violence in child's presence will cease.

- Parent will identify wounds of racial trauma [or other oppression-based wounds] that may impede desired parenting interactions.
- Parent will promote child's racial literacy by speaking about race, racism, and race-related issues.
- Parent will verbally identify for child microaggressions directed at family.
- Parent will verbally identify for child microaggressions that family members direct toward people from other cultures.
- Instances of parent mocking/humiliating child will cease.
- Parent and child will rehearse together empowering retorts they can use when confronted with biased, bigoted, or oppressive remarks or questions about their family from others.
- Child's demonstrated interest in and curiosity about cultural difference will be optimized by parent to promote respectful connections and learning.
- Parent will identify when child engages in disrespectful interactions with others and will demonstrate alternative interactions that are respectful.
- Instances of child making self-disparaging statements will cease.
- Parent will identify the effects of stigma/oppression on family members throughout generations and develop a strategy to interrupt the cycle.
- Parent will verbally identify sources of strength and inspiration in personal/family/cultural history.
- Parent will make representations of family culture (e.g., photographs, food, household traditions) known and available at child care center.
- Parent will verbally describe harmful views of other cultures they were exposed to as a child that they want to avoid passing on to their child.

PCRC 17: Parent is able to act to restore a sense of safety, hope, trust, and well-being for self and child following a distressing, disturbing, or **traumatic event** AND child is able to respond to parent's actions and to calm, restore, and heal.

Sample relationship-focused objectives addressing PCRC 17 include the following:

- Parent's capacity to plan and follow through on behalf of child and family rather than freezing or reacting in panic will increase.
- Parent's trauma-based pattern of placing child and family in harm's way will cease.
- Parent will identify wounds of racial trauma in self, child, and family.
- Parent will identify wounds of historical trauma in self, child, and family.
- Child and parent will engage in joyful interactions for a duration of...
- Child will demonstrate a renewed sense of hope, as reflected in play or drawing themes or pleasurable anticipation of future events.
- Child will demonstrate a renewed sense of trust in parent's protective capacities, as reflected in restored social referencing or refueling behaviors.
- Child and parent will be able to relax and rest, as evidenced by sleeping through the night.
- Parent will be able to articulate the difference between traumatic play and transformative/ growth-promoting play.
- Parent will successfully interrupt child's traumatic play, steering child toward transformative play.
- When child wakes from a nightmare, parent will reassure child that they are safe now.

- Parent will create a developmentally meaningful narrative together with child regarding the traumatic experience.
- Incidents of parent experiencing emotional numbing that prevents attunement to child will decrease.
- Incidents of parent frightening child by talking about traumatic material in a flooded state will cease.

PCRC 18: Parent is able to mourn losses and support child in **mourning** losses AND child is able to make use of parent's support to mourn losses in keeping with developmental level.

Sample relationship-focused objectives addressing PCRC 18 include the following:

- Parent will verbally acknowledge losses suffered by child.
- Parent will create a developmentally meaningful narrative to share with child regarding major losses.
- Parent will create a developmentally meaningful narrative to share with child regarding how things are different now.
- Parent and child will symbolize losses through joint ritual, song, play, or drawing themes.
- Parent and child will engage in remembering activities together to honor losses.
- Parent will help child understand that parent is grieving but will get better.
- Parent will be able to verbally describe child behaviors that may signal experiences of loss or grief.
- Symptoms of depression (e.g., insomnia/hypersomnia, lack of appetite) will decrease.
- Incidents of irritable acting out will decrease.
- Child will demonstrate restored capacity to take pleasure in activities and interactions with parent.

- Parent will demonstrate restored capacity to take pleasure in activities and interactions with child.
- Sense of foreshortened future will abate, as evidenced by shared pleasurable anticipation of a future event.
- Family isolation will be reduced, as evidenced by participation in [activity].

PCRC 19: Parent has the ability to work or otherwise contribute to society/the world AND child shows developmentally expectable signs of a sense of **efficacy**, confidence, and competence.

Sample relationship-focused objectives addressing PCRC 19 include the following:

- Parent will identify impediments to finding employment to provide for child/family.
- Incidents of parent blaming self for employment-related access barriers rooted in systems of oppression will decrease.
- Parent will take steps to address work-related hazards and stressors that undermine family health, safety, and well-being.
- Incidents of parent's work-related stressors negatively impacting family life will decrease.
- Parent will identify an activity that will satisfy their wish to make a positive contribution.
- Parent will take steps to participate in an activity satisfying their wish to make a positive contribution.
- Parent will expose child to pathways for making a positive contribution by pointing out interesting or laudable endeavors others are engaged in.
- Parent will articulate for child mechanisms that facilitate or block access.
- Parent will problem-solve with child overcoming barriers to participation in desired activities.

- Parent will articulate experiencing increased confidence in general, including in parenting capacities.
- Parent will promote in child a sense of success in contributing to family, community, or wider world by...
- Parent will verbally affirm infant's impulses to "help."
- Toddler will contribute to household chores by joining in picking up toys.
- Child will contribute to household projects by...
- Child will evidence pride in accomplishments by clapping hands when done.
- Parent will verbally identify impediments to advocating for child.
- Parent will develop a plan to advocate on child's behalf with school personnel.
- Parent will follow through with advocacy efforts on child's behalf.
- Parent will encourage child to persist rather than abandoning a frustrating task.
- Child will make use of parent's encouragement to persist with challenging tasks.

PCRC 20: Parent is able to **reflect** upon/think about his or her own experience, including how his or her past experiences may be impacting his or her experiences as a parent and can recognize the child's experience as that of a separate person AND child shows developmentally expectable signs of experiencing him- or herself as a unique person with interest in and concern for others as separate people.

Sample relationship-focused objectives addressing PCRC 20 include the following:

- Parent will articulate to child the perceived meaning behind the actions of others.

- Parent will verbally identify aspects of child's personality that are similar to and different from their own.
- Child will demonstrate comfort with differentiation from parent (e.g., preferring different food).
- Parent will demonstrate pride and pleasure in child's differentiation (e.g., a quality the child is in possession of that parent lacks).
- Instances of demonstrating negative capability (e.g., holding one's tongue, waiting) will increase.
- Parent will engage in reflection with child rather than action the next time [X] occurs.
- Child will engage in reflection with parent rather than action the next time [X] occurs.
- Parent will verbally describe how experiences in their past may be affecting their present experiences as a parent.
- Incidents of parent's framing nuanced matters in black-and-white terms will decrease.
- Incidents of parent's globalizing will decrease.
- Incidents of parent's evidencing catastrophic thinking will decrease.
- Incidents of parent offering grossly contradictory accounts of the same material will decrease.
- Incidents of parent entering "freeze/fight/flight" mode will decrease.
- Incidents of child entering "freeze/fight/flight" mode will decrease.
- Parent will cease to say disparaging things in child's presence regarding people representing particular groups.
- Instances of parent verbally blaming child inappropriately will cease.
- Parent will verbally articulate a plausible emotional motivation for child's behavior.

- Parent will verbally articulate to child what they imagine child may be thinking, feeling, imagining, or pondering in a given moment.
- Instances of parent attributing malevolence to child will decrease.
- Parent will pause to identify for themselves their motivation before interrupting/correcting/redirecting/reprimanding child.
- Parent will practice saying out loud to child every fourth thing that occurs to them.
- Child will articulate intention to parent prior to taking action.
- Child will sustain emotional equilibrium despite parent's distress.
- Child will verbally articulate an understanding of parent's point of view.
- Child will express concern for parent without evidence of undue anxiety.
- Child will engage in symbolic play reflecting working through of emotionally salient material.

APPENDIX G

Library of Sample Relationship-Focused, Infant Mental Health (IMH) Intervention Verbs

Three critical cautions when using this appendix include the following:

1. *Know your stuff.* This appendix is merely a list of examples, intended as a memory prompt. Infant mental health (IMH) workers use interventions in keeping with their training and expertise.

2. *Know your context.* Some interventions listed here might not be appropriate within particular practice settings or reimbursable in certain contexts. Many are just fragments of interventions, intended to be fleshed out in meaningful ways by IMH workers in practice. Requirements vary regarding how fine-grained, time-specific, and measurable interventions must be.

3. *Know your family.* IMH workers bring their own orientation and expertise, but intervention approaches must be acceptable and meaningful to families served. Interventions are things that IMH workers *do in collaboration with* and *on behalf of families*, not *to* families. In some instances, interventions are also things that parents will implement as collateral partners to support their child's progress toward meeting goals and objectives.

Interventions are specific things that IMH workers do to address mental health barriers to family well-being: to reduce impairment, restore functioning, promote resiliency, allow developmental progress as appropriate, or prevent significant deterioration in an area of life functioning. These practices may be deemed to be evidence-based or clinical techniques particular to a specific treatment modality. The distinguishing feature is that they are actions taken by the IMH worker, perhaps together with the collateral partner, in service of furthering the family treatment goals and supporting the clients in meeting collaboratively generated, relationship-focused objectives. In many practice settings, the overarching treatment modality (e.g., infant–parent psychotherapy, child–parent psychotherapy, ecosystemic play therapy, DIRFloortime®) will be discussed with parents and included in the collaboratively generated treatment plan of care. In most settings, "strengthen Parent–Child Relationship Competency (PCRC)" would be considered too vague and overarching to count as a specific intervention. Instead, the discreet actions taken by the IMH worker to support the identified client and collateral partner in strengthening the PCRC should be described.

In many systems of care, each progress note bears the responsibility of being meaningful as a "stand-alone" document. This standard means that the IMH worker makes it clear in each instance how the actions they are recording having taken during the session in question addressed the collaboratively generated goals and objectives, which, in turn, follow from the diagnosable condition and related areas of difficulty negatively affecting family well-being.

The following intervention verbs and phrases may be useful in formulating PCRC-informed treatment plans and documenting PCRC-focused interventions in progress notes:

Access resources on behalf of child and family.

Accompany parent and child through unaccustomed interactions/emotional experiences.

Account for puzzling child behavior through the lens of social–emotional development.

Activate parent's caregiving motivational system/child's attachment motivational system.

Adapt interventions to child's/parent's/family's individual needs and sociocultural context.

Address directly issues of historical trauma and systems of oppression that affect the parent's and child's experiences and the IMH worker–family relationship.

Admire out loud potentially unnoticed strengths in parent/child.

Advise parent (nondidactically) regarding developmentally informed understandings of child behavior.

Advocate on client's/family's behalf with pediatric provider/landlord/parole officer.

Affirm parent's goals/priorities/sense of challenge/injustice or child's perception of danger/need for interaction/exploration/understanding/comfort.

Affix words to experience.

Alter protocols to respond to family culture.

Amplify subtle/muted expressions on the part of one relationship partner to help the other apprehend them.

Analyze collaboratively with parent impact on child of....

Anticipate developmentally expectable challenges.

Applaud moments of collaboration/shared understanding/successful limits between parent and child.

Apply Diversity-Informed Tenets in session by....

Apprise parent of new literature/findings regarding child's condition.

Arbitrate in moments of conflict between co-parents toward keeping child's experience in mind.

Articulate understanding of parent–child conflict areas.

Ask for parent's understanding of the meaning of child's behavior/permission to intervene directly with child when such-and-such is happening.

Assess potential safety/danger issues collaboratively with parent.

Assist parent in securing needed resources for family.

Attune to both parent and child, even when they present in very disparate emotional states.

Avert power struggles between child and parent when they appear to be imminent.

Balance attention to child and parent needs in the moment.

Bear and (when the time is right) put into words emotional pain (parent's and child's) that parent may have a hard time thinking about.

Bolster parent's sense of authority.

Brainstorm with parent ways to....

Breathe deeply and with attention together with toddler and parent in moments of dysregulation to support coregulation.

Bridge emotional distance when co-parents are alienated from each other/service systems to pave the way for family.

Broaden the range of pleasurable activities parent and child can engage in together/emotional experiences parent can identify in child.

Broker compromises between co-parents that both can agree are in child's best interests.

Build parent's skill in attuning to child's emotional experience.

Call parent between sessions to check in about....

Calm parent's worries so parent is better able to attend to child.

Capture child's imagination by using ordinary objects in unexpected ways/parent's attention by demonstrating gut-level understanding/the emotional tone/inner state of infant by using evocative feeling language.

Carry out collaboratively generated plan to carve pumpkins during IMH session to enhance parent's comfort with growth-promoting messy play and learning experiences.

Celebrate developmental milestones that might be overlooked, given family stress.

Challenge undermining beliefs/problematic attributions/harmful practices.

Channel parent's anger away from the baby and toward worthy targets.

Check in with parent regarding week's pattern of bedtime/waking up routines.

Circle back to important themes/underexplored content/early concerns.

Clarify child welfare worker's expectations for parents.

Coach parents in practicing unaccustomed interactions with child.

Collaborate with parent regarding....

Collect evidence to present parent with a counternarrative about their parenting/their child/their family.

Combat discriminatory policies and practices harming child/parent/family.

Combine parent's and child's experiences/perspectives into a cohesive narrative.

Communicate with foster mother on a regular monthly basis in collaboration with birth parents regarding child's development and well-being.

Concentrate on details of child's play to explore possible meanings with parent.

Conduct (with parent's permission) a collaborative meeting with other providers to ensure that all are working in a coordinated way on behalf of child and family.

Confer and collaborate with child welfare worker to support reunification.

Confirm (with parent's permission) parent's ongoing sobriety on a monthly basis by telephone with case worker from recovery program.

Confront instances of perceived minimization of impact of trauma on child.

Connect themes in contemporary parent–child relationship with influential experiences from parent's past.

Consider with parent the impact of racism/classism/xenophobia in shaping parenting experiences.

Consolidate learning.

Construct a trauma-focused genogram collaboratively with parent.

Consult to speech therapist with parent's collaboration regarding child's understanding of....

Contact parent's psychiatrist to coordinate family care.

Contribute professional expertise when parent indicates that this feedback is welcome.

Convey developmentally realistic expectations/hope regarding possibilities for the future.

Coordinate early intervention, pediatric, and parent support services.

Coregulate with parent so that parent can coregulate with child.

Correct parent's inaccurate perceptions of IMH worker's scope of practice.

Counsel parent around emotional challenges related to child's medical condition.

Counter patterns that undermine family well-being.

Counteract negative impact of institutionalize oppression by....

Court parent's/child's curiosity by....

Create space in sessions to discuss race and racism to support parent in fostering child's racial literacy.

Cue child when transitions such as session endings are imminent.

Cultivate collaboratively with parent a list of things that help in moments of family stress.

Debrief with parent following stressful encounters with child welfare worker.

Debunk myths and stereotypes arising from systems of oppression.

Deconstruct mythology of good versus bad parents.

Deepen parent's understanding of child's experienced dilemma.

Defer to parent as authority on child and family.

Defuse conflict between parent and child by....

Delineate household boundaries that are meaningful and helpful to parent and child.

Demonstrate therapeutic holding/empathic understanding/flexibility/vulnerability/transparency.

Describe observed problematic/growth-promoting interactions between parent and child.

Desensitize dyad to trauma triggers with reflection and empathy.

Determine collaboratively with parent appropriate duration of sessions.

Develop collaboratively with parent a strategy for managing conflict in public.

Devise bedtime routines for child collaboratively with parent to increase sleep and decrease conflict.

Differentiate collaboratively with parent between past and present/parent's attributions and child's experience/things that can be changed and those that cannot.

[With parent's permission] **Direct** parent to interact with child in calming ways when child is dysregulated.

Disaggregate with parent confounding elements leading to being overwhelmed.

Disclose personal impressions and information in the service of building rapport as clinically indicated.

Discourage activities that might undermine parent's recovery.

Discuss ongoing impact of racism/homophobia/able-ism on family well-being.

Help parent to **disentangle** past experiences from present.

Dislodge parent's erroneous convictions regarding their parenting.

Distribute focus across all family members in the room to develop a holistic understanding of family experience.

Document child's language acquisition progress with parent on refrigerator chart.

Draw attention to mismatched pacing/misread cues/bids for comfort/signs of being overwhelmed.

Draw on family's non-dominant bodies of knowledge in finding solutions to family challenges.

Dwell on details of well-functioning PCRCs to lay foundation for addressing those that need strengthening.

Earn parent's trust by/right to challenge parent by/child's trust by....

Ease parent's burden by conducting telephone inquiries on their behalf.

Eat together with family to learn family culture/support nurturing connections/participate in establishing routines around nutrition desired by parent.

Educate parent regarding system of care.

Elicit family immigration stories.

Elongate intervals of playful interaction between parent and child by slowing parent down.

Empower parent by lifting up their voice rather than speaking for them/child by recognizing them as a person whose experience must be considered.

Encourage parent to prepare for morning routine the night before.

Engage child care consultant at child's center to improve family–center communication.

Engage in medical advocacy efforts on behalf of child/family.

Enhance parent's capacity to "pick their battles."

Enjoy moments of parent's and child's enjoyment of one another.

Enlist grandparent with parent's permission to develop intergenerational understanding of family struggles.

Enter domestic spaces with parent's permission and an eye to what they communicate about the family.

Envision change collaboratively with parent.

Equip parent to advocate for desired outcomes at upcoming Individualized Family Service Plan meeting.

Evaluate impact of therapeutic shadow on child's functioning in the classroom.

Experience discomfort without pressuring family to relieve this experience to learn about family realities.

Explicate parent's emotional state to child (verbal or preverbal).

Explore obstacles to family self-determination.

Expose parent gradually to situations they find intimidating that might be a positive resource for family.

Express concerns directly to parent so they may be addressed in the moment.

Extend intervals of attuned interaction/playful engagement between parent and child.

Facilitate transition to parenthood/mutually pleasurable interactions/reparation following rupture.

File a family safety plan with community immigrants' rights organization on behalf of family.

Find, collaboratively with parent, objects close at hand in home that hold interest for baby.

Form new relational expectations based on reciprocity and mutuality.

Focus on family recovery and self-determination.

Follow parent's lead in speaking with teachers about family challenges/child's lead in play.

Foster parental confidence by identifying growth-promoting interactions.

Frame questions that direct attention to....

Generate ideas collaboratively with parent regarding activities that might calm child at bedtime.

Grant ambivalence, conflict, and multiplicity to develop comprehensive understandings with parent.

Guide parent and child in completing loops of communication.

Handle scheduling dilemmas directly with co-parent so that parent is freed from gatekeeping position.

Harness child's senses to sustain engagement in play/learning.

Have fun with parent and child to support connecting and learning through pleasurable interactions.

Hazard guesses regarding underlying causes of conflict between parent and child.

Heal early wounds for parent by facilitating reparative experience with child.

Help parent formulate questions to ask pediatrician.

Highlight moments of positive connection between parent and child.

Hold parent appropriately accountable while conveying compassion.

Hone parent's skill in discerning meaning of child's behavior.

Honor family self-determination by....

Hypothesize with parent regarding how past experiences may be influencing present moments.

Identify moments when child appears to be attempting to please parent/instances of institutional racism affecting family/natural supports available to family.

Illustrate for parent unintended negative effects of developmentally mismatched expectations.

Implement strategies to increase dyad's capacity for mutual regulation.

Initiate a referral for regional center services/pretend play/ conversations about systems of oppression.

Inoculate dyad against institutional racism by anticipating how it may present itself.

Increase parental awareness of disabilities rights.

Inquire about parent's experiences when child cries or otherwise expresses distress.

Integrate a developmental perspective when discussing relationship stresses.

Interpret for Spanish-speaking parents English-speaking pediatrician's communications regarding child's medical condition with consideration for impact on parental mental health.

Interrupt problematic interactions between parent and child before they escalate.

Introduce developmental principles that may reframe child's behavior.

Invite parent and child to directly express negative thoughts and emotions about IMH worker.

Invoke ancestral traditions that are meaningful for family to meet contemporary challenges.

Involve mental health consultant in resolving discord between parents and child care staff.

Isolate discreet sensory modalities to help parent understand child's overstimulation.

Jabber about innocuous subjects to diffuse parental anxiety and engage child's interest.

Join parent in describing child's needs and strengths/child's developmental level to new child care provider.

Justify sound clinical actions forthrightly and transparently in response to parental questions.

Keep track of moments of mutually pleasurable connection between parent and child.

Kindle parent's/child's interest in....

Label feeling states child is likely experiencing/internalized negative parental images.

Learn from parents what their goals and priorities are/ collaboratively with family what works for them/from child what their individual processing patterns are.

Leverage power and privilege to counter barriers faced by family.

Link parent–child dyad with potentially helpful services including.../past experience with present behavior/parent–child dyad with potentially enjoyable recreational activities including....

List collaboratively with parent examples of child's efforts to cooperate/early warning signs of relapse/supportive people to call on in moments of stress.

Listen to parent's descriptions of challenges.

Locate resources on behalf of child and family.

Look to child's state as a barometer of household climate.

Maintain inclusive interaction with parent and child so both are engaged in session.

Make room for conflict and ambivalence.

Manage conflict among collateral providers to protect family from iatrogenic effects of system difficulties.

Match emotions of child to illustrate how this technique may be done.

Measure progress toward treatment objectives in regular reflective conversations with parent.

Mediate between co-parents while supporting their capacity to collaborate.

Mirror infant's facial expressions and engage parent in imaging what they reflect.

Mitigate adverse child outcomes of parental substance abuse by engaging parent in harm-reduction, decision-making process.

Mix active play with quiet reflection during sessions.

Mobilize service providers to advocate for family/parent's protective impulses/child's innate interests.

[Avoid **"model"** as an intervention verb—this action is often countertherapeutic when seeking to support parental capacities.]

Modify intervention approach to meet individual developmental profile of child.

Modulate sensory and motor stimulation for child collaboratively with parent.

Monitor impact of parent's psychotropic medication on their patience with child.

Name perceived impact of trauma on parent–child interaction patterns.

Narrate child's play activities out loud to support parent's noticing and reflecting.

Negotiate on behalf of family with landlord around environmental issues affecting child.

Normalize parental reactions to/child's behavior at developmental stress points.

Notice out loud when child appears to be seeking parent's approval/when parent seems to be internally preoccupied/when parental conflict seems to be affecting child.

Nurture positive parental identity.

Observe child in child care setting at parent's request.

Obtain parent's permission to contact child's pediatrician.

Offer nondidactic developmental guidance/examples of observed moments of successful parenting.

Open and close circles of communication.

Open new pathways of feeling between parent and child by establishing safety.

Optimize home-visiting context to address potential child-proofing needs.

Organize living space collaboratively with parent to promote infant's safe exploration.

Orient parent to the concept of school readiness.

Outline steps and strategies for selecting a child care that will be a good fit for child and family.

Pace session collaboratively with parent responding to infant's shifting states of alertness and arousal.

Paraphrase statements made by parent into terms child will understand and feel included in.

Parse collaboratively with parent multiple contributions to child's emotional distress.

Participate in Individualized Education Program meeting to represent social–emotional developmental needs.

Pique parent's/child's interest by....

Plan termination phase collaboratively with parent.

Play together with parent and child to support sustained engagement.

Point out ruptures and opportunities for repair in parent–child attunement.

Postulate out loud what infant/child might be experiencing.

Practice inclusive interaction/perspective taking/mutual regulation.

Present mutual regulation techniques such as up- and down-regulating finger games and songs.

Prevent adverse outcomes by helping parent attend to child's experience of stress or trauma.

Prime parent and child for emotional attunement.

Prioritize safety-related issues.

Problem solve collaboratively with parent when....

Promote safety by.../mutuality and reciprocity by....

Prompt parent to set needed limits with child in the moment.

Propose alternate possible meanings of child's behavior when parent is vexed by it.

Provide anticipatory developmental guidance.

Pursue resources on behalf of family/information regarding medical condition/funding for....

Qualify parent's global perceptions of child with observations that provide more nuance and complexity.

Quantify with parent degrees of perceived stress in child.

Question parenting practices that appear to negatively affect child's sense of security.

Quiz parent to prepare for stressful meeting.

Reach consensus among collateral providers regarding markers that the time is right for reunification.

Reaffirm treatment objectives that remain important to parent.

Reassure child that parent will return.

Recapitulate lessons learned, themes identified, and gains made in treatment.

Recast interactions experienced negatively in terms of the hope for meaningful connection that motivated them.

Reciprocate when child signals....

Recognize signs of distress in child and support parent in recognizing these signs.

Recommend additional potentially beneficial services.

Redefine parental authority, distinguishing it from authoritarianism.

Redirect child to make bids for play directly to parent/parent to focus on need signaled by child's behavior.

Reduce conflict between parent and child by suggesting compromises and strategies for collaboration.

Refer child to speech–language specialist/parent for medication evaluation/family to legal aid.

Reference goals and objectives parent has identified.

Reflect with parent on impact of parenting stress on experiences in early recovery.

Reframe self-defeating constructs so that change can be imagined/problematic behavior as survival strategy.

Rehearse with parent speaking with extended family about child's challenges.

Reinforce parental authority with child/growth-promoting interactions/new skills and self-concepts.

Reject pathologizing interpretations of child's behavior/ parent schemas derived from internalized racism.

Rejoice with family when connection, growth, and healing happen.

Relabel child's challenging behaviors in light of the needs they most likely arise from.

Remind parent of progress in moments of feeling overwhelmed or discouraged.

Remind parent of shared understandings of triggers and defenses.

Renew commitment to collaborative efforts on behalf of child/focus on impact of substance use and recovery on parenting.

Repair ruptures in IMH worker–parent and IMH worker– child relationships when they occur.

Report to pediatrician impact of feeding recommendations.

Research historical and cultural contexts that may be meaningful to family to relieve them of the burden of teaching IMH worker.

Respond to infant's cues in ways that include parent/to parent's distress so parent can respond to child's distress.

Reunify separated family members.

Review with parent recent treatment gains.

Revisit parent's early experiences in light of contemporary parent–child relationship.

Reward child collaboratively with parent for clearly expressing feelings/cooperating with limits/reaching developmental achievements.

Rhyme and sing to engage child and narrate parent–child interactions in an arresting/disarming manner.

Role play with parent growth-promoting, limit-setting interactions.

Scaffold growth-promoting play interactions between parent and child.

Secure emergency food resources on family's behalf.

Shake up problematic patterns of relating by....

Shape child's expectations collaboratively with parent.

Share insights regarding.../an expanded vocabulary of emotion/thoughts regarding.../impressions of....

Shift focus away from behavior and toward the feelings that motivate this behavior.

Shore up parent's conviction via reflective conversations in advance of changes to child's environment or routine.

Signal for parent moments when child may need encouragement.

Speak on behalf of child when parent is struggling to consider child's experience.

Speculate collaboratively with parent regarding possible meanings of child's behavior.

State clearly what parenting behaviors seem to be escalating the difficulty.

Stay engaged in moments of conflict and discomfort.

Steer conversation in the direction of family strengths.

Strategize with parent regarding....

Strengthen PCRC [number].../parent's capacity to.../child's ability to....

Stretch parent's tolerance for messy play by participating in clean-up/child's capacity for shared attention by supporting pleasurable interactions.

Strike a balance between challenging attributions to child that may be inaccurate and validating the experiences that contribute to these distortions.

Structure sessions to balance talking, playing, and reflecting activities.

Substitute new, growth-promoting relationship patterns for injurious historical ones.

Suggest new parenting strategies that may be more effective.

Summarize shared understandings of determinants of behavior/progress toward goals.

Support parent's development of patience via positive reinforcement.

Tailor interactions to child's sensory profile.

Take turns in conversation and play to establish contingency and reciprocity.

Talk about things that affect parent and child but that family may avoid acknowledging without help.

Target for change behaviors that put dyad at most risk for family separation.

Teach parent to identify possible miscues in child.

Tease out incremental attainable objectives from parent's description of long-range family goals.

Tell early childhood mental health consultant about family transitions that may be affecting child's behavior in child care.

Testify in court regarding understandings of family experiences.

Think with parent about....

Titrate challenge as parent learns new ways of being with child.

Tolerate ambiguity/conflict/discomfort in the service of building parent's capacity to do so.

Track instances of joyful interaction shared by parent and child/child's development.

Train parent in potentially useful strategies for mindful self-regulation.

Translate between parent and child when their actions are baffling or frustrating to one another.

Treat preverbal infants as legitimate participants in family conversation/parents as experts on their children/family.

Trust the self-righting capacity of parent–child relationships to guide the pace and course of treatment.

Underline historical and political root causes of family instability.

Help parent to **unearth** sustaining memories.

Urge parent to consistently attempt to comfort child despite initial rejection.

Use humor to leaven parent's sense of being frustrated and overwhelmed.

Validate parent's accurate perceptions/child's perceived experience.

Valorize caregiving and child-rearing labor.

Verbalize understanding of impact of historical trauma on family well-being.

Verify eligibility status and availability of sources of medical care.

Visualize together with parent what parent–child relationship satisfaction would look and feel like.

Vitalize parent–child interactions via coaching to secure child's cross-modal engagement.

Wait for infant to signal readiness to engage.

Walk with child and parent to counteract agoraphobia/isolation/energy deficit.

Watch child's play closely together with parent to reflect together.

Witness and attest to family pain/instances of injustice affecting family.

Wonder with parent about possible meanings of child's behavior.

Work through moments of conflict or discomfort with family rather than withdrawing or retaliating.

Write a birth plan collaboratively with parent-to-be.

Yield to parent's authority.

APPENDIX H

Sample DSM-5 and DC:0–5 Diagnoses Affecting Parent–Child Relationship Competencies (PCRCs), as Illustrated by Vignettes

Adjustment Disorder with Anxiety—Vignettes 10.2, 12.2, 19.2

Adjustment Disorder with mixed anxiety and depressed mood—Vignette 8.1

Adjustment Disorder with Depressed Mood—Vignette 16.2

Adjustment Disorder with mixed anxiety and depressed mood—Vignette 5.1

Alcohol Use Disorder—Vignette 6.2

Attention Deficit Hyperactivity Disorder—Vignette 7.1

Autism Spectrum Disorder—Vignette 4.2

Bipolar II Disorder—Vignette 1.2

Borderline Personality Disorder—Vignette 11.2

Complicated Grief Disorder of Infancy/Early Childhood—Vignette 18.1

Dependent Personality Disorder—Vignette 20.2

Depressive Disorder of Early Childhood—Vignette 9.2

Disorder of Dysregulated Anger and Aggression of Early Childhood—Vignette 14.1

Early Atypical Autism Spectrum Disorder—Vignette 12.1

Excessive Crying Disorder—Vignette 11.1

Generalized Anxiety Disorder—Vignettes 2.2, 4.1, 8.2

Intermittent Explosive Disorder—Vignette 13.2

Major Depressive Disorder—Vignette 18.2

APPENDIX I

Questions to Guide Reflection

Working with the Parent–Child Relationship Competencies (PCRCs) often entails a significant conceptual shift for practitioners who have been trained in and are experienced with individually focused assessment and treatment approaches. Even infant mental health (IMH) workers who have long embraced relational approaches usually find that the PCRC framework brings new depths of awareness of relational dynamics and sensitivity to the mechanisms of mutual influence. Such deepened awareness and sensitivity are often accompanied by the stirring of feeling, as aspects of each person's own relationship history are illuminated by the PCRC material.

Diversity-Informed Tenet # 1 (© Irving Harris Foundation; www.diversityinformedtenets.org) reminds us that Self-Awareness Leads to Better Services for Families. The questions that follow were generated to support IMH workers in deepening personal awareness regarding the PCRCs in order to further professional understanding and expand the repertoire of skills. They may be useful in the context of individual reflection, reflective supervision, reflective consultation, or group or team learning and professional development processes. It is recommended that these questions be applied to Chapters 2–21, with Chapter 1 and the Afterword considered first as groundwork for diversity-informed reflection.

> **Tenet # 1:**
> Self-Awareness Leads to Better Services for Families

1. What initially stands out to you when you read this PCRC? Do images come to mind? Are you aware of any particular emotional response? How does it sit with you?

2. Write down a personal memory that demonstrates this PCRC functioning well. Be as detailed as possible. Who were you with? Where were you? What sense memories

---

Find a printable copy of these questions on www.zerotothree.org/PCRCresources

are associated? What is the emotional tone? (If no memory presents itself, write what comes to mind for you and what you are experiencing in this effort to recall something.) Note that you may be positioned as a child or a parent in the memory—or you may be positioned differently. What are your thoughts and feelings about this?

3. Write down a personal memory that demonstrates this PCRC *not* functioning well. Be as detailed as possible. Who were you with? Where were you? What sense memories are associated? What is the emotional tone? (If no memory presents itself, write what comes to mind for you and what you are experiencing in this effort to recall something.) Note that you may be positioned as a child or a parent in the memory—or you may be positioned differently. What are your thoughts and feelings about this?

4. Consider the epigraph that opens the chapter. What part of the PCRC does it seem to illustrate, give voice to, or comment on? What are your thoughts about this?

5. Identify a passage in a piece of literature or a clip from a film or other cultural production that might serve as an alternate epigraph illustrating an aspect of this PCRC. What difference does it introduce?

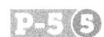

6. Each PCRC may be expressed in a wide range of ways consistent with varying sociocultural contexts. What are your thoughts and feelings about how sociocultural factors might influence the healthy functioning of this PCRC?

7. As you read and consider the paragraphs discussing this PCRC, are there things that surprise you? Things you disagree with? Things that come to mind that ought to be included?

8. When you consider your professional role(s), how do you think you might support the functioning of this PCRC?

9. What personal or systemic impediments might there be to your supporting the functioning of this PCRC?

5 4

10. As you read and consider each vignette, what feelings and thoughts arise for you? Consider specifically:

- Developmental issues for the child

P-5 1

- Psychological issues for the parent

- Relational context more broadly—family and community

P-5 2

P-5 3

- Sociocultural issues, whether these are specified in the vignette or not

P-5 5

- Role issues for the IMH worker, including potential countertransference challenges

- Role issues regarding collateral providers

P-5 8

- The identified diagnosis

11. Consider each vignette in this chapter in light of the Diversity-Informed Tenets. Which Tenets might be especially important to bear in mind in working with this family and why? Which Tenets might be challenging to uphold and why?

12. Imagine that the social location markers of the family members and IMH worker were different than those specified in the vignette. How might this change things?

13. Construct a vignette drawn from your own practice illustrating the need to strengthen this PCRC.

14. Find a current article addressing a topic core to this PCRC and review it in relation to this PCRC. What does it add to your understanding of this PCRC? Does it challenge aspects of the discussion of the PCRC? When viewed through a PCRC and a Diversity-Informed Tenets lens, are there aspects of the article that you find problematic? What best practice or ethical issues does it raise or shed light on?

P-5 7

15. What support would be useful to you—from colleagues, supervisors, or consultants—in relation to this PCRC?

P-5 6

P-5 8

REFERENCES

Abram, J. (1996). *The language of Winnicott: A dictionary of Winnicott's use of words.* London, England: Karnac Books.

American Psychiatric Association. (2013). *Diagnostic and statistical manual of mental disorders* (5th ed.). Arlington, VA: American Psychiatric Publishing.

Americans With Disabilities Act of 1990, Pub. L. 101-336, 42 U.S.C. §§ 12101–12213 (2000).

Andermahr, S. (2016). Decolonizing trauma studies: Trauma and postcolonialism introduction. *Humanities, 4,* 500–505.

Angelou, M. (2008). *Letter to my daughter.* New York, NY: Random House.

Babcock, B., Monthan, G., & Monthan, D. (1986). The *pueblo storyteller.* Tucson: University of Arizona Press.

Baudrillard, J. (1981). *For a critique of the political economy of the sign* (Charles Levin, Trans.). Candor, NY: Telos Press.

Beebe, B., Cohen, P., & Lachmann, F. (2016). *The mother–infant interaction picture book: Origins of attachment.* New York, NY: Norton.

Bernstein, V. J., Harris, E., Long, C. W., Iida, E., & Hans, S. L. (2005). Issues in the multi-cultural assessment of parent–child interaction: An exploratory study from the Starting Early Starting Smart collaboration. *Applied Developmental Psychology, 26,* 241–275.

Boggs, G. L. (2011). *The next American revolution: Sustainable activism for the twenty-first century.* Berkeley: University of California Press.

Bourgeois, P. (1987). *Big Sarah's little boots.* New York, NY: Scholastic.

Bowlby, J. (1980). *Loss, sadness, and depression* (Attachment and Loss, vol. 3). London, England: Basic Books.

Bowlby, J. (1982). *Attachment* (2nd ed.). London, England: Basic Books. (Original work published in 1969)

Brave Heart, M. Y. H. (1999). Gender differences in the historical trauma response among the Lakota. *Journal of Health & Social Policy, 10*(4), 1–21.

Brown, L. B. (2007). *Circles in the nursery: Practicing multiracial family therapy.* Washington, DC: ZERO TO THREE.

Burt, T., Gelnaw, A., & Lesser, L. K. (2010). Do no harm: Creating welcoming and inclusive environments for lesbian, gay, bisexual, and transgender (LGBT) families in early childhood settings. *Young Children, 65,* 97–102.

Butler, J. (1995). Melancholy gender—Refused identification. *Psychoanalytic Dialogues, 5*(2), 165–180.

Carson, R. (1956). *A sense of wonder.* New York, NY: Harper & Row.

Center for Excellence in Children's Mental Health. (2010, October). Historical trauma and microaggressions: A framework for culturally-based practice. *Child Welfare Series e-Review*. Retrieved from https://conservancy.umn.edu/handle/11299/120667

Chabat, A. (Producer), & Balmès, T. (Director). (2010). *Babies* [Motion Picture]. France: Studio Canal.

Coates, T.-N. (2015). *Between the world and me*. New York, NY: Spiegel & Grau.

Collins, P. H. (1991). *Black feminist thought*. New York, NY: Routledge.

Collins, P. H., & Bilge, S. (2016). *Intersectionality: Key concepts*. Malden, MA: Polity Press.

Copeland, M. E. (2000). *Wellness recovery action plan*. Dummerston, VT: Peach Press.

Costa, G., & Noroña, C. R. (2019). The art and science of obtaining a history in infant and early childhood mental health assessment. In K. A. Frankel, J. N. Harrison, & F. M. Wanjiku (Eds.), *Clinical guide to psychiatric assessment of infants and young children* (pp. 21–76). New York, NY: Springer.

Crenshaw, K. (1989). Demarginalizing the intersection of race and sex: A Black feminist critique of antidiscrimination doctrine, feminist theory, and antiracist politics. *University of Chicago Legal Forum, (1989)*, 1, Article 8, 139–167.

Crenshaw, K. W. (2014, December 30). *Black girls matter: Pushed out, overpoliced, and underprotected*. Retrieved from https://www.atlanticphilanthropies.org/wp-content/uploads/2015/09/BlackGirlsMatter_Report.pdf

Culture. (n.d.). In *New World Encyclopedia*. Retrieved from www.newworldencyclopedia.org/entry/Culture

DeGangi, G. (2000). *Pediatric disorders of regulation in affect and behavior: A therapist's guide to assessment and treatment*. San Diego, CA: Academic Press.

DeGruy, J. (2005). *Post traumatic slave syndrome: America's legacy of enduring injury and healing*. Portland, OR: Uptone Press.

Denard, C. (Ed.). (2008). *Toni Morrison: Conversations*. Jackson: University Press of Mississippi.

DiAngelo, R. (2011). White fragility. *International Journal of Critical Pedagogy, 3*(3), 54–70.

Eggbeer, L., Shahmoon-Shanok, R., & Clark, R. (2010). Reaching toward an evidence base for reflective supervision. *ZERO TO THREE Journal, 31*(2), 39–45.

Eng, D., & Han, S. (2000). A dialogue on racial melancholia. *Psychoanalytic Dialogues, 10*(4), 667–700.

Erdrich, L. (1995). *The blue jay's dance: A memoir of early motherhood*. New York, NY: Harper.

Evans-Campbell, T., & Walters, K. L. (2006). Catching our breath: A decolonization framework for healing indigenous families. In F. Fong, R. McRoy, & C. O. Hendricks (Eds.), *Intersecting child welfare, substance abuse, and family violence: Culturally competent approaches* (pp. 266–292). Alexandria, VA: CSWE Publications.

Fadiman, A. (1997). *The spirit catches you and you fall down: A Hmong child, her American doctors, and the collision of two cultures.* New York, NY: Farrar, Straus, & Giroux.

Fanon, F. (2008). *Black skin, white masks.* New York, NY: Grove Press. (Original work published in 1952)

Fonagy, P., Steele, M., Steele, H., Moran, G., & Higgitt, A. (1991). The capacity for understanding mental states: The reflective self in parent and child and its significance for security of attachment. *Infant Mental Health Journal, 12,* 201–218.

Foster, R. P. (2001). When immigration is trauma: Guidelines for the individual and family clinician. *American Journal of Orthopsychiatry, 71,* 153–170.

Fraiberg, S. (1959). *The magic years.* New York, NY: Charles Scribner's Sons.

Fraiberg, S. (1974). Clinical dimension of baby games. *Journal of the American Academy of Child Psychiatry, 13,* 202–220.

Fraiberg, S. (1977). *Insights from the blind.* New York, NY: Basic Books.

Fraiberg, S. (1980). *Clinical studies in infant mental health: The first year of life.* New York, NY: Basic Books.

Frankel, K. A., Harrison, J. N., & Wanjiku, F. M. (Eds.). (2019). *Clinical guide to psychiatric assessment of infants and young children.* New York, NY: Springer.

Frawley-O'Dea, M. G., & Sarnat, J. E. (2001). *The supervisory relationship: A contemporary psychodynamic approach.* New York, NY: Guilford Press.

Freire, P. (2007). *Education for critical consciousness.* London, England: Continuum Books. (Original work published 1974)

Freud, S. (1955). Mourning and melancholia. In J. Strachey (Ed. & Trans.), *The standard edition of the complete psychological works of Sigmund Freud* (Vol. 14, pp. 243–258). London, England: Hogarth Press. (Original work published 1917)

Ghosh-Ippen, C., & Lewis, M. L. (2011). "They just don't get it": A diversity-informed approach to understanding engagement. In J. D. Osofsky (Ed.), *Clinical work with traumatized young children* (pp. 31–52). New York, NY: Guilford Press.

Ghosh Ippen, C., Noroña, C. R., & Thomas, K. (2012). From tenet to practice: Putting diversity-informed services into action. *ZERO TO THREE Journal, 33*(2), 23–28.

Gilliam, W. (2005, May). *Prekindergarteners left behind: Expulsion rates in state prekindergarten programs* (FCD Policy Brief Series No. 3). Retrieved from https://medicine.yale.edu/childstudy/zigler/publications/National%20Prek%20Study_expulsion%20brief_34775_5379_v1.pdf

Gilliam, W. (2008, January). *Implementing policies to reduce the likelihood of preschool expulsion* (FCD Policy Brief Series No. 7). Retrieved from https://medicine.yale.edu/childstudy/zigler/publications/PreKExpulsionBrief2_34772_284_5379_v1.pdf

Gold, L. (2014). DSM–5 and the assessment of functioning: The World Health Organization Disability Assessment Schedule 2.0 (WHODAS 2.0). *The Journal of the American Academy of Psychiatry and the Law, 42*, 173–81.

Graham, A. M., Fisher, P. A., & Pfeifer, J. H. (2013). What sleeping babies hear: A functional MRI study of interparental conflict and infants' emotion processing. *Psychological Science, 24*, 782–789. https://doi.org/10.1177/0956797612458803

Greenspan, S. I., & Greenspan, N. D. (2003). *Clinical interview of the child* (3rd. ed.). Washington, DC: American Psychiatric Publishing.

Greenspan, T., & Lewis, N. B. (1999). *Building healthy minds: Six experiences that create intelligence and emotional growth in babies and young children.* New York, NY: Da Capo Press.

Hanks, A., Solomon, D., & Weller, C. E. (2018, February 21). *Systemic inequality: How America's structural racism helped create the Black/White wealth gap.* Retrieved from https://www.americanprogress.org/issues/race/reports/2018/02/21/447051/systematic-inequality

Hardy, K. V. (2013). Healing the hidden wounds of racial trauma. *Reclaiming Children and Youth, 22*(1), 24–28.

Hardy, K. V., & Bobes, T. (Eds.). (2017). *Promoting cultural sensitivity in supervision: A manual for practitioners.* New York, NY: Routledge.

Hardy, K. V., & Leszloffy, T. A. (1995). The cultural genogram: Key to training culturally competent family therapists. *Journal of Marital and Family Therapy, 21*, 227–237.

Heffron, M. C., & Murch, T. (2010). *Reflective supervision and leadership in infant and early childhood programs.* Washington, DC: ZERO TO THREE.

Heffron, M. C., & Murch, T. (2012). *Finding the words, finding the ways: Exploring reflective supervision and facilitation.* Sacramento: California Center for Infant–Family and Early Childhood Mental Health.

Hernández, P., & McDowell, T. (2010). Intersectionality, power, and relational safety in context: Key concepts in clinical supervision. *Training and Education in Professional Psychology, 4*(1), 29–35.

Hosseini, K. (2007). *A thousand splendid suns*. New York, NY: Riverhead Books.

Jacoby, J. (Ed.). (2009). *Street art San Francisco: Mission muralismo.* New York, NY: Harry N. Abrams.

Johnson, A. (1994). *Joshua's night whispers.* New York, NY: Orchard Books

Juarez-Marazzo, S. (2016). *¡Mamá, cuéntame porqué viniste! Mommy, tell me, why did you come here?* Atlanta, GA: LitFire.

Kozol, J. (2005). *The shame of the nation: The restoration of apartheid schooling in America.* New York, NY: Three Rivers Press.

Lacan, J. (1977). *Écrits: A selection* (B. Fink, Trans.). New York, NY: Norton.

Lahiri, J. (2003). *The namesake.* New York, NY: Mariner Books.

Lerner, C. (2017, March 22). *Just say no to judgment: How judging parents actually leads to worse, not better, outcomes for kids.* Retrieved from https://www.zerotothree.org/resources/1716-just-say-no-to-judgment-how-judging-parents-actually-leads-to-worse-not-better-outcomes-for-kids

Lewis, M. (2005). The cultural context of infant mental health: The developmental niche of infant-caregiver relationships. In C. H. Zeanah (Ed.), *Handbook of infant mental health* (2nd ed., pp. 91–107). New York, NY: Guilford Press.

Lieberman, A. F., Compton, N. C., Van Horn, P., & Ippen, G. (2003). *Losing a parent to death in the early years: Guidelines for the treatment of traumatic bereavement in infancy and early childhood.* Washington, DC: ZERO TO THREE.

Lieberman, A. F., Ghosh Ippen, C., & Van Horn, P. (2015). *Don't hit my mommy: A manual for child–parent psychotherapy with young children exposed to violence and other trauma* (2nd ed.). Washington, DC: ZERO TO THREE.

Lieberman, A. F., & Pawl, J. H. (1993). Infant–parent psychotherapy. In C. H. Zeanah (Ed.), *Handbook of infant mental health* (pp. 427–442). New York, NY: Guilford Press.

Lieberman, A. F., Silverman, R., & Pawl, J. H. (2000). Infant–parent psychotherapy: Core concepts and current approaches. In C. H. Zeanah (Ed.), *Handbook of infant mental health* (2nd ed., pp. 472–484). New York, NY: Guilford Press.

Lieberman, A. F., & Van Horn, P. (2008). *Psychotherapy with infants and young children: Repairing the effects of stress and trauma on early attachment.* New York, NY: Guilford Press.

Martín-Baró, I. (1996). *Writings for a liberation psychology* (A. Aron & S. Corne, Eds.). New York, NY: Harvard University Press.

McHale, J. P. (2007). *Charting the bumpy road of coparenthood: Understanding the challenges of family life.* Washington, DC: ZERO TO THREE.

McHale, J. P., & Fivaz-Depeursinge, E. (2010). Principles of effective coparenting and its assessment in infancy and early childhood. In S. Tyano, M. Keren, H. Herrman, & J. Cox (Eds.), *Parenthood and mental health: A bridge between infant and adult psychiatry* (pp. 357–371). New York, NY: Wiley.

McIntosh, P. (1989, July/August). White privilege: Unpacking the invisible knapsack. *Peace and Freedom Magazine*, 10–12.

Morrison, T. (1973). *Sula*. New York, NY: Random House.

National Center for Children in Poverty. (2018, November). *How states use Medicaid to cover key infant and early childhood mental health services: Results of a 50-state survey.* Retrieved from http://nccp.org/publications/pdf/text_1211.pdf

National Council on Disability. (2012, September 27). *Rocking the cradle: Ensuring the rights of parents with disabilities and their children.* Retrieved from https://www.ncd.gov/sites/default/files/Documents/NCD_Parenting_508_0.pdf

National Research Council & Institute of Medicine. (2000). *From neurons to neighborhoods: The science of early childhood development.* Washington, DC: National Academy Press.

Noroña, C. R. (2011, Fall). *Working with immigrant Latin-American families exposed to trauma.* Los Angeles, CA: National Child Traumatic Stress Network, Spotlight on Culture. Retrieved from https://www.nctsn.org/resources/working-immigrant-latin-american-families-exposed-trauma

Noroña, C. R., Heffron, M., Grunstein, S., & Nalo, A. (2012). Broadening the scope: Next steps in reflective supervision. *ZERO TO THREE Journal, 33*(2), 29–34.

Pawl, J. (1990, February). Infants in day care: Reflections on experience, expectations, and relationships. *ZERO TO THREE, 10*(3), 1–6. Available from https://www.zerotothree.org/resources/114-the-fundamentals-of-infant-early-childhood-mental-health

Pawl, J. (1991). A book is a child's companion. *ZERO TO THREE Journal, 12*(1), 9.

Pawl, J., & St. John, M. (1998). *How you are is as important as what you do...in making a positive difference for infants, toddlers, and their families.* Washington, DC: ZERO TO THREE.

People's Charter for Health. (2000). *People's health movement.* Retrieved from https://www.phmovement.org/sites/www.phmovement.org/files/phm-pch-english.pdf

Piper, W. (2009). *The little engine that could.* New York, NY: Grosset & Dunlap. (Original work published 1930)

Powell, B., Cooper, B., Hoffman, K., & Marvin, B. (2014). *The circle of security intervention: Enhancing attachment in early parent–child relationships.* New York, NY: Guilford Press.

Ra, C., Cho, J., & Stone, M. (2018). Association of digital media use with subsequent symptoms of attention-deficit/hyperactivity disorder among adolescents. *JAMA 320*(3), 255–263.

Reggio Children. (2008). *Dialogues with places: The catalogue.* Reggio Emilia, Italy: Author.

Reschke, K., LeMoine, S., Greene, K., & Macasaet, K. (2017). *ZERO TO THREE Critical Competencies for Infant-Toddler Educators™ course curriculum.* Washington, DC: ZERO TO THREE.

Rich, A. (1986). *Of woman born: Motherhood as experience and institution.* New York, NY: W. W. Norton.

Roberts, D. (2002). *Shattered bonds: The color of child welfare.* New York, NY: Perseus Books.

Sendak, M. (1963). *Where the wild things are.* New York, NY: HarperCollins.

Shaw, F. (1928). *Songs of a baby's day to the tune of a very gentle jog.* Chicago, IL: F. J. & E. M. Schmidt.

Siegel, D. (2001). Toward an interpersonal neurobiology of the developing mind: Attachment relationships, "mindsight," and neural integration. *Infant Mental Health Journal, 22*(1–2), 67–94.

Silverman, K. (1988). *The acoustic mirror: The female voice in psychoanalysis and cinema.* Bloomington: Indiana University Press.

Silverman, R., & Lieberman, A. (1999). Negative maternal attributions, projective identification, and the intergenerational transmission of violent relational patterns. *Psychoanalytic Dialogues, 9*(2), 161–186.

Singleton, G. E. (2015). *Courageous conversations about race: A field guide for achieving equity in the schools* (2nd ed.). Thousand Oaks, CA: Corwin.

Slade, A. (2005). Parental reflective functioning: An introduction. *Attachment and Human Development, 7*, 269–281.

Solomon, D. (2018, April 18). *Racism: The evergreen toxin killing Black mothers and children* (Center for American Progress Issue Brief). Retrieved from https://www.americanprogress.org/issues/race/reports/2018/04/18/449774/racism-evergreen-toxin-killing-black-mothers-infants/

Speranza, A. M., & Mayes, L. (2017). Mental health and developmental disorders in infancy and early childhood. In V. Lingiardi & N. McWilliams (Eds.), *Psychodynamic diagnostic manual* (2nd ed., pp. 625–747). New York, NY: Guilford Press.

Stevenson, H. C. (2014). *Promoting racial literacy in schools: Differences that make a difference.* New York, NY: Teachers College Press.

Stevenson, R. L. (1885). Block city. *A children's garden of verses.* New York, NY: D. Appleton.

St. John, M. S., & Nalo, A. (2016, November 28). *The Diversity-Informed Infant Mental Health Tenets in California*. Retrieved from http://cacenter-ecmh.org/wp/the-diversity-informed-infant-mental-health-tenets-in-california

St. John, M. S., & Pawl, J. H. (2000). Inclusive interaction in infant–parent psychotherapy. In J. H. Pawl, C. A. Ahern, C. Grandison, K. Johnston, M. S. St. John, & A. Waldstein (Eds.), *Responding to infants and parents: Inclusive interaction in assessment, consultation, and treatment in infant/family practice* (pp. 8–14). Washington, DC: ZERO TO THREE.

St. John, M. S., Thomas, K., & Noroña, C. R. (2012). Infant mental health professional development: Together in the struggle for social justice. *ZERO TO THREE Journal, 33*(2), 13–22.

Strayed, C. (2012). *Wild: From lost to found on the Pacific Crest Trail*. New York, NY: Alfred A. Knopf.

Sue, D. W., Capodilupo, C. M., Torino, G. C., Buccerin, J. M., Holder, A. M. B., Nadal, K. L., & Esquilin, M. (2007). Racial microaggressions in everyday life: Implications for clinical practice. *American Psychologist, 62*, 271–286.

Sweet Honey in the Rock. (1983). More than a paycheck. On *We all... Everyone of us* (CD). London, England: Cooking Vinyl.

Tandon, M., Cardeli, E., & Luby, J. (2009). Internalizing disorders in early childhood: A review of depressive and anxiety disorders. *Child and Adolescent Psychiatry Clinics of North America*, (18)3, 593–610.

Taubman, S. (2007). *The BTA treatment plan documentation guide for use in California's public behavioral health care services*. Berkeley, CA: Berkeley Training Associates.

Thomas, D. (1978). *A child's Christmas in Wales*. Boston, MA: David R. Godine. (Original work published 1954)

Thomas, K. (2019). *Prevalence and potential buffers of intergenerational trauma in African American and Latinx parent-child dyads* (Doctoral dissertation). Loyola University Chicago, Chicago, Illinois, USA.

Thomas, K., Noroña, C. R., & St. John, M. S. (2019). Cross-sector allies together in the struggle for social justice: The Diversity-Informed Tenets for Work With Infants, Children, and Families. *ZERO TO THREE Journal, 39*(3), 44–54.

Tronick, E. (2007). *The neurobehavioral and social-emotional development of infants and children*. New York, NY: W. W. Norton.

Uchida, Y. (1971). *Journey to Topaz*. Berkeley, CA: Heyday.

U.S. Department of Health and Human Services. (2016, May 11). Maternal depression screening and treatment: A critical role for Medicaid in the care of mothers and children. *CMCS Informational Bulletin.* Retrieved from https://www.medicaid.gov/federal-policy-guidance/downloads/cib051116.pdf

Visser, I. (2015). Decolonizing trauma theory: Retrospect and prospects. *Humanities, 4,* 250–265.

Winnicott, D. W. (1949). Hate in the counter-transference. *The International Journal of Psychoanalysis, 30,* 69–74.

Winnicott, D. W. (1956). Primary maternal preoccupation. In *Collected papers: Through paediatrics to psycho-analysis* (pp. 300–305). London, UK: Tavistock.

Winnicott, D. W. (1958). Anxiety associated with insecurity. In *Collected papers: Through pediatrics to psychoanalysis* (pp. 97–100). London, England: Tavistock. (Original work published 1952)

Winnicott, D. W. (1965a). Development of the capacity for concern. In *The maturational processes and the facilitating environment: Studies in the theory of emotional development* (pp. 73–82). Madison, CT: International Universities Press. (Original work published 1963)

Winnicott, D. W. (1965b). Integrative and disruptive factors in family life. In *The maturational processes and the facilitating environment: Studies in the theory of emotional development* (pp. 40–49). Madison, CT: International Universities Press. (Original work published 1957)

Winnicott, D. W. (1965c). *The maturational processes and the facilitating environment: Studies in the theory of emotional development.* Madison, CT: International Universities Press.

Winnicott, D. W. (1966). The ordinary devoted mother. In C. Winnicott, R. Shepherd, & M. Davis, (Eds,), *Babies and their mothers* (pp. 3–14). London, UK: Free Association Books.

Winnicott, D. W. (1971). The location of cultural experience. In *Playing and reality* (pp. 95–103). London, England: Tavistock. (Original work published 1967)

Winnicott, D. W. (1987) The ordinary devoted mother. In C. Winnicott, R. Shepherd, & M. Davis (Eds.), *Babies and their mothers* (pp. 3–14). London, England: Free Association Books. (Original work published 1966)

Wolff, T. (1989). *This boy's life: A memoir.* New York, NY: Grove Press.

World Association for Infant Mental Health. (2016, May 13). *WAIMH position paper on the rights of infants.* Amended version. University of Tampere, Finland: Author.

World Health Organization. (1992). *The ICD–10 classification of mental and behavioural disorders: Clinical descriptions and diagnostic guidelines.* Geneva, Switzerland: Author.

Wright, B. M. (1992). Treatment of infants and their families. In J. R. Brandell (Ed.), *Countertransference in psychotherapy with children and adolescents* (pp. 127–139). Northvale, NJ: Jason Aronson.

Zadra, J. R., & Clore, G. L. (2011). Emotion and perception: The role of affective information. *Wiley Interdisciplinary Reviews: Cognitive Science, 2*, 676–685.

ZERO TO THREE. (2016). *DC:0–5™: Diagnostic classification of mental health and developmental disorders of infancy and early childhood.* Washington, DC: Author.

ZERO TO THREE. (2017, September 26). *Cross-sector core competencies for the prenatal to age 5 field.* Available from https://www.zerotothree.org/resources/2059-cross-sector-core-competencies-for-the-prenatal-to-age-five-field

ZERO TO THREE Journal. (2018). Infants and the opioid epidemic, *38*(5).

Zheng, F., Gao, P., He, M., Li, M., Wang, C., Zeng, Q.,...Zhang, L. (2014). Association between mobile phone use and inattention in 7102 Chinese adolescents: A population-based cross-sectional study. *BMC Public Health, 14*(1022), 1–7.

REPRINT PERMISSIONS